ADOLESCENT MEDICINE: STATE OF THE ART REVIEWS

Adolescent Gynecology

GUEST EDITORS

Martin M. Fisher, MD

Eduardo Lara-Torre, MD

April 2012 • Volume 23 • Number 1

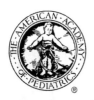

ADOLESCENT MEDICINE:
STATE OF THE ART REVIEWS
April 2012
Editor: Diane E. Lundquist, MS
Marketing Manager: Marirose Russo
Production Manager: Shannan Martin
eBook Developer: Mark Ruthman
eBook Production Coordinator: Linda J. Atteo

Volume 23, Number 1
ISBN 978-1-58110-601-5
ISSN 1934-4287
MA0593
SUB1006

Adolescent Medicine: State of the Art Reviews is published three times per year by the American Academy of Pediatrics, 141 Northwest Point Blvd, Elk Grove Village, IL 60007-1019. Periodicals postage paid at Arlington Heights, IL.

POSTMASTER: Send address changes to American Academy of Pediatrics, Department of Marketing and Publications, Attn: AM:STARs, 141 Northwest Point Blvd, Elk Grove Village, IL 60007-1019.

Subscriptions: Subscriptions to *Adolescent Medicine: State of the Art Reviews* (AM:STARs) are provided to members of the American Academy of Pediatrics' Section on Adolescent Health as part of annual section membership dues. All others, please contact the AAP Customer Service Center at 866/843-2271 (7:00 am–5:30 pm Central Time, Monday–Friday) for pricing and information.

Adolescent Medicine: State of the Art Reviews

Official Journal of the American Academy of Pediatrics
Section on Adolescent Health

EDITORS-IN-CHIEF

VICTOR C. STRASBURGER, MD, Professor of Pediatrics, Division of Adolescent Medicine, University of New Mexico, School of Medicine, Albuquerque, New Mexico

DONALD E. GREYDANUS, MD, Professor of Pediatrics, Michigan State University; and Pediatrics Program Director, Kalamazoo Center for Medical Studies, Kalamazoo, Michigan

GUEST EDITORS

MARTIN M. FISHER, MD, Division of Adolescent Medicine, Stephen and Alexandra Cohen Children's Medical Center of New York, North Shore-Long Island Jewish Health System, Hofstra North Shore-LIJ School of Medicine, New Hyde Park, New York

EDUARDO LARA-TORRE, MD, Associate Professor, Residency Program Director, Department of Obstetrics and Gynecology, Virginia Tech-Carilion School of Medicine, Carilion Clinic Medical Center, Roanoke, Virginia

CONTRIBUTORS

LISA M. ALLEN, MD, FRCSC, Section Head, Pediatric Gynecology, Hospital for Sick Children; Head, Gynecology, Mt. Sinai Hospital; Site Chief, Department of Obstetrics and Gynecology, Women's College Hospital; Associate Professor, Departments of Obstetrics and Gynecology and Pediatrics, University of Toronto, Toronto, Ontario, Canada

HEATHER APPELBAUM, MD, Department of Obstetrics and Gynecology, Division of Pediatric and Adolescent Gynecology, Long Island Jewish Medical Center and Cohen Children's Medical Center of New York, Hofstra North Shore LIJ School of Medicine, North Shore-LIJ Health System, New Hyde Park, New York

AMANDA Y. BLACK, MD, MPH, Department of Obstetrics, Gynecology, and Newborn Care, The Ottawa Hospital; Division of Pediatric and Adolescent Gynecology, The Children's Hospital of Eastern Ontario, Ottawa, Ontario, Canada

ELLEN LANCON CONNOR, MD, Associate Professor of Pediatric Endocrinology, University of Wisconsin, Madison, Wisconsin

SUSAN M. COUPEY, MD, Chief, Adolescent Medicine, Professor of Pediatrics, Children's Hospital at Montefiore, Albert Einstein College of Medicine, Bronx, New York

NIRUPAMA K. DE SILVA, MD, Assistant Professor, Pediatric and Adolescent Gynecology, University of Oklahoma–Tulsa, Department of Obstetrics and Gynecology, Tulsa, Oklahoma

JONATHAN D. FISH, MD, Section Head, Survivors Facing Forward Program, Hematology/Oncology and Stem Cell Transplantation, Steven and Alexandra Cohen Children's Medical Center of New York, New Hyde Park, New York

NATHALIE A. FLEMING, MD, Department of Obstetrics, Gynecology, and Newborn Care, The Ottawa Hospital; Chief, Division of Pediatric and Adolescent Gynecology, The Children's Hospital of Eastern Ontario, Ottawa, Ontario, Canada

FAREEDA HAAMID, DO, Section of Adolescent Medicine, Department of Pediatrics, Assistant Professor of Clinical Pediatrics, The Ohio State University College of Medicine, Nationwide Children's Hospital, Columbus, Ohio

CYNTHIA HOLLAND-HALL, MD, MPH, Associate Professor of Clinical Pediatrics, The Ohio State University College of Medicine, Columbus, Ohio

YOLANDA A. KIRKHAM, MA, MD, FRCSC, Section of Pediatric Gynaecology, Hospital for Sick Children, University of Toronto, Toronto, Ontario, Canada

SARI KIVES, MD, MSc, FRCSC, Section of Pediatric Gynaecology, Hospital for Sick Children, University of Toronto, Toronto, Ontario, Canada

ALEXANDRA C. NEVIN LAM, MD, FRCSC, North York General Hospital, Hospital for Sick Children; Lecturer, Department of Obstetrics and Gynecology, University of Toronto, Toronto, Ontario, Canada

SHILPA MALHOTRA, MD, Department of Obstetrics and Gynecology, Division of Pediatric and Adolescent Gynecology, Long Island Jewish Medical Center and Cohen Children's Medical Center of New York, Hofstra North Shore LIJ School of Medicine, North Shore-LIJ Health System, New Hyde Park, New York

PAMELA MURRAY, MD, MHP, West Virginia University Department of Pediatrics, Morgantown, West Virginia

ELLEN S. ROME, MD, MPH, Head, Section of Adolescent Medicine, Cleveland Clinic Children's Hospital, Cleveland, Ohio

SHON PATRICK ROWAN, MD, West Virginia University Department of Obstetrics and Gynecology, Morgantown, West Virginia

JEAN SOMESHWAR, MD, West Virginia University Department of Pediatrics, Morgantown, West Virginia

VICTOR C. STRASBURGER, MD, Professor of Pediatrics, Professor of Family & Community Medicine, University of New Mexico School of Medicine, Albuquerque, New Mexico

HINA J. TALIB, MD, Postdoctoral Fellow, Adolescent Medicine, Children's Hospital at Montefiore, Albert Einstein College of Medicine, Bronx, New York

LEA E. WIDDICE, MD, Division of Adolescent Medicine, Cincinnati Children's Hospital Medical Center, University of Cincinnati College of Medicine, Cincinnati, Ohio

CONTENTS

Puberty is the biological transition from childhood to adulthood. The process involves the coordination of hormonal, physical, psychosocial, and cognitive systems to result in physiologic change. Although most adolescents follow a predictable path through pubertal maturation, the timing and sequence of pubertal development can be variable. Genetic predisposition to the initiation and duration of pubertal maturation is influenced by environmental exposures and overall health. An insult to the hypothalamic-pituitary-ovarian (HPO) axis can lead to significant deviation in terms of normal pubertal development. Early activation of the HPO axis results in precocious puberty, whereas impaired activation of the HPO axis causes delayed puberty. The spectrum of abnormal pubertal development is addressed in this article, and current recommendations concerning the diagnosis and treatment of early, delayed, and incomplete puberty are reviewed.

In the absence of effective sex education in the United States, the media have arguably become the leading sex educator for children and teenagers. Considerable research now exists that attests to the ability of the media to influence adolescents' attitudes and beliefs about sex and sexuality. In addition, new research has found a significant link between exposure to sexual content in the media and earlier onset of sexual intercourse. Although there is little research on the behavioral effects of "new" media, they are discussed as well. Suggestions for clinicians, parents, the federal government, and the entertainment industry are provided.

health services, including contraception. The consistent use of both condoms and hormonal contraception are recommended for STI and pregnancy prevention. A range of hormonal contraception is available, varying in drug, dose, and delivery mechanisms. Long-acting reversible contraception use is encouraged to decrease the teen pregnancy rate.

As the cure rate for adolescents with cancer has improved, the focus on future reproductive potential has increased. Despite a concerted effort to reduce the impact of cancer treatment on fertility through the alteration of therapy and the implementation of protective measures, many adolescent women with cancer remain at risk for impaired reproductive potential. Although the only standard-of-care approach to fertility preservation in this population remains embryo cryopreservation, there has been intense development of oocyte and ovarian cryopreservation as viable alternatives. This article focuses on the developing modalities of fertility preservation for adolescent women diagnosed with cancer.

Adolescent pregnancy remains a public health issue with significant medical, emotional, and societal consequences for the adolescent mother, her child, and her family. Teenage pregnancies are at higher risk of many adverse outcomes, including preterm delivery, low birth weight, and neonatal and infant mortality. Teen pregnancy and motherhood may have detrimental effects on the teen mother and her child; antenatal and postpartum care need to be adapted to meet the special needs of pregnant adolescents because standard obstetrical environments may not do so. This comprehensive review of adolescent pregnancy will highlight global statistics, factors contributing to adolescent pregnancy, social implications of adolescent pregnancy, obstetrical and neonatal outcomes, and the importance of multidisciplinary antenatal and postnatal care.

Menstrual dysfunction and symptoms commonly affect adolescents. Premenstrual syndrome/premenstrual dysphoric disorder (PMS/PMDD) is a pervasive problem with a significant impact on the quality of life of affected individuals. This condition most often begins in adolescence with the establishment of normal ovulatory menstrual cycles; however, the underlying pathophysiology has yet to be delineated. Dysmenorrhea is common in adolescents, affecting up to 93%. Although most cases are primary, health care providers (HCPs) must be vigilant to allow for early diagnosis and treatment of secondary causes, thereby preventing long-term sequelae of delayed diagnosis. With PMS/PMDD, prospective evaluation is key to the confirmation of the diagnosis before the initiation of pharmacotherapy, especially psychotropic therapies, due to the possibly harmful side effect profile for adolescents compared to adults. This review focuses on the pathophysiology, diagnosis, and management of premenstrual syndrome and dysmenorrhea, both primary and secondary.

Polycystic ovary syndrome (PCOS) can be identified in the adolescent years but is a process with genetic and epigenetic origins. Intrauterine growth retardation and premature adrenarche may precede the presentation of hyperandrogenism and oligo/anovulation. Other causes of hyperandrogenism and ovulatory dysfunction must be ruled out before PCOS is diagnosed. Obesity and insulin resistance often are associated features and greatly increase a girl's risk of developing metabolic syndrome and type 2 diabetes mellitus. Oral contraceptives, metformin, antiandrogens, and lifestyle modifications can have roles in alleviating the symptoms of PCOS and are reviewed in this article.

Contemporary management of ovarian cysts in the adolescent consists of conservative management, whether expectant, medical, or surgical. An understanding of ovarian physiology in the perimenarcheal and postpubertal patient supports ovarian preservation surgery, as the rate of malignancy is low and the alternative can be devastating. The most common ovarian cysts in adolescents are functional and often regress without further treatment. Symptomatic ovarian cysts warrant further investigation. Endometriomas arising from endometriosis are extremely uncommon. Tubo-ovarian abscesses are managed medically and rarely by drainage or surgery. Ovarian torsion is a surgical emergency, and prompt conservative operative management is indicated. Consideration of additional imaging, tumor markers, and surgical management of persistent or complex masses with ultrasound findings suspicious for malignancy is appropriate. This article reviews all these conditions and conservative management using laparoscopy as the preferred method if surgical intervention is needed. Unilateral removal of malignancies is advocated when possible.

Human papillomaviruses (HPV) are a family of viruses that infect the epithelium of many parts of the body. Persistent infection with high-risk HPV is necessary but insufficient to cause cervical cancer. High-risk HPV types are increasingly recognized as a risk factor for cancers other than cervical cancer. A large proportion of vulvar, vaginal, anal, penile, and oropharyngeal cancers are associated with HPV. Low-risk HPV types cause genital warts. Recent advancement in the prevention of HPV infection, genital warts, and HPV-associated precancers and cancers include vaccination. Until the full potential of vaccination can be attained, cervical cancer screening remains an important component of prevention.

Preface

Adolescent Gynecology

In the summer of 2009, the editors of AM:STARS approached the leadership of the North American Society for Pediatric and Adolescent Gynecology (NASPAG) about developing an issue on the topic of Adolescent Gynecology. Founded in the 1980s as an organization that combines the expertise of specialists in adolescent medicine with obstetricians and gynecologists who have a particular interest in pediatric and adolescent gynecology, NASPAG today has over 400 members: approximately one-third specialists in adolescent medicine and two-thirds obstetricians and gynecologists.

In keeping with the philosophy and makeup of NASPAG, this issue represents a combined effort of editors and authors, most of whom are NASPAG members, from the fields of adolescent medicine and obstetrics and gynecology. The articles cover a full range of topics in adolescent gynecology. While focusing mainly on the medical aspects of adolescent patient care shared by both pediatricians and obstetricians and gynecologists, they also include psychosocial aspects of care most commonly associated with the field of adolescent medicine and the surgical components of care as practiced by obstetricians and gynecologists. A review article summarizing the information presented in this issue of AM:STARS will be published in the *Journal of Pediatric and Adolescent Gynecology,* the official journal of NASPAG.

As editors of this issue of AM:STARS, we appreciate the opportunity to have worked together, and thank both the American Academy of Pediatrics and the North American Society for Pediatric and Adolescent Gynecology for their support. We applaud the efforts of the authors of the articles and hope that the information proves useful to readers in both the fields of pediatrics and gynecology.

Martin M. Fisher, MD
Division of Adolescent Medicine
Stephen and Alexandra Cohen
Children's Medical Center of New York
North Shore-Long Island Jewish Health System
Hofstra North Shore-LIJ School of Medicine

Eduardo Lara-Torre, MD
Associate Professor
Residency Program Director
Department of Obstetrics and Gynecology
Virginia Tech-Carilion School of Medicine
Carilion Clinic Medical Center

Adolesc Med 23 (2012) 1–14

A Comprehensive Approach to the Spectrum of Abnormal Pubertal Development

Heather Appelbaum, MD[a]*, Shilpa Malhotra, MD[a]

[a]*Department of Obstetrics and Gynecology, Division of Pediatric and Adolescent Gynecology, Long Island Jewish Medical Center and Cohen Children's Medical Center of New York, Hofstra North Shore LIJ School of Medicine, North Shore-LIJ Health System, New Hyde Park, New York*

INTRODUCTION

Puberty is the biological transition from childhood to adulthood. The process involves the coordination of hormonal, physical, psychosocial, and cognitive systems to result in physiologic change. Although most adolescents follow a predictable path through pubertal maturation, the timing and sequence of pubertal development can be variable. The average onset of pubertal development in girls is 12 years, but genetic predisposition is influenced by environmental exposures and overall health. An insult to the hypothalamic-pituitary-ovarian (HPO) axis can lead to significant deviation of normal pubertal development. Early activation of the HPO axis results in precocious puberty, whereas impaired activation of the HPO axis causes delayed puberty. Secondary sexual development before the age of 8 years may be indicative of precocious puberty, whereas puberty is considered delayed in girls who do not have signs of development by age 13 years. There is a spectrum of aberrant pubertal development that includes incomplete precocious puberty, where girls show evidence of early partial development, and a variation of delayed puberty, which includes prolonged sexual maturation (Figure 1).

NORMAL PUBERTY

Normal puberty is initiated centrally, with ovarian function being driven by gonadotropin-releasing hormone (GnRH) from the hypothalamus and gonadotropin secretion from the pituitary gland. Activation of the GnRH pulse genera-

---

*Corresponding author.
E-mail address: happelba@nshs.edu (H. Appelbaum).

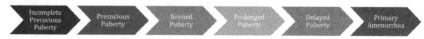

Figure 1. Spectrum of Pubertal Development

tor is dependent on many factors, leading to predictable events. The pulsatile release of GnRH is obligatory to sustain normal gonadotropin synthesis and secretion, which is essential for pubertal development. The initial sign of pubertal development in most girls is breast development, although some will have pubic hair as the earliest manifestation of puberty.[1] Thelarche is the initial appearance of breast tissue. The normal age range for this event is between 8 and 13 years.[2] Adrenarche is the activation of the adrenal glands, resulting in development of axillary and pubic hair. Pubarche is the appearance of pubic hair. Gonadarche marks the activation of the ovaries by the pituitary hormones, follicle stimulating hormone (FSH), and luteinizing hormone (LH). Menarche is the age of onset of the first menstrual period. Growth hormone and insulin-like growth factor-1 levels increase markedly during puberty in response to rising estrogen levels. Approximately 18% of overall growth occurs during puberty[3] and peak height velocity occurs on average 6 months before menarche.[4] According to a recent longitudinal study, adrenarche follows the presence of breast tissue in 66% of girls[2] and typically starts between the ages of 9 and 11 years.[1]

Other studies have defined the average onset of breast and pubic hair development for black girls at ages 8.8 and 8.9 years, respectively. The average age of menarche reported by the National Health and Nutrition Examination Survey (NHANES) from 1999 to 2002 was 12.34 years, with a variance from 12.06 years in black girls to 12.52 years in non-Hispanic white girls.[6] The median length of time between the onset of development of secondary sexual characteristics and menarche is 2.6 years.[4] Based on 17,000 healthy girls in the United States, the Pediatric Research in Office Settings (PROS) Network defined the mean age of breast development at 10 years and the mean age of pubic hair growth at 10.5 years for white girls.[5]

The timing and duration of the pubertal process may be modified by body composition, social milieu, and environmental exposures. Critical body weight and nutritional status play a significant role in the onset of puberty.[7,8] Body mass index (BMI) is an important factor in determining the age of onset of puberty, and leptin levels may play a significant role in mediating gonadotropin secretion.[9,10] In fact, studies have demonstrated that providing leptin to leptin deficient mice potentiates the onset of puberty.[11] Nutritional deficits and low BMI can delay pubertal development, whereas obesity is associated with early maturation. Insulin may be a codeterminant of pubertal tempo.[12,13] Peripubertal obesity is associated with an insulin induced reduction of sex hormone binding globulin, which increases the bioavailability of sex steroids, including estradiol.[14] Chronic illnesses, acute infections, and therapeutic modalities, including antipsychotic medications, chemotherapeutic agents, and radiation therapy, can also affect the onset and duration of the pubertal process.

Endocrine disruptors are natural or synthetic environmental chemicals or pollutants that can alter or affect the normal physiologic endocrine processes. Endocrine disruptors accumulate in the environment and are introduced into the body through water, air, foods, and plastics or can be transferred from mother to fetus via the placenta or breast milk.[7,15,16] Endocrine disruptors exert their effects by binding to hormone receptors and affecting cell signaling pathways, resulting in suppression or activation of relevant hormonal activities.[17] Many chemicals used in agriculture, as well as cleaning substances, cosmetic and hygienic products, dyes, plastic compounds (phthalates), and solvents, contain endocrine disruptors. These substances are stored in fat tissue, and the cumulative effect of long-term exposures may cause detrimental effects. Certain pesticides, phthalates, bisphenol A, and plant-derived phytoestrogens have been implicated in driving a recent trend toward earlier puberty in girls.[18]

EARLY PUBERTAL DEVELOPMENT

Precocious Puberty

Precocious puberty is defined as pubertal development beginning earlier than expected based on normal standards. The standards must take into consideration race and other environmental factors. Abnormal or early pubertal development is defined by children entering puberty more than 2.5 to 3.0 standard deviations earlier than the median age. Breast development and linear growth before the age of 8 years may be indicative of precocious puberty. The Lawson Wilkins Pediatric Endocrine Society (LWPES) recommends evaluation for white girls with signs of precocious development before the age of 7 and black girls before the age of 6[19]; however, these guidelines have been disputed because the lower age may fail to identify a significant number of patients with treatable pathologic processes.[20]

Early development of secondary sexual characteristics may be attributable to androgen or estrogen excess via centrally mediated processes influencing the HPO axis. Alternatively, hormonal activation may originate from peripheral or exogenous sources. Gonadotropin dependent precocious puberty or central precocious puberty (true precocious puberty) is caused by early maturation of the HPO axis. Gonadotropin independent precocious puberty or peripheral precocious puberty (pseudo-precocious puberty) is caused by excess sex hormones. These hormones can be secreted from the ovaries or adrenal glands, or they may originate from external inadvertent or intentional exposures (Table 1).

Nutritional status and an increase in adiposity in obese girls leads to early signs of puberty via several mechanisms. Obese girls have lower levels of sex hormone–binding globulin, which leads to greater bioavailability of circulating sex steroid hormones. Storage of estrogens and aromatization of estrogen precursors is increased in girls with a high index of fat cells. Furthermore, the per-

Table 1.
Differential Diagnosis of Precocious Puberty

Gonadotropin Dependent Precocious Puberty/Central Precocious Puberty	Gonadotropin Independent Precocious Puberty/Peripheral Precocious Puberty
CNS tumors	Follicular cysts
CNS irradiation	Gonadoblastoma
Hydrocephalus	Granulosa-cell tumors
Head trauma	McCune-Albright syndrome
CNS inflammatory disease	Adrenal tumors
Midline CNS congenital malformations	Congenital adrenal hyperplasia
Genetic mutations	Exogenous hormonal exposures
High serum levels of androgens	
Primary hypothyroidism	

CNS, central nervous system

missive action of leptin on the GnRH pulse generator may lead to earlier activation of the HPO axis in obese girls.[8]

Gonadotropin Dependent Precocious Puberty/Central Precocious Puberty/True Precocious Puberty

Early maturation of the HPO axis leads to accelerated linear growth for age, advanced bone age, and hormonal levels consistent with a pubertal state. The majority of girls with gonadotropin dependent precocious puberty have no identifiable cause. However, there may be an association in some cases with central nervous system injury, an intracranial disturbance, hormonal imbalance, or genetic mutations that lead to the release of gonadotropin-releasing hormones that result in early activation of the HPO axis. For example, hamartomas contain GnRH neurons that act as ectopic hypothalamic tissue, and mutations in G protein receptor complexes involving the GPR54-kisspeptin complex responsible for the initiation of normal puberty may undergo early activation.[21,22,23] Girls exposed to high serum levels of androgens from exogenous sources, androgen secreting tumors, or poorly controlled congenital adrenal hyperplasia may have advanced maturation of the hypothalamus. Furthermore, chronic elevation of thyroid stimulating hormone (TSH) associated with hypothyroidism may result in early activation of FSH receptors due to cross-reactivity. The treatment for gonadotropin dependent precocious puberty is cause specific. Treatment of the underlying disorder is paramount, but GnRH agonists can be used to delay pubertal advancement.

Gonadotropin Independent Precocious Puberty/Peripheral Precocious Puberty/ Pseudo-Precocious Puberty

Precocious puberty that is independent of gonadotropin-releasing hormone is caused by exogenous hormones or excess secretion of sex hormones from the gonads or adrenal glands. Examples of gonadotropin independent precocious puberty include ovarian cysts, granulosa-cell tumors or gonadoblastomas, adrenal tumors, enzymatic defects in adrenal steroidogenesis, and exogenous exposure to estrogens or androgens. The peripheral sources of hormone excess lead to suppression of gonadotropins, rendering GnRH agonists ineffective.

Incomplete Precocious Puberty

Rarely, children present with incomplete precocious puberty. In these cases, one or more signs of puberty may exist in isolation. Isolated premature thelarche or adrenarche is usually a normal variant but may result in precocious puberty in 18–20% of girls, with early variable development of secondary sexual characteristics.[1] In the United States, black girls may be two to three times more likely than white girls to have an early appearance of pubic hair.[1] The hormonal basis of early adrenarche is premature activation of adrenal sources of androgens. Typically the etiology of early activation is unknown, and most cases are idiopathic. Alternatively, premature adrenarche can be a sign of congenital adrenal hyperplasia or may be indicative of an adrenal tumor. Additionally, low birth weight increases the risk of developing premature adrenarche. The mechanism by which this occurs may be mediated by the influence of prenatal malnutrition on the development of insulin resistance or by in utero effects of altered secretion of cortisol associated with low birth weight infants.[13] More commonly, premature adrenarche is associated with obesity and may be a marker for future development of polycystic ovarian syndrome or metabolic syndrome.[13,24,25]

According to a longitudinal study in Israel, premature thelarche is present in 43% of girls between 1 and 24 months and 15% of girls aged 2–8 years. In the same study, 51% of all cases of premature thelarche regressed, 36% persisted, and only 3% progressed.[26] Alternatively, estrogens from any source can promote breast tissue development. Therefore, it is possible that premature thelarche with or without premature adrenarche may not reflect true activation of the HPO axis, but more likely represents the influence of peripheral sources, including aromatization of adrenal androgens or an increased bioavailability of estrogens in obese girls, with reduced sex hormone binding globulin.[8]

Isolated premature menarche presents a diagnostic quandary. Nonmenstrual sources of vaginal bleeding must be considered including tumors, vulvovaginal infections or dermatoses, vaginal foreign bodies, or trauma. There are case reports that identify girls with normal physical findings, normal pelvic ultrasounds, and routine hormonal levels who present with cyclic or sporadic vaginal bleeding in the absence of signs of secondary sexual development. However, there is no literature that clearly defines the mechanism of this paradox.

Evaluation of Early Pubertal Development

Evaluation in girls younger than the age of 8 years who present with signs of secondary sexual characteristics is warranted (Figure 2). A detailed history and physical examination guides further testing. The history should focus on when the initial

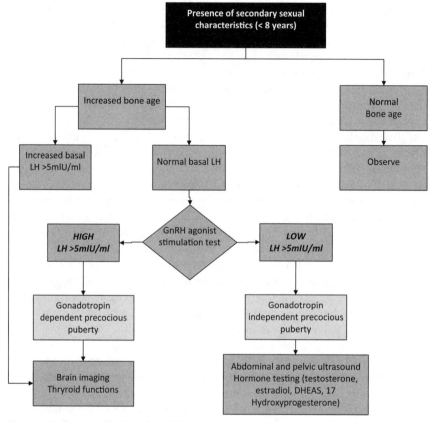

Figure 2. Evaluation of Early Pubertal Development

signs of pubertal development began. Family history of pubertal onset should be elicited. A history of head trauma or an intracranial insult should be assessed, along with a focused review of systems for headaches, visual changes, seizures, nausea and vomiting, or abdominal pain. A linear growth chart should be reviewed, and height velocity (cm/year) should be assessed. It is important to assess breast development not only by inspection, but careful palpation is essential to avoid confusion with adipose tissue under the nipple and areola. A fundoscopic examination for papilledema indicating increased intracranial pressure, assessment of visual fields, an appropriate abdominal examination for masses, and a thorough dermatologic examination to evaluate for café-au-lait spots indicative of McCune-Albright syndrome should be performed. Tanner staging for breast development should be assessed. The presence of signs of androgen excess should be identified and evidence of acanthosis nigricans suggestive of chronic insulin resistance should be documented. Examination of the external genitalia can provide useful information on hormonal status. Evidence of genital ambiguity or estrogenization of mucosal membranes can be elucidated by inspection of the external genitalia.

Assessment of skeletal maturation is indicated if there are early secondary sexual findings on examination. An x-ray of the nondominant hand indicates bone age, and results can be compared with chronological age. Advanced bone age in the presence of secondary sexual characteristic development requires further evaluation with hormonal testing.

Baseline LH and FSH levels should be measured. High basal levels of LH exceeding 5 mIU/mL are indicative of gonadotropin dependent precocious puberty. Girls with low baseline levels of gonadotropins should undergo a GnRH agonist stimulation test by administering a single dose of leuprolide acetate 20 mcg/kg. Peak levels of LH above 5 mIU/mL after 1 to 3 hours are suggestive of gonadotropin dependent precocious puberty, whereas gonadotropin levels do not increase following GnRH stimulation in gonadotropin independent precocious puberty.

Girls with elevated basal or stimulated levels of LH indicative of gonadotropin dependent precocious puberty require brain imaging. Magnetic resonance imaging (MRI) is useful to determine a hypothalamic lesion.

Alternatively, if gonadotropin independent precocious puberty is suspected, a pelvic and abdominal ultrasound to assess for ovarian or adrenal tumors should be performed, along with hormonal testing that includes testosterone, estradiol, dehydroepiandrosterone sulfate (DHEAS), and 17-hydroxyprogesterone. The reliability of androgen laboratory testing is improved with the availability of standardized tests using tandem mass spectrometry and liquid chromatography assays.[27] Thyroid function should be assessed if there is clinical evidence of hypothyroidism.

Treatment of Early Pubertal Development

Treatment is dictated by the etiology and the rate of sexual maturation. Therapy should be directed to the underlying pathology. In cases where there is an unidentifiable cause for early maturation, treatment is dependent on the estimated adult height. Treatment should be offered to prevent early fusion of the epiphyseal plates to avoid unnecessary short stature and should not be based on the perceived psychosocial consequences of early puberty. Palmert et al[28] found that some girls with slowly progressive central precocious puberty achieve a normal adult height without treatment. However, girls with a compromised height prediction can benefit from the use of a GnRH agonist to slow growth velocity and delay epiphyseal fusion to attain slow but progressive increases in height. If the predicted adult height based on measurements of height velocity is greater than 150 cm, a more conservative approach is warranted. Studies suggest that the benefit of treatment with a GnRH agonist is greatest for girls who have the onset of central precocious puberty before 6 years of age.[29] Treatment is less effective in children with substantially advanced bone age.

GnRH agonists, when administered chronically, blunt the natural pulsatile secretion of GnRH from the hypothalamus and thus inhibit pituitary production of gonadotropins. Treatment is continued until 10 to 11 years of age. GnRH treatment is safe, and menstrual cycles resume on an average of 16 months from the end of treatment. Bone mineral density may be decreased during treatment, but it normalizes without any long-term effect on peak bone mass. Furthermore, there are no reports in the literature of compromise to reproductive function or increase in the rate of infertility following GnRH therapy.[19]

There are several different formulations of GnRH available for commercial use. These preparations have not been directly compared in randomized clinical trials and therefore preference for 1 month, 3 month, or 12 month sustained release administration is not evidence based. One prospective study evaluated low birth weight girls who entered early puberty and found that metformin therapy prolonged pubertal progression, resulting in increased height gains.[12] The use of aromatase inhibitors has been the subject of investigation to treat selective forms of precocious puberty, but its efficacy in girls remains debatable.[30]

The efficacy of treatment is monitored by the periodic assessment of pubertal development and bone age. Breast development, growth velocity, and further advancement of bone age should decline. GnRH stimulation tests can be used to assess the adequacy of GnRH agonist dosing. However, this test requires multiple blood sampling. Alternatively, 3-hour LH values can be used for monitoring therapy in patients with gonadotropin dependent precocious puberty.[31]

DELAYED PUBERTY

Delayed Pubertal Development

Delayed puberty is the absence or incomplete development of secondary sexual characteristics. The distinction between delayed puberty and primary amenorrhea may be arbitrary, although primary amenorrhea implies a more permanent dysfunction of the HPO axis. A delay in pubertal progression from onset to menarche of greater than 4–5 years is considered prolonged. An arrest of maturation or interruption in pubertal development may be due to genetic, organic, or psychosocial influences on the GnRH pulse generator responsible for pubertal advancement. Inappropriate gonadal steroid secretion may result from intrinsic gonadal disease, an insult to the anterior pituitary resulting in inadequate levels of gonadotropins, or hypothalamic dysfunction causing an alteration in the secretion of GnRH (Table 2).

According to one small retrospective study, 30% of girls with a delayed onset of puberty resulted from constitutional delay.[32] These girls are slow to mature, as evidenced by delayed bone age. Ultimately, puberty ensues without any compromise to adult height or future fertility.

Table 2.
Differential Diagnosis of Delayed Puberty

Hypogonadotropic Hypogonadism	Hypergonadotropic Hypogonadism
Physiological/constitutional delay	Oophorectomy
Malnutrition	Gonadal dysgenesis
Excessive exercise	Radiation or chemotherapy
Genetic mutation syndromes	Autoimmune or infectious oophoritis
Physiologic or psychological stress	Congenital adrenal hyperplasia
Chronic systemic disorders	Aromatase deficiency
Endocrinopathies	Antiovarian antibodies
Infiltrative or infectious diseases	Genetic mutation syndromes
Traumatic brain injury	Receptor mutations
CNS radiation	
Empty sella	

CNS, central nervous system

Primary Hypogonadism/Hypergonadotropic Hypogonadism

Primary hypogonadism (hypergonadotropic hypogonadism) or ovarian insufficiency may be genetic or acquired. Acquired causes include the presence of anti-ovarian antibodies or gonadotropin autoantibodies,[33,34,35] exposure to radiation or chemotherapy, an inflammatory insult, surgical removal of the gonads, or functional amputation from ovarian torsion. Genetic causes include Turner syndrome, gonadal dysgenesis, and receptor mutations. Ovarian insufficiency is marked by high levels of gonadotropins.

Secondary Hypogonadism/Hypogonadotropic Hypogonadism

Secondary hypogonadism (hypogonadotropic hypogonadism) is usually due to hypothalamic dysfunction, resulting in impaired secretion of GnRH. Hypothalamic dysfunction can be functional, as in constitutional delay of puberty, or due to organic causes that include chronic illness, malnutrition, excessive exercise, stress, central nervous system tumors, infiltrative diseases, hormonal imbalances such as hypothyroidism or hyperprolactinemia, or genetic mutations. Children and adolescents with acute Glasgow coma scale scores of less than or equal to 8 have a greater risk of hypothalamic or pituitary dysfunction related to traumatic brain injury.[36] FGFR1 gene mutations, leptin receptor deficiency mutations, mutations in GPR54 regulation of GnRH release, GNRHR gene mutations (receptor mutations), X-linked Kallmann syndrome (GnRH deficiency), and transcription factor mutations such as PROP1, HESX1, and LHX3 are all genetic sources for hypothalamic dysfunction.[37] Some medications, particularly antipsychotic drugs, can also disrupt the normal function of the HPO axis.

Caloric restriction, excessive exercise, or energy imbalance can suppress GnRH pulsatility, thereby disrupting normal pubertal development. The mechanism by which this occurs is poorly understood but may be related to the physiologic effect of leptin suppression on the hypothalamus.[8] In girls with hypothalamic amenorrhea resulting from negative energy balance, leptin treatment restores the pulse frequency of GnRH.[38] Negative energy balance modulates the hypothalamic pituitary mechanism, prolongs the prepubertal stage, and delays pubertal progression.[39] A critical percentage of body fat is necessary to maintain a metabolic balance to allow for HPO axis activation.

Adverse environmental situations can induce an exaggerated neuroendocrine response that can result in a delay or interruption of pubertal development. Stress, for example, causes the release of corticotrophin-releasing hormone (CRH) from the hypothalamus. In addition to causing an increase in circulating levels of cortisol, CRH inhibits the GnRH pulse generator and ultimately prevents adequate estrogen production.[40]

Incomplete Pubertal Development

Occasionally, adolescents present with arrested or prolonged pubertal development. Restoration of pubertal progression is dependent on the mechanism of interruption, and further maturation is contingent on the nature of the insult to the HPO axis. Genetic and acquired causes may be irreversible, whereas environmental exposures, hormonal disturbances, and metabolic processes may be mutable.

Evaluation of Delayed Puberty

The history and physical examination are particularly useful in elucidating the etiology of delayed puberty. A detailed history should assess for congenital abnormalities, including midline defects that may suggest congenital GnRH deficiency, the family history of timing of pubertal onset, nutritional and exercise habits, psychosocial stressors, use of medications and exposures to radiation or chemotherapeutic agents, and a complete review of systems to assess for other metabolic or hormonal imbalances or chronic illnesses. Neurologic symptoms such as headache, visual changes, anosmia, seizures, and mental retardation are pertinent and may suggest hypothalamic dysfunction.

General assessment includes height and weight, blood pressure, palpation of the thyroid gland, and rating of sexual maturity based on breast and pubic hair assessment. Fundoscopic examination and a thorough neurologic evaluation are essential. Distribution and extent of hair growth should be evaluated using the modified Ferrimen-Gallaway score, and severity of acne should be documented. The presence of acanthosis nigricans should be noted. Evaluation of the vulvovaginal structures can reveal signs of immaturity or virilization and the degree of pubertal mucosal maturation and physiologic discharge in response to increasing intrinsic or extrinsic estrogenic stimulation.

Growth velocity should be assessed, and bone age evaluation is indicated to determine skeletal maturation. Weight is compromised more than height in conditions related to nutrition and caloric intake like anorexia nervosa, celiac disease, or inflammatory bowel disease, rendering underweight girls of normal to slightly diminished stature. On the other hand, height and weight are both affected with endocrinopathies or genetic defects and affected girls tend to have short stature and be overweight.[41] Laboratory evaluation should include hormonal and metabolic screening including FSH, estradiol, thyroid function, and prolactin levels; transglutaminase IgA to assess for celiac disease; a complete blood count; and liver function tests to assess for chronic illnesses. Hypothalamic dysfunction can be distinguished from primary hypogonadism by the presence of low levels of gonadotropins (Figure 3).

Patients with elevated gonadotropins should have a karyotype determined. Pelvic ultrasound can be performed to assess for ovarian volume and the presence of appropriate Müllerian structures. MRI of the head is critical if neurologic symptoms exist or there is impairment in olfactory function.

Treatment of Delayed Puberty

Treatment for delayed puberty is dictated by the underlying disorder. However, the ability to distinguish between congenital GnRH deficiency and constitutional delay of puberty remains challenging. Short-term usage of exogenous estrogens to initiate pubertal development is indicated in girls without evidence of secondary sexual characteristics by the age of 12 years but may result in some loss of adult height due to premature epiphyseal closure. Estrogen therapy can be administered orally or transdermally. Low dose estrogen is warranted for the induction of breast development. Several different formulations of estrogens are

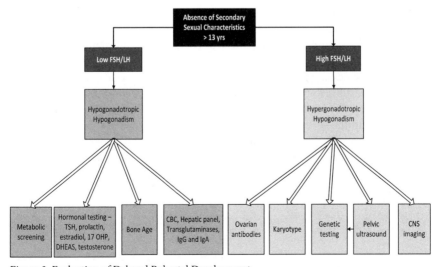

Figure 3. Evaluation of Delayed Pubertal Development

available. These include 0.3 mg of conjugated estrogen, 0.5 mg of micronized estrogen, 10 μg of ethinyl estradiol, or a 25 μg/d estradiol patch; these can all be used for 6 to 12 months with similar efficacy. The dose of estrogen should then be doubled for 6 months. Progesterone should be added at the completion of breast development to protect the endometrial lining from overgrowth, which can result from unopposed estrogen stimulation.[41,42] If constitutional delay is a consideration, a holiday from exogenous hormones should be advised intermittently to determine if spontaneous menstruation occurs. Regardless of the etiology, the long-term goal for patients with inadequate GnRH stimulation is to maintain the serum concentration of sex steroids within the normal adult range to prevent premature bone loss and ultimately to induce fertility when indicated.

SUMMARY

- Puberty is the biological transition from childhood to adulthood. The process involves the coordination of hormonal, physical, psychosocial, and cognitive systems to result in physiologic change.
- Precocious puberty is defined as pubertal development beginning earlier than expected based on normal standards.
- Gonadotropin dependent precocious puberty is caused by premature activation of the hypothalamus resulting in pulsatile secretion of GnRH.
- Gonadotropin independent precocious puberty is caused by excess sex hormones from peripheral or external sources.
- Treatment with GnRH agonists should be offered to prevent early fusion of the epiphyseal plates to avoid unnecessary short stature and should not be based on perceived psychosocial consequences of early puberty.
- Delayed puberty is the absence of or incomplete development of secondary sexual characteristics.
- Hypergonadotropic hypogonadism or primary hypogonadism may result from genetic mutation syndromes or can be acquired from antiovarian antibodies, exposure to radiation or chemotherapy, inflammatory insult, or surgical removal of the gonads.
- Hypogonadotropic hypogonadism or secondary hypogonadism is due to hypothalamic dysfunction resulting in impaired secretion of GnRH.
- The long-term goal for patients with inadequate estrogen stimulation is to maintain the serum concentration of sex steroids within the normal adult range to promote the development of secondary sexual characteristics, prevent premature bone loss, and ultimately to induce fertility when indicated.

References

1. Susman EJ, Houts RM, Steinberg L, et al. Longitudinal development of secondary sexual characteristics in girls and boys between ages 9 ½ and 15 ½ years. *Arch Pediatr Adolesc Med.* 2010;164 (2):164–173
2. Kaplowitz P. Update on precocious puberty: girls are showing signs of puberty earlier, but most do not require treatment. *Adv Pediatr.* 2011;58:243–258

3. Abassi V. Growth and normal puberty. *Pediatrics.* 1998;102:507
4. Biro FM, Galvez MP, Greenspan LC. Pubertal assessment method and baseline characteristics in a mixed longitudinal study of girls. *Pediatrics.* 2010;126(3):583–590
5. Hermman-Giddens ME, Slora EJ, Wasserman RC. Secondary sexual characteristics and menses in young girls seen in office practice: a study from the Pediatric Research in Office Settings network. *Pediatrics.* 1997;99(4):505–512
6. Wu T, Mendola P, Buck GM. Ethnic differences in the presence of secondary sex characteristics and menarche among US girls: the Third National Health and Nutrition Examination Survey, 1988–1994. *Pediatrics.* 2002;110(4):752–757
7. Buck Louis GM, Gray LE, Marcus M. Environmental factors and puberty timing: expert panel research needs. *Pediatrics.* 2008;121:192–207
8. Burt Solorzano CM, McCartney CR. Obesity and the pubertal transition in girls and boys. *Reproduction.* 2010;140(3):399–410
9. Donato J, Cravo R, Frazao R. Hypothalamic sites of leptin action linking metabolism and reproduction. *Neuroendocrinology.* 2011;93:9–18
10. Quennell JH, Mulligan AC, Tups A. Leptin indirectly regulates gonadotropin-releasing hormone neuronal function. *Neuroendocrinology.* 2009;150(6):2805–28012
11. Chehab FF, Lim ME, Lu R. Correction of the sterility defect in homozygous obese female mice by treatment with the human recombinant leptin. *Nat Genet.* 1996;12:318–320
12. Ibanez L, Valls C, Ong K. Metformin therapy during puberty delays menarche, prolongs pubertal growth, and augments adult height: a randomized study in low birth weight girls with early-normal onset of puberty. *J Clin Endocrinol Metab.* 2006;91(6):2068–2073
13. Idkowaik J, Lavery GG, Dir V. Premature adrenarche: novel lessons from early onset androgen excess. *Eur J Endocrinol.* 2011;165:189–207
14. Ahmed ML, Ong KK, Dunger DB. Childhood obesity and the timing of puberty. *Trends Endocrinol Metab.* 2009;20:237–242
15. McLachlan JA, Simpson I, Martin M. Endocrine disruptors and female reproductive health. *Best Pract Res Clin Endocrinol Metab.* 2006;20:63–75
16. Jacobson-Dickeran I, Le MM. Influence of endocrine disruptors on pubertal timing. *Curr Opin Endocrinol Diabetes Obes.* 2009;16:25–30
17. Ozen S, Darcan S. Effects of environmental endocrine disruptors on pubertal development. *J Clin Res Pediatr Endocrinol.* 2011;3(1):1–6
18. Nebesio TD, Pescovitz OH. Historical perspectives: endocrine disruptors and the timing of puberty. *Endocrinology.* 2005;15(1):44–48
19. Carel JC, Eugster E, Rogol A. Consensus statement on the use of gonadotropin-releasing hormone analogs in children. *Pediatrics.* 2009;123(4):752–762
20. Midyett LK, Moore WV, Jacobson JD. Are pubertal changes in girls before age 8 benign? *Pediatrics.* 2003;111:47
21. Teles MG, Bianco SD, Brito VN. A GPR54-activating mutation in a patient with central precocious puberty. *N Engl J Med.* 2008;358(7):709–715
22. Sills ES, Walsh AP. The GPR54-Kisspeptin complex in reproductive biology: neuroendocrine significance and implications for ovulation induction and contraception. *Neuro Endocrinol Lett.* 2008;29(6):846–851
23. Pineda R, Garcia-Galiano D, Roseweir A. Critical roles of kisspeptins in female puberty and preovulatory gonadotropin surges as revealed by a novel antagonist. *Endocrinology.* 2010;151(2):722–730
24. Rosenfield RL, Lipton RB, Drum ML. Thelarche, pubarche, and menarche attainment in children with normal and elevated body mass index. *Pediatrics.* 2009;123(1):84–88
25. Van Weissenbruch MM. Premature adrenarche, polycystic ovary syndrome and intrauterine growth retardation: does a relationship exist? *Curr Opin Endocrinol Diabetes Obes.* 2007;14(1):35–40
26. DeVries L, Guz-Mark A, Lazar L. Premature thelarche: age at presentation affects clinical course but not clinical characteristics or risk to progress to precocious puberty. *J Pediatr.* 2010;156(3):466–471
27. Kushnir MM, Rockwood AL, Roberts WL. Development and performance evaluation of tandem mass spectrometry assay for four androgen steroids. *Clin Chem.* 52:159–167

28. Palmert MFR, Malin HV, Boepple PA. Unsustained or slowly progressive puberty in young girls; initial presentation in long-term follow up of 20 untreated patients. *J Clin Endocrinol Metab.* 1999;84(2):415–423

29. Lazar L, Kauli R, Pertzelan A. Gonadotropin-suppressive therapy in girls with early and fast puberty affects the pace of puberty but not total pubertal growth or final height. *J Clin Endocrinol Metab.* 2002;87(5):2090–2094

30. Eugster EA. Aromatase inhibitors in precocious puberty: rationale and experience to date. *Treat Endocrinol.* 2004;3(3):141–151

31. Acharya SV, Gopal RA, George J. Utility of single luteinizing hormone determination 3h after depot leuprolide in monitoring therapy of gonadotropin-dependent precocious puberty. *Pituitary.* 2009;12:335–338

32. Sedlemeyer IL, Palmert MR. Delayed puberty: analysis of a case series from an academic center. *J Clin Endocrinol Metab.* 2002;87:1613

33. Shatavi SV, Llanes G, Luborsky J. Association of unexplained infertility with gonadotropin and ovarian antibodies. *Am J Reprod Immunol.* 2006;56(5):286–291

34. Meyer WR, Lavy G, DecCherney AH. Evidence of gonadal and gonadotropin antibodies in women with a suboptimal ovarian response to exogenous gonadotropin. *Obstet Gynecol.* 1990;75:795–799

35. Luborsky JL, VisintinI, Boyers S. Ovarian antibodies detected by immobilized antigen immunoassay in patients with premature ovarian failure. *J Clin Endocrinol Metab.* 1990;70:69–75

36. Acerini CL, Tasker, RC, Bellone S. Hypopituitarism in childhood and adolescence following traumatic brain injury: the case for prospective endocrine investigation. *Eur J Endocrinol.* 2006;155:663–669

37. Caronia LM, Martin C, Welt, C. A genetic basis for functional hypothalamic amenorrhea. *N Engl J Med.* 2011;364(3):215–225

38. Welt CK, Chan JL, Bullen J. Recombinant human leptin in women with hypothalamic amenorrhea. *N Engl J Med.* 2004;351:987–997

39. Georgopoulos NA. Growth in athletes. *Ann NY Acad Sci.* 2010;1205:39–44

40. Edozien LC. Mind over matter: psychological factors and the menstrual cycle. *Curr Opin Obstet Gynecol.* 2006;18:452–456

41. Emans SJ. Delayed Puberty. In: Emans SJ, Laufer MR, Goldstein DP. *Pediatric and Adolescent Gynecology.* 5th ed. Baltimore, MD: Lippincott Williams and Wilkins; 2005:181–213

42. Benjamin I, Block RE. Endometrial response to estrogen and progesterone therapy in patients with gonadal dysgenesis. *Obstet Gynecol.* 1977;50:136

Adolesc Med 23 (2012) 15–33

Adolescents, Sex, and the Media

Victor C. Strasburger, MD*

*Professor of Pediatrics, Professor of Family & Community Medicine,
University of New Mexico School of Medicine, MSC 10 5590,
1 Univ. of New Mexico, Albuquerque, New Mexico 87131*

Something's in the air, and I wouldn't call it love. Like never before, our kids are being bombarded by images of oversexed, underdressed celebrities who can't seem to step out of a car without displaying their well-waxed private parts to photographers.[1]

One erect penis on a U.S. screen is more incendiary than a thousand guns.[2p66]

[My doctor's] only gone to one medical school, but if you go online, you can get advice from all over the world.[3p17]

In the absence of effective sex education in the United States, the media have arguably become the leading sex educator for children and teenagers (Figure 1). Given the fact that American media are extremely suggestive and rarely responsible, this is not a healthy situation. Previous research was convincing in showing that the media contribute to teenagers' sexual attitudes and beliefs about sex and sexuality.[4] Now, new research is beginning to show that the media may contribute substantially in a cause-and-effect manner to the risk of early intercourse and even pregnancy among teenagers.[5,6] Given the risks of early sexual activity—teen pregnancy, sexually transmitted infections (STIs), HIV and AIDS, and so forth—any factor that might have an impact and that could be lessened is important to consider.[7]

WHY IS THIS AN ISSUE?

Although the teenage pregnancy rate in the United States has declined significantly in the past 2 decades—34% between its peak in 1991 and 2005[8]—it

---

*Corresponding author.
E-mail address: VStrasburger@salud.unm.edu (V. C. Strasburger).

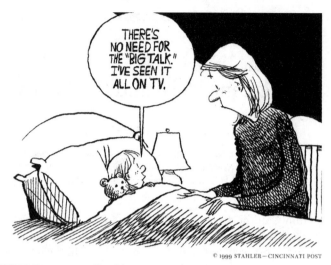

Figure 1. STAHLER. © 1999 Jeff Stahler. Reprinted by permission of Universal Uclick for UFS. All rights reserved.

remains the highest in the Western world. It is 10–15 times higher than in other developed countries with the lowest birth rates.[9] In 2009, approximately 410,000 15–19-year-old female teens—4% of all female teens in that age group—gave birth.[10] Most of these are unintended pregnancies,[11] and the total cost of all such pregnancies in women of childbearing age is an estimated $11 billion a year.[12] Approximately 18% of women having abortions in the United States are teenagers, and one-third are young adults, ages 20–24 years.[13]

Similarly, rates of adolescent sexual activity have leveled off but remain problematic. According to the 2009 Youth Risk Behavior Survey (YRBS)[14]:

- In 2009, nearly half (46%) of all high school students reported ever having had sexual intercourse. This represents a decline from 54% in 1991.
- More than one-third had had sex in the previous 3 months. Six percent said that they had first had sex before age 13. Fourteen percent reported having had 4 or more sexual partners.
- Condom use at last intercourse has increased since 1991 but has plateaued at 61%; birth control pill use has decreased to 20%.

Rates of other sexual activities, especially oral sex, are less well investigated. The YRBS, for example, does not ask about oral sex. One study of 580 ninth graders found that 20% had had oral sex.[15] A large 2002 study that included 10,000 15–19-year-olds found that 55% had had oral sex by age 19.[16]

With sexual activity obviously comes the risk of STIs, and teenagers and young adults have a disproportionate percentage. Of the 18 million STIs diagnosed annually in the United States, approximately half occur in young people aged 15–24 years, even though they represent only 25% of the sexually experienced population.[17]

One might think that with all of these risks to young people's health, there might be a public health impetus to educate teenagers in an intensive and comprehensive way about sex.[18] In the United States, however, that has not been the case.[19] The first 8 years of the new millennium were devoted to abstinence-only sex education, which has been shown to be ineffective [20,21] except with 12-year-old black boys in inner city Philadelphia.[22] Congress has spent $1.5 billion on programs that don't work and are ineffective.[19] Comprehensive sex education—which *does* work[21]—has been marginalized.[23] Although most of the nearly 2800 15–19-year-olds surveyed in the 2006–2008 National Survey of Family Growth reported receiving sex education, 30% of females and 38% of males reported receiving no information on methods of birth control.[24]

Research shows that parent-child communication can clearly be effective in preventing early sexual activity among teenagers.[25] But parents seem to be caught in the middle. Although the majority of parents favor sex education in schools—90% say it is very or somewhat important in one national survey of parents in 2004[26]—half of parents of 10–12-year-olds have not talked about peer pressure to have sex or how to prevent pregnancy and STIs.[27] In a separate Kaiser survey, two-thirds of parents said they are very concerned about their children being exposed to too much inappropriate content in the media, and 55% said that sex in the media was contributing a lot to teenagers' behavior.[28] As the senior vice president of the Kaiser Family Foundation noted, "The 'big talk' isn't what it used to be. It now needs to be 'supersized.' "[29]

"NEW" MEDIA VERSUS "OLD" MEDIA

Despite the seeming tidal wave of "new" media in the past decade (Internet, cell phones, iPads, social networking sites, etc.) (Figure 2), "old" media—TV, movies, and videos—still predominate among children and adolescents. The 2009 Kaiser survey of more than 2000 8–18-year-olds found that they spent an average of more than 7 hours a day with a variety of different media, but TV remains predominant (Figures 3 and 4).[30] What has changed is that TV and movies may no longer be viewed on a TV set but rather on a computer, cell phone, or iPad.[31] Nielsen reports that time spent watching TV and video online rose 45% from 2010 to 2011.[32] TV viewing is actually at an all-time high. Although teens watch less TV than adults (who average nearly 35 hours/week), they still watch an average of nearly 24 hours per week.[33]

But there is no question that the topography of the media landscape is changing, particularly among teenagers[34-36]:

- Teenagers watch an average of more than 7 hours of TV a month on mobile devices.

Teen gadget ownership

The percent of all teens 12-17 who own each of the following devices, as of September 2009.

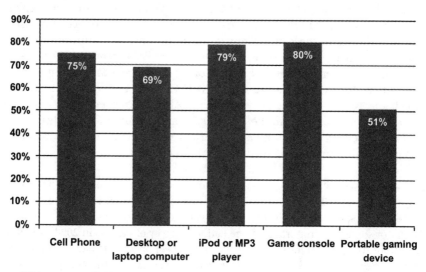

n=800 teens ages 12-17
(including 245 cell phone interviews)

Figure 2. Source: The Pew Research Center. The Pew Internet & American Life Project 2009. Trend Data for Teens: Teen gadget ownership. Reprinted with permission. Available at: http://pewinternet.org/Trend-Data-for-Teens/Teen-Gadget-Ownership.aspx

- Teens ages 13–17 send an average of 3364 texts per month and spend more time texting than talking on the phone. Although adults have caught up to teens in social networking, teens are still heavier users—more than three-fourths of 12–17-year-olds have accessed social networks or blogs.
- American 18-year-olds average nearly 40 hours a week online from their home computers, including 5½ hours of streaming video.
- 93% of teenagers now use the Internet. In a 2009 survey, 7% of 12–17-year-olds owned a cell phone and 80% owned an iPod and a game console.

HOW MUCH SEXUAL CONTENT IS THERE IN THE MEDIA?

Clearly, media and teens' use of them are in a state of flux. Unfortunately, the last content analysis of sexual content on American TV was 7 years ago, but its findings are probably still relevant. More than 75% of primetime TV programs contain sexual content, yet only 14% of sexual references mention risks or responsibilities of sexual activity (Figures 5 and 6).[37] Talk about sex on TV can occur as often as 8–10 times per hour, and the amount of sexual content continues to

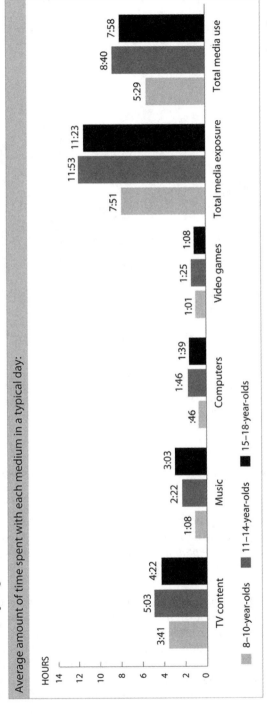

Figure 3. Source: *Report: Generation M²: Media in the Lives of 8- to 18-Year-olds.* (#8010), The Henry J. Kaiser Family Foundation, January 2010. This information was reprinted with permission from the Henry J. Kaiser Family Foundation. The Kaiser Family Foundation, a leader in health policy analysis, health journalism and communication, is dedicated to filling the need for trusted, independent information on the biggest health issues facing our nation and its people. The Foundation is a non-profit private operating foundation, based in Menlo Park, California.

Media Exposure, by TV Environment and Rules

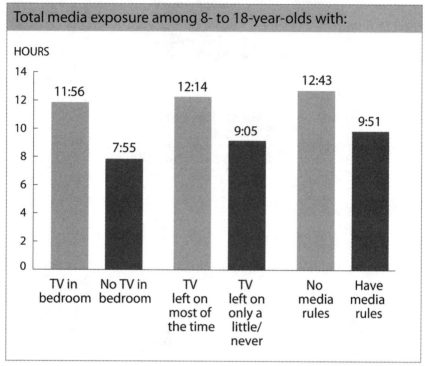

Figure 4. Source: *Report: Generation M²: Media in the Lives of 8- to 18-Year-olds.* (#8010). The Henry J. Kaiser Family Foundation, January 2010. This information was reprinted with permission from the Henry J. Kaiser Family Foundation.

rise.[38] Remarkably, shows targeted at teens actually have more sexual content than adult shows.[37]

Reality TV is also becoming more common and is often filled with sexual innuendo. In 1997, there were only 3 reality dating shows; by 2004 there were more than 30.[39] Shows such as *Temptation Island* brought contestants together with the sole purpose of seeing who "hooks up."

Several other "old" media popular with teenagers are also rife with sexual innuendo: In popular music, an analysis of the 279 most popular songs in 2005 revealed that 37% contained sexual references, many of which were degrading to women.[40] Virtually *every* R-rated teen movie since the 1980s has contained at least 1 nude scene and often several references to intercourse.[4] Teen magazines devote an average of 2.5 pages per issue to sexual topics, but the primary focus seems to be on when to lose one's virginity.[41,42] In mainstream advertising,

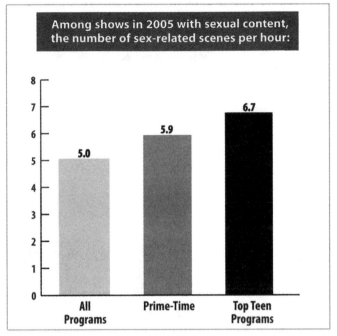

Figure 5. Source: *Sex on TV 4: A Biennial Report to the Kaiser Family Foundation.* (#7399). The Henry J. Kaiser Family Foundation, November 2005. This information was reprinted with permission from the Henry J. Kaiser Family Foundation.

women are as likely to be shown in suggestive clothing (30%), partially clothed (13%), or nude (6%) as they are to be fully clothed.[43]

"New" media have brought new concerns to the forefront—among them, pornography, "sexting," and displays of risky behavior on social networking sites. One national sample of 1500 10–17-year-olds found that nearly half of the Internet users had been exposed to online pornography in the previous year.[44] One recent study of MySpace profiles revealed that nearly one-fourth of them referenced sexual behaviors.[45] "Sexting"—or the transmission of nude pictures via text message—may not be as common as previously thought, however. A national survey of nearly 1300 teens in 2008 put the figure at 20%.[46] However, a very recent national study of 1560 Internet users ages 10–17 puts the figure at 1% of youth who reported sending sexual images of themselves and 5.9% of youth who reported that they had received sexual images.[47]

WHAT DOES THE RESEARCH SHOW?

Abundant research documents that the media can exert a powerful influence on children and teenagers.[4] Probably the two main mechanisms are giving young people "scripts" of how to behave in novel situations (script theory)[48] and by

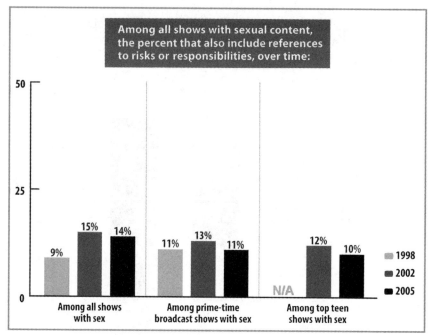

Figure 6. Source: *Sex on TV 4: A Biennial Report to the Kaiser Family Foundation.* (#7399). The Henry J. Kaiser Family Foundation, November 2005. This information was reprinted with permission from the Henry J. Kaiser Family Foundation.

making certain risky behaviors seem normative ("super-peer theory").[49,50] Dozens of studies show that teenagers learn information and attitudes about sex and sexuality from the media (Figures 7 and 8), and that heavy consumers of media are more likely to think that real human behavior mimics behavior seen on TV and in movies (the "cultivation hypothesis").[42,51,52]

But most studies of teenagers and media are correlational—taking a sample at one point in time and investigating if heavily exposed subjects are affected more than lightly exposed subjects. Such research yields possible associations but not cause-and-effect. There are now 17 longitudinal correlational studies that allow cause-and-effect conclusions to be drawn, and virtually all of them show an impact of sexual content in the media on adolescents' sexual behavior (Table 1).[6,53-69] No study is perfect, however. The best study[55] looked at the total media diet of teenagers (TV, movies, music, magazines) but omitted the Internet. Studies range from 1–3 years in follow-up and control for a whole host of other factors known to be associated with early sexual intercourse (eg, household composition, socioeconomic status, parental education, academic achievement, gender, pubertal status, parental styles, religiosity, etc.). Overall, the findings show a doubled risk for early sexual intercourse for teens exposed to more sexual content.[6] Several studies have

ISIS/thinktank survey:

Which of the following online sites have you visited to learn about sex and health related issues, such as sexually transmitted diseases, birth control, pregnancy, or menstruation?

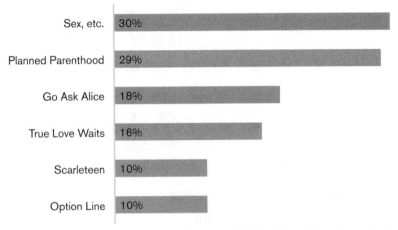

Figure 7. Source: Boyar R, Levine D, Zensius N. *TECHsex USA: Youth Sexuality and Reproductive Health in the Digital Age.* Oakland, CA: ISIS, Inc; 2011. Available at: http://www.isis-inc.org/

found that whites are affected and blacks are not, but the studies typically start assessing teenagers at age 14 and may miss the onset of sexual intercourse in blacks. Studies have also found a relationship between sexual content and noncoital behavior,[53,55] multiple sexual partners,[52] STIs,[52] teen pregnancy,[57] and sexual aggression.[66]

The 17 studies vary in which media they assess. Most have assessed TV,[53,54,57,58,63,65] a few have examined a variety of different media,[55,59,64] two have examined rock music and music videos,[52,56] one examined the protective role of parental coviewing,[59] and only three have examined Internet pornography and other X-rated material.[61,62,66] To date, there are no longitudinal studies on the behavioral impact of sexting or displays of risky behaviors on teenagers' social networking profiles.

This is difficult research to do, and it is instructive that there are more than 2000 studies on media violence but less than 100 on sexual content and adolescents' attitudes and behavior. Parents and schools are shy about allowing access to adolescents, particularly young adolescents, for studies about sex, and both the federal government and private foundations have almost completely ignored funding for such research.

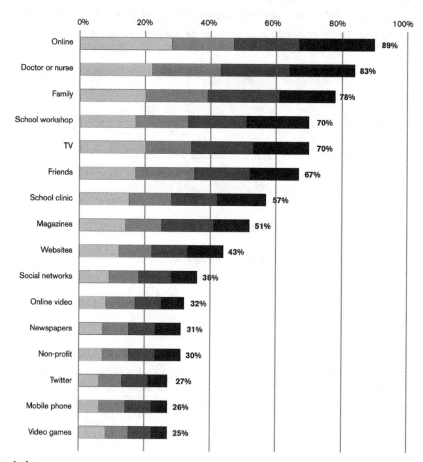

ISIS/thinktank survey:

How do you learn about each of the following topics? (*Check all that apply.*)

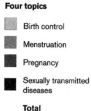

Four topics

- Birth control
- Menstruation
- Pregnancy
- Sexually transmitted diseases

Total

Figure 8. Source: Boyar R, Levine D, Zensius N. *TECHsex USA: Youth Sexuality and Reproductive Health in the Digital Age.* Oakland, CA: ISIS, Inc; 2011. Available at: http://www.isis-inc.org/

Table 1.
Recent Longitudinal Studies of the Impact of Sexual Content on Sexual Behavior

Study	N	Media Type	Duration	Findings
Wingood (2003)	480 14–18 years old	Rap videos	1 year	Exposure to sexual rap videos predicted multiple partners females
Collins (2004)	1792 12–17 years old	TV	1 year	Sexual media exposure strongly predicted intercourse a year later
Martino (2005)	1292 12–17 years old	TV	1 year	Exposure to popular teen shows with sexual content increased risk of intercourse 1 year later
Ashby (2006)	4808 Seventh-twelfth grades	TV	1 year	> 2 hours TV/day increased risk of intercourse by 1.35 times
Brown (2006)	1107 12–14 year olds	Sexual media diet (TV, movies, magazines, music)	2 years	2 times increased risk of sexual intercourse for white teens with high sexual media diet
Martino (2006)	1242 12–17 year olds	Music	3 years	Degrading sexual content predicted earlier intercourse
Bersamin (2008)	887 12–16 years old	TV	1 year	Parental coviewing of TV protective against early intercourse and oral sex
Bleakley (2008)	501 14–16 years old	TV, movies, magazines, music, video games	1 year	Positive and reciprocal relationship between media exposure and intercourse
Chandra (2008)	744 12–20 years old	TV	3 years	Sexual media exposure is a strong predictor of teen pregnancy
L'Engle (2008)	854 12–14 years old	Sexual media diet, including Internet	2 years	Peer and media exposure increased risk of early sex; stronger connection to parents and schools was protective
Peter (2008)	962 13–20 years old	Internet	1 year	Exposure to sexual content on the Internet increased sexual preoccupation
Brown (2009)	967 Seventh-eighth graders	X-rated movies, magazines, Internet pornography	2 years	Early exposure to X-rated media predicts earlier onset of sexual intercourse and oral sex
Delgado (2009)	754 7–18 years old	TV, movies	5 years	Watching adult-targeted TV increases the risk of intercourse by 33% for every hr/day viewed at a young age
Hennessy (2009)	506 14–18 years old	TV, movies, magazines, music, video games, and media	2 years	Increased risk of intercourse for white teens
Bersamin (2010)	824 14–18 years old	TV	1 year	Premium cable TV viewing associated with casual sex
Gottfried (2011)	474 14–16 years old	TV—varying genres	1 year	No impact of overall sexual content found on sexual intercourse, but exposure to TV sitcoms did predict earlier sex
Ybarra (2011)	1159 10–15 years old	X-rated media (movies, magazines, Internet pornography)	3 years	Intentional exposure to violent X-rated material predicted a nearly 6 times risk of sexually aggressive behavior

CONTRACEPTIVE ADVERTISING

One of the great paradoxes of American television is that sex is used to advertise everything from cars and shampoos to the new fall line-up of TV shows, but advertising contraceptives is nearly *verboten*.[42] The United States is the only Western country that still subscribes to the myth that giving teenagers access to birth control—and media are one way of doing that—makes them more sexually active. In fact, one recent study found that 86% of the recent decline in teen pregnancies could be attributed to increased contraceptive use; only 14% was attributable to increased abstinence.[70] There are now 8 peer-reviewed clinical studies that have found that giving teenagers freer access to condoms does not increase their sexual activity but does increase the use of condoms among those who are already sexually active.[71-78] In 2007, both CBS and FOX refused to air a condom advertisement because it specifically mentioned preventing pregnancy rather than preventing HIV/AIDS.[79] Two of the 6 major networks refuse to air condom ads, and 3 others air them only after 9 PM or 11 PM. Several networks also refuse to air ads for birth control pills, and the ones that do refuse to allow the words "prevent pregnancy" in such ads.[80] This, despite the fact that a majority of American adults *favor* the advertising of condom ads on TV (71% of 1142 adults surveyed in a national sample done by Kaiser). In fact, more adults oppose beer ads (34%) than condom ads (25%).[81]

CAN MEDIA HAVE A POSITIVE IMPACT?

Media represent just one avenue for sex education, but a potentially powerful one. The disconnect between sexual content and responsible sexual information seen in the 2005 Kaiser report (see Figure 6) is remediable. In fact, there have been several notable attempts by writers and producers to embed socially responsible information into mainstream programming (so-called "edutainment"):

- In 2002, *Friends* aired an episode about condoms. Twenty-seven percent of a national sample of teenagers reported seeing the episode, and many talked with an adult about contraception as a result.[82]
- The hit show *ER* featured storylines on emergency contraception and on HPV.[83]
- A 2008 episode of *Grey's Anatomy* explored the issue of treating HIV-positive women who are pregnant.[84]
- Media giant Viacom has partnered with MTV to air public service announcements (PSAs) concerning HIV/AIDS and condom use.[85]

Mass media have also been used to try to increase parent-child discussions about sex. In North Carolina, an intensive campaign of PSAs on radio, TV, and billboards delivered the message, "Talk to your kids about sex. Everyone else is." A follow-up study found it to be effective.[86]

SOLUTIONS

If the United States and other Western countries are serious about lowering rates of teen pregnancy and nurturing sexually healthy adolescents, then the media and society's use of media must change dramatically.

Clinicians

Clinicians are weighed down by many financial and time constraints. Nevertheless, the media have an impact on *virtually every concern* they have about teenagers: sex, drugs, aggressive behavior, obesity, eating disorders, sleep, and school performance.[87] Clinicians need to ask 2 media-related questions at every well-child and well-teen visit: (1) How much entertainment screen time do you spend, per day, on all possible screens? (2) Is there an Internet connection, TV, cell phone, or iPad in your bedroom? Research has shown that the presence of a bedroom TV increases the risk of substance use and early sexual activity by teens.[88] According to a recent office-based study, just a minute or two of counseling about media could result in nearly 1 million more children and teenagers limiting their total media time.[89] Clinicians can also use new media to access their patients in new ways: A $2 million grant from the National Institutes of Health is being used to produce twelve 20-minute soap opera vignettes that women can watch on their cell phones.[90] Cell phone texts, social networking sites, and teen-friendly Web sites can be used to connect teenagers to much-needed health services.[91,92]

Parents

On a list of 100 problems parents want to fight with their children about, media usually would rank at about 112. Parents think their children and teenagers are "safe" if they are in their bedroom, watching TV or surfing online. The research says otherwise.[87] Having clear rules about media, setting limits on screen time, and keeping media out of the bedroom are associated with fewer hours of media time for adolescents.[93] Parents of younger children, especially preteens, need to understand that letting their children see PG-13 and R-rated movies may lead to harmful consequences.[94-96] Parents also need to be more aware of social networking sites and maintain some vigilance.[36,97,98]

Parents also need to understand that sex education is not just a one-semester course taught in high school. It is a lifelong process—much of it nonverbal—and it includes how young parents refer to their baby's genitalia when changing a diaper, whether there is an "open bathroom door policy," how parents are affectionate with each other, and how they react to something sexy on TV. Parents who understand media effects can use TV and movies wisely to replace "the big talk" with questions about what sexual content is being watched together (co-viewing).

Schools

With rare exceptions, schools have become relatively clueless in how to deal with "new" media and have done a poor job of sex education.[99] Administrators seem to fear the aftershocks of permitting comprehensive sex education, yet the majority of American adults favor such programs over abstinence-only sex education.[26] Schools also need to create intelligent rules to deal with Internet abuse and sexting. In particular, media literacy programs have been shown to be effective with both "old" media[100,101] and "new" media.[102]

Entertainment Industry

With the billions of dollars it rakes in every year, Hollywood needs to be more responsible in how it deals with the sensitive issues of sex and sexuality (Figure 9). Embedding prosocial health messages into mainstream programming does not interfere with anyone's First Amendment or creative rights, yet it could potentially have major positive health consequences (Table 2).[103] A dialogue between adolescent medicine clinicians; pediatricians; family practitioners; public health activists; and Hollywood writers, directors, and producers could be very useful.

Federal Government

From 2000–2008, the US government spent $1.5 billion on abstinence-only sex education, despite the fact that (1) multiple research studies showed it to be ineffective[5] and (2) the media are hardly abstinence-only, and they have become an increasingly powerful sex educator in young people's lives. Congress and the

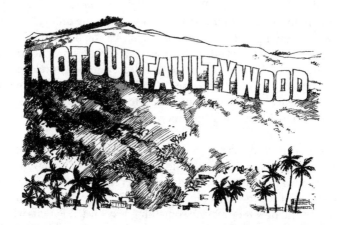

© 1999 BORGMAN – CINCINNATI ENQUIRER

Figure 9. BORGMAN ©1999 Cincinnati Enquirer. Used by permission of Universal Uclick. All rights reserved.

Table 2.
Guide to Responsible Sexual Content in TV, Films, and Music

- Recognize sex as a healthy part of life
- Parent-child conversations about sex should be encouraged
- Demonstrate that not only the young, unmarried, and beautiful have sexual relationships
- Not all affection and touching must culminate in sexual intercourse
- Portray couples having sexual relationships with feelings of love and respect for each other
- Consequences of unprotected sex should be discussed or shown
- Use of contraceptives should be shown as a normal part of a sexual relationship
- Avoid associating violence with sex or love
- Miscarriage should not be used as a dramatic prop for resolving an unwanted pregnancy
- The ability to say "no" should be respected

Adapted from Haffner DW, Kelly M. Adolescent sexuality in the media. *SIECUS Rep.* March/April, 1987:9–12. Reprinted with permission.

Federal Communications Commission (FCC) need to encourage the advertising of condoms, birth control pills, and even emergency contraception. Congress also needs to provide funding for more research into media effects. To date, there has been very little federal funding for media research and virtually no funding from private foundations. Given the impact that media have on young people's lives, this lack of funding is extremely short-sighted.

Recommended Readings

Brown JD, ed. *Managing the Media Monster: The Influence of Media (From Television to Text Messages) on Teen Sexual Behavior and Attitudes.* Washington, DC: The National Campaign to Prevent Teen and Unplanned Pregnancy; 2008

Levin DE, Kilbourne J. *So Sexy So Soon: The New Sexualized Childhood and What Parents Can Do to Protect Their Kids.* New York, NY: Ballantine; 2009

References

1. Deveny K, Kelley R. Girls gone wild: what are celebs teaching kids? *Newsweek.* February 12, 2007:40–47
2. Ansen D. A handful of tangos in Paris. *Newsweek.* September 12, 1999: 66
3. Boyar R, Levine D, Zensius N. *TECHsex USA: Youth Sexuality and Reproductive Health in the Digital Age.* Oakland, CA: ISIS, Inc; 2011
4. Strasburger VC, Wilson BJ, Jordan AB. *Children, Adolescents, and the Media.* 2nd ed. Thousand Oaks, CA: Sage; 2009
5. Strasburger VC and Council on Communications and Media. Sexuality, contraception, and the media (policy statement). *Pediatrics.* 2010;126:576–582
6. Wright PJ. Mass media effects on youth sexual behavior: assessing the claim for causality. *Communication Yearbook.* 2011;35:343–386
7. Christakis DA, Zimmerman FJ. Media as a public health issue. *Arch Pediatr Adolesc Med.* 2006;160: 445–446
8. National Campaign to Prevent Teen and Unplanned Pregnancy. Teen childbearing in the United States, final 2008 birth data. Washington, DC: National Campaign to Prevent Teen and Unplanned Pregnancy; 2010

9. United Nations. *2008 Demographic Yearbook.* New York, NY: United Nations; 2010

10. Centers for Disease Control and Prevention. Vital signs: teen pregnancy—United States, 1991–2009. *MMWR.* 2011;60(13):414–420

11. Kaiser Family Foundation. *Sexual Health of Adolescents and Young Adults in the United States.* Menlo Park, CA: Kaiser Family Foundation; 2011

12. Monea E, Thomas A. Unintended pregnancy and taxpayer spending. *Perspect Sex Reprod Health.* 2011;43:88–93

13. Kost K, Henshaw S, Carlin L. *US Teenage Pregnancies, Births and Abortions: National and State Trends and Trends by Race and Ethnicity.* New York, NY: Guttmacher Institute; 2010

14. Centers for Disease Control and Prevention. Youth risk behavior surveillance—United States, 2009, Surveillance Summaries, June 4, 2010. *MMWR.* 2010;59(No. SS-5)

15. Halpern-Felsher BL, Cornell JL, Kropp RY, Tschann JM. Oral versus vaginal sex among adolescents: perceptions, attitudes, and behavior. *Pediatrics.* 2005;115:845–851

16. Mosher WD, Chandra A, Jones J. Sexual behavior and selected health measures: men and women 15–44 years of age, United States, 2002. *Advance Data.* 2005;362:1–55

17. Centers for Disease Control and Prevention. *Sexually Transmitted Disease Surveillance 2009.* Atlanta, GA: U.S. Department of Health and Human Services; 2010

18. Strasburger VC. Is there an unconscious conspiracy against teenagers in the United States? *Clin Pediatr.* 2006;45(8):714–717

19. Quindlen A. Let's talk about sex. *Newsweek.* March 16, 2009:62

20. Santelli J, Ott MA, Lyon M, Rogers J, Summers D, Schleifer R. Abstinence and abstinence-only education: a review of U.S. policies and programs. *J Adolesc Health.* 2006;38:72–81

21. Kirby D, Laris BA. Effective curriculum-based sex and STD/HIV programs for adolescents. *Child Dev Perspect.* 2009;3:21–29

22. Jemmott JB III, Jemmott LS, Fong GT. Efficacy of a theory-based abstinence-only intervention over 24 months. *Arch Pediatr Adolesc Med.* 2010;164:152–159

23. Lindberg LD, Santelli JS, Singh S. Changes in formal sex education: 1995–2002. *J Adolesc Health.* 2006;38:182–189

24. Martinez G, Abma J, Copen C. Educating teenagers about sex in the United States. NCHS data brief, no. 44. Hyattsville, MD: National Center for Health Statistics; 2010

25. Martino SC, Elliott MN, Corona R, Kanouse DE, Schuster MA. Beyond the "big talk": the roles of breadth and repetition in parent-adolescent communication about sexual topics. *Pediatrics.* 2008;121:e612–e618

26. National Public Radio/Kaiser Family Foundation/Kennedy School of Government. *Sex Education in America.* Menlo Park, CA: Kaiser Family Foundation; 2004

27. The Kaiser Family Foundation/Children Now. *Talking with Kids About Tough Issues: A National Survey of Parents and Kids.* Menlo Park, CA: Kaiser Family Foundation; 1999

28. Rideout V. *Parents, Children & Media.* Menlo Park, CA: Kaiser Family Foundation; 2007

29. Kaiser Family Foundation. New national survey finds kids in families who talk openly about sex and relationships more likely to say would turn to parent first if faced with crisis (new release). March 1, 1999. http://www.kff.org/youthhivstds/1460-kids.cfm. Accessed June 13, 2011

30. Rideout VJ, Foehr UG, Roberts DF. *Generation M²: Media in the Lives of 8- to 18-Year-olds.* Menlo Park, CA: Kaiser Family Foundation; 2010

31. Battaglio S. The future of TV is now. *TV Guide.* October 4–10, 2010:22–23

32. Worden N. Online video viewing jumps, bolstering Netflix. *Wall Street Journal.* February 14, 2011 http://online.wsj.com/article/SB10001424052748703584804576144371093782778.html. Accessed June 13, 2011

33. Nielsen Company. State of the media: TV usage trends: Q3 and Q4 2010. March 10, 2011. http://blog.nielsen.com/nielsenwire/media_entertainment/tv-usage-trends-q3-and-q4-2010/. Accessed June 13, 2011

34. Nielsen Company. How the class of 2011 engages with media. June 8, 2011. http://blog.nielsen.com/nielsenwire/consumer/kids-today-how-the-class-of-2011-engages-with-media/. Accessed June 13, 2011

35. Pew Foundation. Trend data for teens 2011. http://www.pewinternet.org/Static-Pages/Trend-Data-for-Teens.aspx. Accessed June 13, 2011
36. O'Keefe GS, Clarke-Pearson K, Council on Communications and Media. Clinical report: the impact of social media on children, adolescents, and families. *Pediatrics.* 2011;127:800–804
37. Kunkel D, Eyal K, Finnerty K, Biely E, Donnerstein E. *Sex on TV 4: A Biennial Report to the Kaiser Family Foundation.* Menlo Park, CA: Kaiser Family Foundation; 2005
38. Kunkel D, Eyal K, Donnerstein E, Farrar KM, Biely E, Rideout V. Sexual socialization messages on entertainment television: comparing content trends 1997–2002. *Media Psychol.* 2007;9:595–622
39. Zurbriggen EL, Morgan EM. Who wants to marry a millionaire? Reality dating television programs, attitudes towards sex, and sexual behaviors. *Sex Roles.* 2006;54:1–17
40. Primack BA, Gold MA, Schwarz EB, Dalton MA. Degrading and non-degrading sex in popular music: a content analysis. *Public Health Rep.* 2008;123:593–600
41. Walsh-Childers K, Gotthoffer A, Lepre CR. From "just the facts" to "downright salacious:" teens' and women's magazines' coverage of sex and sexual health. In: Brown JD, Steele JR, Walsh-Childers K, eds. *Sexual Teens, Sexual Media.* Hillsdale, NJ: Lawrence Erlbaum; 2002:153–171
42. Brown JD, Strasburger VC. From Calvin Klein to Paris Hilton and MySpace: adolescents, sex and the media. *Adolesc Med State Art Rev.* 2007;18:484–507
43. Reichert T, Carpenter C. An update on sex in magazine advertising: 1983 to 2003. *J Mass Communic Q.* 2004;81:823–837
44. Mitchell KJ, Wolak J, Finkelhor D. Trends in youth reports of sexual solicitations, harassment and unwanted exposure to pornography on the Internet. *J Adolesc Health.* 2007;40:116–126
45. Moreno MA, Parks MR, Zimmerman FJ, Brito TE, Christakis DA. Display of health risk behavior on MySpace by adolescents. *Arch Pediatr Adolesc Med.* 2009;163:27–34
46. National Campaign to Prevent Teen and Unplanned Pregnancy. *Sex and Tech.* Washington, DC: National Campaign to Prevent Teen and Unplanned Pregnancy; 2008
47. Mitchell K, Finkelhor D, Jones L, Wolak J. Prevalence and characteristics of youth sexting: a national study. *Pediatrics.* 2012;129:13–20
48. Huesmann LR. The role of social information processing and cognitive schema in the acquisition and maintenance of habitual aggressive behavior. In: Geen RG, Donnerstein E, eds. *Human Aggression: Theories, Research, and Implications for Policy.* New York, NY: Academic Press;1998: 73–109
49. Strasburger VC. *Adolescents and the Media: Medical and Psychological Impact.* Newbury Park, CA: Sage, 1995
50. Brown JD, Halpern CT, L'Engle KL. Mass media as a sexual super peer for early maturing girls. *J Adolesc Health.* 2005;36:420–427
51. Fisher DA, Hill DL, Grube JW, Bersamin MM, Walker S, Gruber EL. Televised sexual content and parental mediation: influences on adolescent sexuality. *Media Psychol.* 2009;12:121–147
52. Wright PJ, Malamuth NM, Donnerstein E. Research on sex in the media: what do we know about effects on children and adolescents. In: Singer DG, Singer JL, eds. *Handbook of Children and the Media.* 2nd ed. Thousand Oaks, CA: Sage; 2012, pp. 273–302
53. Wingood GM, DiClemente RJ, Bernhardt JM, Harrington K, Davies SL, Robillard A, Hook EW. A prospective study of exposure to rap music videos and African American female adolescents' health. *Am J Public Health.* 2003;93:437–439
54. Collins RL, Elliott MN, Berry SH, Kanouse D, Kunkel D, Hunter S, et al. Watching sex on television predicts adolescent initiation of sexual behavior. *Pediatrics.* 2004;114:e280–e289
55. Ashby SL, Arcari CM, Edmonson MB. Television viewing and risk of sexual initiation by young adolescents. *Arch Pediatr Adolesc Med.* 2006;160:375–380
56. Brown JD, L'Engle K, Pardun CJ, Guo G, Kenneavy K, Jackson C. Sexy media matter: exposure to sexual content in music, movies, television, and magazines predicts black and white adolescents' sexual behavior. *Pediatrics.* 2006;117:1018–1027
57. Martino SC, Collins RL, Elliott MN, Strachman A, Kanouse DE, Berry SH. Exposure to degrading versus nondegrading music lyrics and sexual behavior among youth. *Pediatrics.* 2006;118:e430–e441

58. Chandra A, Martino SC, Collins RL, et al. Does watching sex on television predict teen pregnancy? Findings from a National Longitudinal Survey of Youth. *Pediatrics.* 2008;122:1047–1054
59. Bersamin M, Todd M, Fisher DA, Hill DL, Grube JW, Walker S. Parenting practices and adolescent sexual behavior: a longitudinal study. *J Marriage Fam.* 2008;70:97–112
60. Bleakley A, Hennessy M, Fishbein M, Jordan A. It works both ways: the relationship between exposure to sexual content in the media and adolescent sexual behavior. *Media Psychol.* 2008;11:443–461
61. Peter J, Valkenburg PM. Adolescents' exposure to sexually explicit Internet material and sexual preoccupancy: a three-wave panel study. *Media Psychol.* 2008;11:207–234
62. Brown JD, L'Engle KL. X-rated: sexual attitudes and behaviors associated with U.S. early adolescents' exposure to sexually explicit media. *Communic Res.* 2009;36:129–151
63. Delgado H, Austin SB, Rich M, Bickham D. Exposure to adult-targeted television and movies during childhood increases risk of initiation of early intercourse (abstract). Paper presented at: Pediatric Academic Societies Meeting; May 4, 2009; Baltimore, MD
64. Hennessy M, Bleakley A, Fishbein M, Jordan A. Estimating the longitudinal association between adolescent sexual behavior and exposure to sexual media content. *J Sex Res.* 2009;46:586–596
65. Bersamin MM, Bourdeau B, Fisher DA, Grube JW. Television use, sexual behavior, and relationship status at last oral sex and vaginal intercourse. *Sex Cult.* 2010;14:157–168
66. Ybarra ML, Mitchell KJ, Hamburger M, Diener-West M, Leaf PJ. X-rated material and perpetration of sexually aggressive behavior among children and adolescents: is there a link? *Aggress Behav.* 2011;37:1–18
67. Martino SC, Collins RL, Kanouse DE, Elliott M, Berry SH. Social cognitive processes mediating the relationship between exposure to television's sexual content and adolescents' sexual behavior. *J Pers Soc Psychol.* 2005;89:914–924
68. L'Engle KL, Jackson C. Socialization influences on early adolescents' cognitive susceptibility and transition to sexual intercourse. *J Res Adolesc.* 2008;18:353–378
69. Gottfried JA, Vaala SE, Bleakley A, Hennessy M, Jordan A. Does the effect of exposure to TV sex on adolescent sexual behavior vary by genre? *Commun Res.* First published on July 17, 2011. doi:10.1177/0093650211415399
70. Santelli JS Lindberg LD, Finer LB, Singh S. Explaining recent declines in adolescent pregnancy in the United States: the contribution of abstinence and increased contraceptive use. *Am J Public Health.* 2007;97:150–156
71. Wolk LI, Rosenbaum R. The benefits of school-based condom availability: cross-sectional analysis of a comprehensive high school-based program. *J Adolesc Health.* 1995;17:184–188
72. Furstenberg FF Jr, Geitz LM, Teitler JO, Weiss CC. Does condom availability make a difference? An evaluation of Philadelphia's health resource centers. *Fam Plann Perspect.* 1997;29:123–127
73. Guttmacher S, Lieberman L, Ward D, Freudenberg N, Radosh A, Des Jarlais D. Condom availability in New York City public high schools: relationships to condom use and sexual behavior. *Am J Public Health.* 1997;87:1427–1433
74. Jemmott JB III, Jemmott LS, Fong GT. Abstinence and safer sex: HIV risk-reduction interventions for African American adolescents. *JAMA.* 1998;279:1529–1536
75. Schuster MA, Bell RM, Berry SH, Kanouse DE. Impact of a high-school condom availability program on sexual attitudes and behaviors. *Fam Plan Perspect.* 1998;30:67–72
76. Kirby D, Brener ND, Brown NL, Peterfreund N, Hillard P, Harrist R. The impact of condom distribution in Seattle schools on sexual behavior and condom use. *Am J Public Health.* 1999;89:182–187
77. Blake SM, Ledsky R, Goodenow C, Sawyer R, Lohrmann D, Windsor R. Condom availability programs in Massachusetts high schools: relationships with condom use and sexual behavior. *Am J Public Health.* 2003;93:955–962
78. Sellers DE, McGraw SA, McKinlay JB. Does the promotion and distribution of condoms increase sexual activity? Evidence from an HIV prevention program for Latino youth. *Am J Public Health.* 1994;84:1952–1959
79. Kristof N. Beyond chastity belts. *New York Times.* May 2, 2006: A25
80. Espey E, Cosgrove E, Ogburn T. Family planning American style: why it's so hard to control birth in the US. *Obstet Gynecol Clin N Am.* 2007;34:1–17

81. Kaiser Family Foundation. *A Survey Snapshot: Condom Advertising on Television*. Menlo Park, CA: Kaiser Family Foundation; 2001

82. Collins RL, Elliott MN, Berry SH, Kanouse DE, Hunter SB. Entertainment television as a healthy sex educator: the impact of condom-efficacy information in an episode of *Friends*. *Pediatrics*. 2003;112:1115–1121

83. Brodie M, Foehr U, Rideout V, et al. Communicating health information through the entertainment media. *Health Aff (Millwood)*. 2001;20:192–199

84. Rideout V. *Television as a Health Educator: A Case Study of Grey's Anatomy*. Menlo Park, CA: Kaiser Family Foundation; 2008

85. Tannen T. Media giant and foundation team up to fight HIV/AIDS. *Lancet*. 2003;361:1440–1441

86. DuRant RH, Wolfson M, LaFrance B, Balkrishnan R, Altman D. An evaluation of a mass media campaign to encourage parents of adolescents to talk to their children about sex. *J Adolesc Health*. 2006;38:298.e1–298.e9

87. Strasburger VC, Jordan AB, Donnerstein E. Child and adolescent health and the media. *Pediatrics*. 2010;125:756–767

88. Gruber EL, Wang PH, Christensen JS, Grube JW, Fisher DA. Private television viewing, parental supervision, and sexual and substance use risk behaviors in adolescents (abstr). *J Adolesc Health*. 2005;36:107

89. Barkin SL, Finch SA, Ip EH, et al. Is office-based counseling about media use, timeouts, and firearm storage effective? Results from a cluster-randomized, controlled trial. *Pediatrics*. 2008;122:e15–e25

90. Delli Santi A. Cell phone soap operas deliver safe-sex message. *Associated Press*. January 4, 2009. http://www.foxnews.com/story/0,2933,475630,00.html. Accessed February 13, 2012

91. Ralph LJ, Berglas NF, Schwartz SL, Brindis CD. Finding teens in TheirSpace: using social networking sites to connect youth to sexual health services. *Sex Res Soc Policy*. 2011;8:38–49

92. Borzekowski DLG, McCarthy C, Rosenfeld W. Ten years of TeenHealthFX.com – a case study of an adolescent health website. *Pediatr Clin North Am*. 2012; in press

93. Ramirez ER, Norman GH, Rosenberg DE, Kerr J, Saelens BE, Durant N, Sallis JF. Adolescent screen time and rules to limit screen time in the home. *J Adolesc Health*. 2011;48:379–385

94. Dalton MA, Adachi-Mejia AM, Longacre MR et al. Parental rules and monitoring of children's movie viewing associated with children's risk for smoking and drinking. *Pediatrics*. 2006;118:1932–1942

95. Jackson C, Brown JD, L'Engle KL. R-rated movies, bedroom televisions, and initiation of smoking by White and Black adolescents. *Arch Pediatr Adolesc Med*. 2007;161:260–268

96. Sisson SB, Broyles ST, Newton RL Jr, Baker BL, Chernausek SD. TVs in the bedrooms of children: does it impact health and behavior? *Prev Med*. 2011;52:104–108

97. Mitchell KJ, Ybarra M. Social networking sites: finding a balance between their risks and their benefits. *Arch Pediatr Adolesc Med*. 2009;163:87–89

98. Collins RL, Martino SC, Shaw R. *Influence of New Media on Adolescent Sexual Health: Evidence and Opportunities*. Santa Monica, CA: RAND; 2011

99. Strasburger VC. Why are teachers and schools so clueless about the media? *Liberal Opinion Week*. January 27, 2010: 24

100. McCannon B. Media literacy/media education: solution to big media? In: Strasburger VC, Wilson BJ, Jordan A. *Children, Adolescents, and the Media*. 2nd ed. Thousand Oaks, CA: Sage; 2009:519–569

101. Pinkleton BE, Austin EW, Cohen M, Chen Y-C, Fitzgerald E. Effects of a peer-led media literacy curriculum on adolescents' knowledge and attitudes toward sexual behavior and media portrayals of sex. *Health Commun*. 2008;23:462–472

102. Moreno MA, Vanderstoep A, Parks MR, Zimmerman FJ, Kurth A, Christakis DA. Reducing at-risk adolescents' display of risk behavior on a social networking web site. *Arch Pediatr Adolesc Med*. 2009;163:35–41

103. Murphy ST, Hether HJ, Rideout V. *How Healthy is Prime Time? An Analysis of Health Content in Popular Prime Time Television Programs*. Menlo Park, CA: Kaiser Family Foundation; 2008

Adolesc Med 23 (2012) 34–52

Breast Disorders in the Female Adolescent

Nirupama K. De Silva, MD*

Assistant Professor, Pediatric and Adolescent Gynecology, University of Oklahoma–Tulsa, Department of Obstetrics and Gynecology, 4502 E 41st Street, Room 2HO7, Tulsa, OK 74135-2512

INTRODUCTION

Initiation of breast development in the adolescent female marks a significant time of change in the female body. As females go through this transition, any deviations from what is perceived as "normal" by the adolescent can be a source of significant concern.

Risk factors for development of benign breast disease include thinner girls, taller girls, and those with rapid growth.[1] An appropriate history, physical examination, and testing should be performed, and the most appropriate safe and conservative management plan should be implemented. The fact that benign disease dominates the differential diagnosis of breast disorders in adolescents should be of paramount consideration as treatment plans are made.

NORMAL BREAST DEVELOPMENT

Development of the breast begins around 4–6 weeks of gestation, when the ectodermal cells on the anterior body wall thicken into a ridge known as the "milk line" or "milk ridge." This ridge runs the length of the axilla to the groin. The areas of the ridge above and below the pectoralis muscle recede while in utero, leaving the mammary primordium, which is the origin of the breast tissue.[2] The lactiferous ducts and mammary glands develop from this tissue. The developing mesenchyme that surrounds this becomes the fibrous and fatty portions of the breast.[3] The nipple appears at 8 months gestation. The breast bud, under the stimulation of maternal estrogen, becomes palpable at 34 weeks of gestation.[3] This bud regresses within the first months of life, as the estrogen stimulation is no longer present.

---

*Corresponding author.
E-mail address: rupadesilva73@gmail.com (N. K. De Silva).

The breast tissue remains dormant until puberty is initiated. Thelarche, or the onset of pubertal breast development, normally occurs between the ages of 8 and 13 years, with an average age of 10.3 years, and is hormonally mediated.[4] Race also plays a role in the timing of thelarche, with black girls experiencing thelarche on average at 8.8 years and white girls experiencing thelarche on average at 10.2 years.[4,5] Lack of development by age 13 is considered delayed and warrants evaluation.

Once thelarche is initiated, adipose tissue and ductal tissue grow in response to estrogen. Progesterone stimulation results in lobular growth and alveolar budding.[2] The normal development of the breast, which occurs over a period of 2–4 years, is classified by the Sexual Maturity Rating into 5 stages (Figure 1).

BREAST SELF-EXAMINATION

Historically, experts have recommended teaching adolescents to perform breast self-examination for a variety of reasons, including cancer detection, teaching self-detection for future application, and contributing to greater understanding and comfort with their changing bodies. There are currently no data to support these rationales as experts now believe that girls who identify a breast mass themselves may experience multiple physician visits, invasive testing, and perhaps unwarranted surgery. The American Congress of Obstetricians and Gynecologists (ACOG) recommends breast self-examination beginning at age 19 years.[6] Women with previous exposure to therapeutic chest radiation therapy are advised to begin breast self-examination 10 years after exposure.[7]

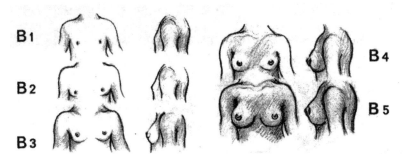

Figure 1. Tanner Stages of the Breast
Stage B1: elevation of the papilla only
Stage B2: elevation of the breast and papilla as a small mound, enlargement of the areolar diameter
Stage B3: further enlargement of the breast and areola with no separation of their contours
Stage B4: further enlargement with projection of the areola and papilla to form a secondary mound above the level of the breast
Stage B5: projection of the papilla only due to recession of the areola to the general contour of the breast (Source: Laufer MR, Goldstein DP. The breast: examination and lesions. In: Emans SJ, Laufer MR, Goldstein DP, eds. *Pediatric and Adolescent Gynecology*. 5th ed. Philadelphia, PA: Lippincott Williams & Wilkins; 2005:130. Reprinted with permission.)

ABNORMALITIES IN DEVELOPMENT OF THE ADOLESCENT BREAST

Amastia and Hypomastia

Complete absence of the breast, or amastia, is rare and occurs from lack of formation or obliteration of the milk line during embryogenesis.[8] Amastia can be associated with syndromes such as congenital ectodermal dysplasia or anomalies in which there is congenital underdevelopment or absence of the chest muscle on one side of the body as seen in Poland syndrome. Bilateral amastia can be associated with systemic disorders (eg, malnutrition, Crohn's disease) and/or endocrine disorders (eg, congenital adrenal hyperplasia, gonadal dysgenesis, hypogonadotropic hypogonadism).[9] Because the nipple complex does not normally develop until the eighth month of gestation, it can be quite difficult to identify in the premature infant. As a result, placement of chest tubes or central lines can inadvertently injure the developing breast, resulting in amastia or hypomastia. Such a condition can also result from injuries sustained during thoracotomy, inappropriate biopsy of the breast bud, radiotherapy, or severe burns.[3] Breast hypoplasia and amastia require reconstruction with implants.[10] In order to maximize the cosmetic result, reconstruction for hypoplasia and unilateral amastia should be performed after the breast has acquired full growth potential (on or around age 18). In this way, the chances of asymmetry are decreased.

Polymastia and Polythelia

Supernumerary breast tissue occurs in approximately 1% of the population and is the most common anomaly of the pediatric breast.[2,10] The abnormally placed tissue is almost always located in the axilla or just inferior to the normally positioned breast along the embryonic milk line (Figure 2). Breast tissue found outside the normal milk line is exceedingly rare but has been reported on the face, back, perineum, and in the midline of the anterior torso.[8,11,12] Sixty-five percent of children with supernumerary breast tissue have a single accessory nipple (polythelia) or breast (polymastia), and 30–35% have two nipples.[8] No treatment is needed unless resection of accessory nipples is desired for cosmetic reasons or if there is concern that there will be painful swelling of polymastia during pregnancy.

Polythelia has been associated with abnormalities of the kidney or urinary tract,[13] and accessory breast tissue has also been linked to cardiovascular disorders, although this relationship is not definite.[14] Clinicians may consider evaluation of affected patients for renal or cardiovascular disorders.

Breast Hypertrophy

Idiopathic breast hypertrophy in adolescents, referred to as "juvenile" or "virginal" breast hypertrophy, involves the uncontrolled overgrowth of breast tissue. The breasts initially develop normally during puberty but then continue to grow.

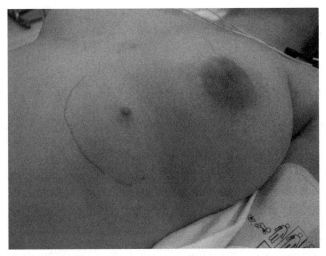

Figure 2. Polythelia. Extra nipple located along the "milk line." (Source: DeSilva NK, Brandt ML. Breast disorders in children and adolescents. In: Sanfilippo JS, Lara-Torre E, Edmonds DK, Templeman C (eds). *Clinical Pediatric and Adolescent Gynecology*. New York: Informa Healthcare USA, Inc; 2009:199. Reprinted with permission.)

This rapid growth can be unilateral or bilateral and usually occurs shortly after thelarche. It is thought to be the result of excessive end-organ sensitivity to gonadal hormones.[15] However, the number of hormonal receptors in the hypertrophic breast tissue is normal, as are serum estradiol levels.[3] An autoimmune etiology has been suggested by some authors because of an occasional association with Hashimoto's thyroiditis, rheumatoid arthritis, and myasthenia gravis.[3]

For many adolescents, breast hypertrophy and/or persistent significant asymmetry may result in both psychological and physical consequences. These adolescents may receive unwanted attention from boys, experience difficulties with physical activities, and have socialization problems that lead to poor self-esteem.[2] Treatment via breast reduction surgery should be deferred until breast growth has been completed. If it is not possible to wait until complete growth is finished, progesterone or tamoxifen can be used in conjunction with surgery to control breast growth and prevent recurrences.[16] Patients should be aware that recurrences are common.

Breast Asymmetry

Maturation can sometimes occur asymmetrically due to fluctuation of the hormonal environment and variable end-organ sensitivity.[17] It most commonly resolves with normal development, although visible asymmetry persists in 25% of women.[5,18] The differential diagnosis includes unilateral hypoplasia or amastia, unilateral hypertrophy, large breast mass or abscess, and Poland syndrome. Diagnosis is established through the medical history and physical examination, looking for skeletal abnormalities and skin changes of the breast. Ultrasound is a useful option to rule out a mass or abscess.[5] If no pathology is found, expectant management is warranted. If the asymmetry persists, treatment is through surgical intervention after development is complete.

BREAST MASSES IN THE ADOLESCENT

Of all breast masses diagnosed in adolescents, recent retrospective chart reviews demonstrate that approximately 67% are fibroadenomas, 15% are fibrocystic changes (most often associated with mastalgia), and 3% are an abscess or mastitis[9] (Table 1). Almost all breast masses in the adolescent are benign, with one study noting that less than 1% of lesions are malignant.[19] However, any mass warrants obtaining a history and performing an examination. The history should include questions about risk factors for breast cancer, the family history and any personal history of prior malignancy or radiation exposure, age of menarche, and any prior pregnancies.[19] Imaging is warranted when the diagnosis is uncertain with examination alone. The American College of Radiology Appropriateness Criteria recommends ultrasound as the first imaging test for women younger than age 30 with focal signs of the breast. Mammography is not routinely indicated in asymptomatic, low-risk adolescents due to the risk of radiation, the decreased sensitivity given the dense nature of adolescent breast tissue, and the low prevalence of cancer in this population.[20] The combination of palpation, imaging, and biopsy is called the "triple test" of breast evaluation.[2] Sonography can delineate solid versus cystic masses but cannot distinguish benign versus malignant disease. Masses may be evaluated with fine needle aspiration (FNA) or core needle biopsy (CNB). FNA has been shown to lack accuracy due to dependence on the cytology obtained, and it has a false negative rate of up to 20%.[19] While FNA is not commonly used in the adolescent population, one study has noted it to be a reliable tool in evaluation and management of breast masses to reduce anxiety, obtain a diagnosis, and avoid surgery on the growing breast.[21]

Fibroadenomas/Giant Fibroadenomas

Fibroadenomas are extremely common in the adolescent breast and are most often located in the upper outer quadrant. They may enlarge slightly during the menstrual cycle and are bilateral in 10–15% of cases.[2,22] They are thought to be due to an exaggerated response to local estrogen stimulation.[2] Physical examination is usually diagnostic because these lesions are well circumscribed, "rubbery," mobile, and nontender, with an average size of 2–3 cm. The combined estrogen-progesterone oral contraceptive pill appears to be protective of fibroadenomas.[22]

Given the low risk of malignancy, high likelihood of spontaneous resolution, and risks of deformity due to surgery in the growing breast, conservative, non-surgical management is most often appropriate. Fibroadenomas less than 5 cm

Table 1.
Breast Masses in the Adolescent Female

Benign
Fibroadenoma
Fibrocystic changes or cysts
Unilateral thelarche
Hemangioma
Intramammary lymph node
Fat necrosis
Abscess
Mastitis
Lipoma
Hematoma
Hamartoma
Macromastia (juvenile hypertrophy)
Galactocele
Intraductal papilloma
Juvenile papillomatosis
Lymphangioma

Malignant
Malignant cystosarcoma phyllodes
Breast carcinoma
Metastatic disease
-Lymphoma
-Neuroblastoma
-Sarcoma
-Rhabdomyosarcoma
-Acute leukemia

without concerning features can be observed over 1–2 month intervals for growth or regression. When the mass regresses, observation at 3–4 month intervals (with increasingly longer intervals each time) are appropriate for up to 2 years while the mass is regressing.[22] Ultrasound is helpful in equivocal cases, and findings typically include a hypoechoic pattern with an oval shape and circumscribed margins.[23] FNA or CNB should be reserved for those desiring confirmation of the diagnosis.[24] The complete regression of a clinically detectable breast mass in an adolescent is between 10 and 40%.[22]

Significant growth of the mass at any time warrants further evaluation. Giant fibroadenomas are a variant of fibroadenoma that accounts for 2–10% of all fibroadenomas of the breast.[25] They are fibroadenomas that have progressive growth to greater than 5 cm (Figure 3). The differential diagnosis should include hamartomas, lipomas, virginal juvenile hypertrophy, inflammatory masses, and phyllodes tumors with or without associated malignancy.[22] Excisional biopsy and surgery should be reserved for breast masses that are larger than 5 cm; enlarging or without regression; in bilateral breasts or multiple in quantity; associated with overlying skin changes or suspicious imaging findings; abscesses not responding to medical therapy; or suspicious masses presenting in an adolescent with a personal history of a previous malignancy or a high risk genetic mutation or syndrome.[22] The decision to proceed with excision is based on family anxiety, size of the tumor, history of breast cancer, and the patient's age. Families should be counseled that in addition to the common risks of breast surgery, the biopsy or excision may result in cosmetic changes to a growing breast.

Juvenile Papillomatosis

Juvenile papillomatosis usually presents with a firm, well-defined mass in one breast. Tumors range in size from 1–8 cm, and sonography can be helpful in delineating the diagnosis.[24] When resected, this is a well-demarcated mass with multiple cysts separated by fibrous stroma, giving it a "Swiss cheese" appearance.[26] Juvenile papillomatosis is considered a marker for an increased breast cancer risk in family members. In situ or invasive carcinoma in the patient, which is usually a juvenile secretory carcinoma, has been reported in up to 15% of patients with juvenile papillomatosis.[26] The treatment of juvenile papillomatosis is total resection, with preservation of the normal breast.

Retroareolar Cysts

Montgomery tubercles are the small papular projections located on the edge of the areola; they are related to the glands of Montgomery, which may serve a role

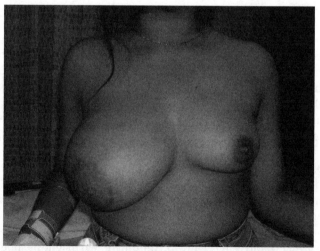

Figure 3. Giant Fibroadenoma in an Adolescent Female. The breast growth must be distinguished from juvenile hypertrophy. (Source: DeSilva NK, Brandt ML. Breast disorders in children and adolescents. In: Sanfilippo JS, Lara-Torre E, Edmonds DK, Templeman C (eds). *Clinical Pediatric and Adolescent Gynecology.* New York: Informa Healthcare USA, Inc; 2009:204. Reprinted with permission.)

during lactation. In adolescents, these glands can obstruct and then present either asymptomatically (38%) or as a mass associated with inflammation, pain, and erythema (62%).[27] Patients may describe a brownish discharge from one of Montgomery tubercles, particularly with compression of the mass. The diagnosis of these retroareolar cysts, also referred to as cysts of Montgomery, is primarily clinical, but it can be confirmed with ultrasound. Ultrasound most commonly demonstrates a single cystic lesion, usually unilocular, located in the expected retroareolar location.

The most common presentation of patients with retroareolar cysts is acute inflammation with localized tenderness, erythema, and swelling under the areola, extending into the breast tissue.[27] Conservative treatment, oral antibiotics directed at *Staphylococcus* along with nonsteroidal anti-inflammatory agents, usually results in resolution of the acute inflammation within 7 days.[27] Following this nonoperative treatment, an asymptomatic mass is usually present. In the absence of persistent infection or other complications, the treatment of retroareolar cysts is observation with serial physical examinations and, if needed, repeat ultrasound examination. More than 80% of these cysts resolve spontaneously, although this may take up to 2 years.[27] Patients should be instructed to not compress the area, because this may prevent resolution of the mass. Only rarely is drainage of a persistent abscess necessary. Resection may be indicated if the mass persists or if the diagnosis is in question.

Other Benign Breast Masses

A variety of rare benign tumors of the breast have been described in adolescents and young adults, including hamartomas, adenomas of the nipple, tubular adenomas, and erosive adenomatosis. Consequences of trauma to the breast can also be confused with a mass.

Hamartomas of the breast are rare tumors composed of the normal components of the breast that can present as unilateral macromastia. Only 8 cases have been reported in women younger than 20 years of age.[28] Treatment of a hamartoma is total excision.

Adenomas of the nipple have been reported to occur in children and adolescents.[29] Tubular adenomas cannot be distinguished from fibroadenomas by history or examination and the diagnosis is usually obtained on pathologic evaluation. No further treatment is necessary after local excision.

Erosive adenomatosis is a tumor that presents with erythema, erosion, and crusting of the nipple.[30] Serosanguineous discharge may occur and a nodule may or may not be palpable. Treatment is local excision of the lesion, which may be delayed until breast growth is complete. Successful treatment with cryosurgery has also been reported.[30]

Trauma can result in lesions that resemble either an infection or a mass in adolescents. This has been reported following seat belt injuries, as well as with other direct blows to the breast.[37] Contusions and abrasions can develop, which are usually mild and resolve spontaneously with time.[2] If a laceration occurs, this should be sutured as needed and monitored for infection. A hematoma can also develop and usually resolves spontaneously. Healing may promote fat necrosis with associated induration, scarring, and calcification that can last for years and these changes can be confused with breast carcinoma.[2]

MALIGNANT MASSES

Phyllodes Tumors

Phyllodes tumors are stromal tumors that are histologically classified as benign, intermediate, or malignant. Despite this distinction, benign lesions can metastasize and may recur locally. Phyllodes tumors have been reported to occur in girls as young as 10 years of age.[32] These tumors occur more frequently in black adolescents.

The diagnosis is difficult to make before biopsy, as the tumor may resemble a giant fibroadenoma on examination and large tumors may cause skin stretching, venous distention, and skin ulceration. Ultrasound findings that are suggestive, but not diagnostic, of cystosarcoma phyllodes include lobulations, a heterogeneous echo pattern, and an absence of microcalcifications.[33]

The treatment of benign cystosarcoma phyllodes is total surgical excision. Patients with histologically malignant cystosarcoma phyllodes traditionally have undergone mastectomy.[33] However, some authors have reported that adolescents with malignant phyllodes tumors have a more "benign" course than adults and have suggested that the breast can be preserved in these patients.[32] In such situations, treatment is resection of the tumor with clear margins. Efforts should be taken to preserve as much breast tissue as possible.

Local recurrence occurs in up to 20% of patients with phyllodes tumors and is treated with re-excision or mastectomy.[32] Metastases are via hematogenous spread and can occur in the lung, pleura, soft tissue, bone, pancreas, and central nervous system.[32] Overall, the 5 year survival rate for malignant phyllodes tumors in adults is approximately 80%. Because adolescents with phyllodes tumors may have biologically less aggressive tumors than adults, the prognosis in the adolescent may be better, although definitive data are not available.[32]

Cancer

Primary breast cancer occurs rarely in the adolescent patient. The National Cancer Institute's Surveillance and End Results (SEER) data from 1975–2006 lists no incident cases of breast cancer in situ in females younger than 20 years of age and publishes an incidence of invasive breast cancer of 0.2/100,000 for females between 15–19 years of age.[34] Due to its rarity, there are minimal data on adolescents with primary breast cancer. One study noted that most breast cancer cases in this population were adenocarcinoma of the breast (juvenile secretory, invasive intraductal, invasive intralobular, and signet ring) or cystosarcoma phyllodes.[35] The treatment of these primary breast cancers in adolescents is complete surgical excision, by local excision or by mastectomy. Adjuvant therapy for juvenile secretory carcinoma is rarely used, and prognosis for these patients is excellent following local excision. Adjuvant therapy for intraductal carcinoma is based on the nodal status and hormone receptors, with most oncologists using modified adult protocols for the treatment of adolescents with this tumor. Before treatment with radiation or chemotherapy for breast cancer or other malignancies in an adolescent, the practitioner should consider options for fertility preservation if the patient and family desire. In single females, oocyte cryopreservation should be considered and can be carried out with the help of a reproductive medicine specialist.[36] An article on this topic, Fertility Preservation for Adolescent Women with Cancer, is included in this current issue of *Adolescent Medicine: State of the Art Reviews.*

Metastatic Disease to the Breast

Cancer metastatic to the breast has been reported most commonly in adolescents with primary Hodgkin lymphoma, non-Hodgkin lymphoma, neuroblastoma, and rhabdomyosarcoma.[24] Rhabdomyosarcoma is one of the most common to metastasize to the breast, occurring in 6% of female patients with rhabdomyosarcoma.[24] In a patient with a known malignancy and an enlarging breast mass, even one with a benign ultrasound appearance, the mass should be investigated promptly with FNA or CNB.[24]

Risk Factors for Malignancy

Although primary breast cancer is uncommon, risk factors for malignancy of the breast should be assessed. Malignancies that occur in the adolescent breast are more likely metastatic from another primary malignancy. Clinical evidence demonstrates that chest radiation exposure to the prepubertal and pubertal breast of females between the ages of 10 and 30 years is associated with the greatest risk of radiation-induced breast cancer later in life.[37] Women with previous exposure to therapeutic chest radiation therapy ($\geq$20 gy) are considered to be high risk and the Children's Oncology Group recommends annual mammography starting 8 years after radiation or age 25, whichever is second.[38]

Effective and accurate counseling for adolescents and their parents regarding breast cancer prevention should be a routine component of preventive health services for female adolescents. Smoking, alcohol consumption, and sun exposure during adolescence have all been associated with an increased risk of breast cancer in adulthood.[39] It is prudent to advise adolescents to avoid these exposures. Additional preventive health guidance in all adolescents should include encouraging exercise in young women because physical activity has been shown to significantly reduce the risk of breast cancer. Intake of fat and red meat in adolescence has also been linked to an increased risk of breast cancer, although the data are conflicting and further research in this area is needed.[40,41,42]

Studies have not found a significantly increased risk of breast cancer with the use of oral contraceptives.[43] Further, a positive family history of breast cancer, including those families with a *BRCA1* or *BRCA2* mutation, should not be regarded as a contraindication to oral contraceptive use.[44]

OTHER BREAST CHANGES THAT MAY PROVOKE ANXIETY IN THE ADOLESCENT

Mastalgia/Fibrocystic Changes

Breast pain, or mastalgia, is a common symptom in the adolescent. Symptoms can be associated with exercise or fibrocystic changes. One study found that 31% of breast discomfort was exercise induced and that approximately half of female athletes had exercise-induced injuries to the breast.[18]

Fibrocystic changes represent a physiologic alteration of the breast associated with mild, cyclic swelling and palpable nodularity. Symptoms associated with fibrocystic changes are seen most often in the upper outer quadrant, are typically cyclic, and are worse premenstrually. When adolescents are noted to have fibrocystic changes, they should be reassured that these are normal and informed that the findings usually vary with the hormonal changes of the menstrual cycle.

For breast pain, evaluation and treatment involves a careful history and physical examination. Ultrasound may be helpful if the diagnosis is equivocal. As mastalgia can be an early sign of pregnancy, pregnancy should be ruled out in the sexually active adolescent. Supportive measures and reassurance are the best treatment for those with mild pain. Smoking cessation should be encouraged, as nicotine has been shown to increase breast pain. Decreasing fat intake in the diet and eliminating caffeine can also reduce breast pain. Treatments with vitamin E and evening primrose oil are unproven but popular.[45] A well fitting bra, particularly a "sports bra" during exercise, has also been shown to reduce pain during movement.[18] Analgesics such as naproxen sodium or non-steroidal anti-inflammatory drugs (NSAIDS) can help alleviate the symptoms. Oral contraceptives have been reported to improve symptoms in some, but they can promote symptoms in others.[18]

Nipple Discharge

Nipple discharge in the adolescent can be milky, purulent, serous, serosanguineous, or bloody and is usually nonmalignant in nature.[9] A purulent discharge suggests infection, whereas a sticky green, serosanguineous or multicolored discharge can be associated with duct ectasia, intraductal papilloma, fibrocystic changes, or (rarely) cancer (Table 2).

Galactorrhea is a milky discharge that can be found after thoracotomy, burns, injuries to the chest wall, herpes zoster, or chronic stimulation of the nipple. Pituitary tumors, especially prolactinomas, are the most common hypothalamic cause of galactorrhea, whereas the most common endocrine cause of galactorrhea in adolescents is hypothyroidism. A wide variety of drugs have also been implicated in causing galactorrhea. The most common of these are dopamine receptor blockers and catecholamine-depleting agents, although oral contraceptive pills can cause this symptom as well.[2] Other common causes of galactorrhea in the adolescent include trauma, suckling, or self-manipulation. Idiopathic or benign galactorrhea is a diagnosis of exclusion.

Table 2.
Common Causes of Nipple Discharge

Pregnancy
Medicines
-Hormones (ie, oral contraceptives, estrogen, progesterone)
-Blood pressure drugs (ie, methyldopa, verapamil)
-Tricyclic antidepressants
-Tranquilizers (antipsychotics)
-Anti-nausea drugs (ie, metoclopramide)
-Herbs (nettle, fennel, blessed thistle, anise, fenugreek seed)
-Illicit drugs (marijuana, opiates)
Stimulation of the breast (sexual or due to lifestyle)
Thyroid abnormalities
Chronic emotional stress
Hypothalamic tumors
Chest wall conditions
-Herpes zoster
-Trauma
-Burns
-Tumors
Breast conditions
-Mammary duct ectasia
-Chronic cystic mastitis
-Intraductal cysts
-Intraductal papillomas
Hypothyroidism

Source: DeSilva NK, Merritt DF. Breast concerns. In: Kliegman RM, et al (eds). *Nelson Textbook of Pediatrics.* 19th ed. Philadelphia, PA: Elsevier Saunders; 2011. Reprinted with permission.

In regards to bloody discharge, the differential diagnosis in adolescents includes mammary ductal ectasia, chronic cystic mastitis, intraductal cysts or papillomas, an infarcted fibroadenoma, and a benign phyllodes tumor. In adolescent athletes, bloody discharge may also be due to chronic nipple irritation (jogger's nipple) or cold trauma (cyclist's nipple).[46] Another important cause of bloody or brownish discharge in adolescents is discharge from the ducts of Montgomery (on the edge of the areola), as described previously.

A proper history and physical examination is essential. The discharge should be examined and cultured if possible. Appropriate laboratory and imaging studies should be ordered in the evaluation process. A ductogram may be warranted to evaluate for underlying pathologic changes in the breast.[2] Treatment of nipple discharge is directed by the results of the findings. Use of any offending drugs should be stopped, antibiotic use initiated if warranted, hypothyroidism treated, and prolactin tumors managed medically or surgically. The patient should be educated regarding behavioral changes to avoid nipple stimulation.

Mammary Duct Ectasia

Mammary duct ectasia refers to an inflammatory dilation of the mammary duct with cells that are not atypical. It is a benign and common cause of bloody discharge when there is an associated cystic lesion in the developing breast.[47] The patient presents with a discharge from one or both breasts, tenderness in the nipple or surrounding breast tissue, redness, and a lump or thickening in the breast. The blocked ducts can predispose to infection, leading to mastitis or a breast abscess. Duct ectasia is commonly associated with nipple inversion.[2] Antibiotics should be used if there is a suspicion of infection or culture results are positive. Once improved, duct ectasia often leaves a residual subareolar nodule. If the patient has continued symptoms of discharge or pain from a persistent mass, treatment with local excision is an option.[2] The possibility of long term breast deformity in the developing breast should be considered if excision is performed.[47]

Intraductal Papilloma

A bloody nipple discharge, when associated with a mass, can also be seen with a papilloma or with papillomatosis and should be evaluated because of the malignant potential of the latter condition. An intraductal papilloma is a growth in breast tissue that punctures a duct. These benign tumors are composed of fibrous tissue and blood vessels and can cause benign nipple discharge. Papillomatosis is a progression of this growth into hyperplastic cells. Referral to a specialist who can excise the mass is warranted.[9]

BREAST INFECTIONS

Mastitis and Breast Abscesses

Mastitis is the most common infection of the breast, especially in lactating females. It can also occur in nonlactating females, but rarely. Nonlactating adolescents may develop nonpuerperal mastitis or a breast abscess as a result of irritation of the skin (through shaving, plucking hair, or nipple stimulation), a foreign body (eg, piercing), or metaplasia of the duct epithelium in the breast.[48]

The initial therapy for all breast infections is use of antibiotics and analgesics for 7–10 days. In nonlactating infections, *Staphylococcus aureus* or anaerobic bacilli (*bacteroides*) are the offending organism in most cases.[49] The clinician might also consider treatment that includes coverage against methicillin-resistant *Staphylococcus aureus* (MRSA), as this has become a significant organism in most communities. Microbial culture should be obtained to promote targeted antimicrobial therapy whenever possible.[49]

Sonography may be utilized to determine if the indurated breast tissue has developed an abscess. Small abscesses should initially be aspirated with a needle, using ultrasound guidance if necessary, while antibiotic therapy is continued. Larger or persistent abscesses should be evaluated for inflammatory breast cancer, although this is rare in the adolescent population.[48] Large abscesses may also need incision and drainage in addition to antibiotic therapy. If incision and drainage is performed, a small, peri-areolar incision is recommended for cosmetic reasons.

ELECTIVE MODIFICATIONS TO THE BREAST

Nipple Piercing

Given the increasing popularity of piercing, clinicians should routinely screen adolescents for intent to undergo a piercing. The most common reasons adolescents give for getting piercings include making a personal statement, reasons of fashion or self acceptance, an improved perception of appearance and thus self-esteem, or as a rite of passage.[50] Multiple piercings in an adolescent has been associated with high risk behaviors or deviant activities, and thus piercing may be a warning sign to practitioners.[50] The most common health risks associated with piercing include infections, pain, bleeding, hematomas, cyst formation, allergic reactions, and keloid formation.[51,52,53] Nipple piercing has also been associated with a transmission risk for human immunodeficiency virus (HIV).[54]

The time from piercing to abscess formation has been shown to vary from 3 to 9 months.[55] Major complications associated with an abscess after nipple piercing can include endocarditis, heart valve injury, cardiac prosthesis infection, metal foreign body reaction in the breast tissue, or recurrent infections. The most common pathogen in nonlactating breasts is *Staphylococcus aureus* (including MRSA), although many abscesses can be polymicrobial.[55] Based on current data, clinical recommendations for patients with postpiercing infections should include oral antibiotic treatment. The piercing should not be removed during active infection as this may close the wound and prevent drainage, thus increasing the risk of abscess formation.[50] If the piercing must be removed, a sterile replacement can be inserted. Screening for hepatitis B, hepatitis C, HIV, and elevated glucose (to exclude diabetes mellitus with its risk of increased infection rate) is important in patients with a postpiercing infection.[51] For those who intend to undergo a piercing, education should be provided regarding safer piercing strategies, such as immunization against hepatitis B and tetanus before the piercing, if they are not already immune.[56]

ELECTIVE SURGICAL ALTERATIONS TO THE BREAST OF ADOLESCENTS

Breast Reduction

Reduction mammoplasty for breast hypertrophy should be addressed when enlarged breasts cause back, shoulder, and/or neck pain or strain, promote a kyphotic posture, create negative attention from others, or cause psychological problems or difficulties with desired activities[57] (Table 3). Surgical correction of breast tissue has been shown to improve self-esteem and increase functional capacity.[58] In a study of satisfaction following reduction mammoplasty in adolescents, the most common reason for recommending the procedure to a peer was to improve self esteem.[16]

There is no definitive guideline for when breast reduction should be suggested. Several recommendations regarding the timing of surgery have been made, including postponing surgery until breast maturity is reached, waiting for 6 months with no change in bra size, or after the age of 18 years. Surgery can be considered earlier when severe symptoms are encountered.[59] The incidence of

Table 3.
Common Noncosmetic Reasons for Requesting Surgical Alterations to the Breast

Breast Augmentation	Breast Reduction
Amastia	Breast asymmetry
Poland syndrome	Juvenile/virginal hypertrophy
Breast asymmetry	Giant fibroadenoma
Gonadal dysgenesis	Phyllodes tumor
Tuberous breasts	

Source: DeSilva N. Plastic surgery and the adolescent breast: preliminary patient counseling. *J Pediatr Adolesc Gynecol.* 2010;23(3):184–6. Reprinted with permission from Elsevier.

breast regrowth after initial reduction during adolescence is not known, but it has been reported.[60]

An assessment of the adolescent's emotional, psychological, and physical maturity is recommended to guide the decision to perform breast reduction surgery so that the surgeon can fully understand the motivation and psychosocial and emotional attributes of the patient seeking the surgery. The surgeon should be confident that the adolescent has realistic expectations and fully understands the risks and benefits, including the limitations of breast surgery.[59]

Postoperatively, adolescent patients have the same short- and long-term potential complications as adult patients. Overall, the most commonly cited short-term complication is pain; long-term complications most often are related to scarring. Lactation success after reduction mammoplasty is similar to that of women who have had other major breast surgeries, and differing surgical techniques have not been associated with improved success. One study of adolescent patients who underwent reduction mammoplasty between the ages of 15 and 17 years found that such patients subsequently breastfed their infants with complication rates similar to those in the general population.[60]

Breast Augmentation

Plastic surgery involving augmentation of adolescent breasts should be performed only after careful consideration and with the highest of ethical standards. Over the past several years, the number of cosmetic surgical procedures performed on the breast in patients aged 18 years or younger has increased substantially.[61] Although sometimes augmentation is due to noncosmetic reasons (see Table 3), purely cosmetic reasons are becoming more common in the adolescent population. This can be attributed to factors such as media influence and distorted perceptions of an ideal body type. In response to this trend, the American Society for Plastic Surgery has adopted guidelines for the appropriate selection of adolescents for aesthetic breast surgery.[62] The guidelines acknowledge that the United States Food and Drug Administration considers the use of saline implants for aesthetic breast augmentation in patients younger than 18 years of age to be an off-label use. They state that adolescent candidates for purely aesthetic breast augmentation should be at least 18 years of age, and they emphasize that aesthetic breast surgery in the adolescent female encompasses unique mental and physical components. As with timing of breast reduction surgery, the emotional maturity and motivation of the adolescent making the request should be assessed. Extensive counseling allows the adolescent and family to have clear expectations of the results of the surgery and allows the surgeon time to assess the patient's mental development to help ensure that the timing of the surgery is appropriate for maximizing the potential of a positive outcome. The adolescent and her parents should be counseled that although breast implants are not typically associated with breastfeeding difficulties, women who undergo breast augmentation surgery can have a greater incidence of lactation insufficiency.[63] There is no increased risk of breast cancer with breast augmentation, although the surgery may make future mammography screening more difficult, and complications caused by breast implants, including possible development of rheumatologic diseases, have been reported.

References

1. Berkey CS, Willett WC, Frazier AL, Rosner B, Tamimi RM, Colditz GA Prospective study of growth and development in older girls and risk of benign breast disease in young women. *Cancer.* 2011;117:1612–1620
2. Greydanus DE, Matytsina L, Gains M. Breast disorders in children and adolescents. *Prim Care.* 2006;33:455–502
3. Duflos C, et al. Breast diseases in adolescents. In: Sultan C, ed. *Pediatric and Adolescent Gynecology.* Basel, Switzerland: S Karger AG; 2004:183–196
4. Gordon CM, Laufer MR. The physiology of puberty. In: Emans SJ, Laufer MR, Goldstein DP, eds. *Pediatric and Adolescent Gynecology.* Philadelphia, PA: Lippincott Williams & Wilkins; 2005:120–155
5. Eidlitz-Markus T, Mukamel M, Haimi-Cohen Y, Amir J, Zeharia A. Breast asymmetry during adolescence: physiologic and non-physiologic causes. *Isr Med Assoc J.* 2010;12:203–206
6. American College of Obstetricians and Gynecologists. Primary and preventive care: periodic assessments: Committee Opinion No. 452. *Obstet Gynecol.* 2009;114:1444–1451
7. De Silva NK (primary author), Adolescent Health Committee. Breast concerns in adolescents. In: *American College of Obstetricians Gynecologists Guidelines for Adolescent Healthcare.* Washington, DC: ACOG; 2011:119–133
8. Skandalakis JE, Gray SW, Ricketts R, Skandalakis LJ. The anterior body wall. In: Skandalakis JE, Gray SW, eds. *Embryology for Surgeons: The Embryological Basis for the Treatment of Congenital Anomalies.* Baltimore, MD: Lippincott Williams & Wilkins; 2004:552–559
9. Laufer MR, Goldstein DP. The breast: examination and lesions. In: Emans SJ, Laufer MR, Goldstein DP, eds. *Pediatric and Adolescent Gynecology.* Philadelphia, PA: Lippincott Williams & Wilkins; 2005:729–759
10. Sadove AM, van Aalst JA. Congenital and acquired pediatric breast anomalies: a review of 20 years' experience. *Plast Reconstr Surg.* 2005;115:1039–1050
11. Koltuksuz U, Aydin E. Supernumerary breast tissue: a case of pseudomamma on the face. *J Pediatr Surg.* 1997;32:1377–1378
12. Leung W, Heaton JP, Morales A. An uncommon urologic presentation of a supernumerary breast. *Urology.* 1997;50:122–124
13. Ferrara P, Giorgio V, Vitelli O, Gatto A, Romano V, Bugalo FD, et al. Polythelia: still a marker of urinary tract anomalies in children? *Scand J Urol Nephrol.* 2009;43:47–50
14. Loukas M, Clarke P, Tubbs RS. Accessory breasts: a historical and current perspective. *Am Surg.* 2007;73:525–528
15. O'Hare PM, Frieden IJ. Virginal breast hypertrophy. *Pediatr Dermatol.* 2000;17:277–281
16. Hoppe IC, Patel PP, Singer-Granick CJ, Granick MS. Virginal mammary hypertrophy: a meta-analysis and treatment algorithm. *Plast Reconstr Surg.* 2011;127:2224–2231
17. Bock K, Duda VF, Hadji P, Ramaswamy A, Schulz-Wendtland R, Klose KJ, et al. Pathologic breast conditions in childhood and adolescence: evaluation by sonographic diagnosis. *J Ultrasound Med.* 2005;24:1347–1354
18. Greydanus DE, Omar H, Pratt HD. The adolescent female athlete: current concepts and conundrums. *Eur J Cancer.* 2010;46:2275–2284
19. Chang DS, McGrath MH. Management of benign tumors of the adolescent breast. *Plast Reconstr Surg.* 2007;120:13e–19e

20. Loving VA, DeMartini WB, Eby PR, Gutierrez RL, Peacock S, Lehman CD. Targeted ultrasound in women younger than 30 years with focal breast signs or symptoms: outcomes analyses and management implications. *Am J Roentgenol.* 2010;195:1472–1477

21. Pacinda SJ, Ramzy I. J Fine-needle aspiration of breast masses. A review of its role in diagnosis and management in adolescent patients. *Adolesc Health.* 1998;23:3–6

22. Jayasinghe Y, Simmons PS. Fibroadenomas in adolescence. *Curr Opin Obstet Gynecol.* 2009;21:402–406

23. Sanchez R, Ladino-Torres MF, Bernat JA, Joe A, DiPietro MA. Breast fibroadenomas in the pediatric population: common and uncommon sonographic findings. *Pediatr Radiol.* 2010;40:1681–1689

24. Chung EM, Cube R, Hall GJ, Gonzalez C, Stocker JT, Glassman LM. From the archives of the AFIP: breast masses in children and adolescents: radiologic-pathologic correlation. *Radiographics.* 2009;29:907–931

25. Gobbi D, Dall'Igna P, Alaggio R, Nitti D, Cecchetto G. Giant fibroadenoma of the breast in adolescents: report of 2 cases. *J Pediatr Surg.* 2009;44:e39–e41

26. Dehner LP, Hill DA, Deschryver K. Pathology of the breast in children, adolescents, and young adults. *Semin Diagn Pathol.* 1999;16:235–247

27. Huneeus A, Schilling A, Horvath E, Pinochet M, Carrasco O. Retroareolar cysts in the adolescent. *J Pediatr Adolesc Gynecol.* 2003;16:45–49

28. Weinzweig N, Botts J, Marcus E. Giant hamartoma of the breast. *Plast Reconstr Surg.* 2001;107:1216–1220

29. Sugai M, Murata K, Kimura N, et al. Adenoma of the nipple in an adolescent. *Breast Cancer.* 2002;9:254–256

30. Albers SE, Barnard M, Thorner P, Krafchik BR. Erosive adenomatosis of the nipple in an eight year-old girl. *J Am Acad Dermatol.* 1999;40:834–837

31. Williams HJ, Hejmadi RK, England DW, et al. Imaging features of breast trauma: a pictorial review. *Breast.* 2002;11:107–115

32. Parker SJ, Harries SA. Phyllodes tumours. *Postgrad Med J.* 2001;77:428–435

33. Chao TC, Lo YF, Chen SC, Chen MF. Sonographic features of phyllodes tumors of the breast. *Ultrasound Obstet Gynecol.* 2002;20:64–71

34. The National Cancer Institute. The SEER cancer statistics review, 1975–2008. http://seer.cancer.gov/csr/1975_2008/browse_csr.php?section=4&page=sect_04_table.12.html. Accessed August 4, 2011

35. Corpron CA, Black CT, Singletary SE, Andrassy RJ. Breast cancer in adolescent females. *J Pediatr Surg.* 1995;30:322–324

36. Sonmezer M, Oktay K. Fertility preservation in young women undergoing breast cancer therapy. *Oncologist.* 2006;11:422–434

37. Goss PE, Sierra S. Current perspectives on radiation-induced breast cancer. *J Clin Oncol.* 1998;16:338–347

38. Nathan PC, Ness KK, Mahoney MC, Li Z, Hudson MM, Ford JS, et al. Screening and surveillance for second malignant neoplasms in adult survivors of childhood cancer: a report from the childhood cancer survivor study. *Ann Intern Med.* 2010;153:442–451

39. Berkey CS, Willett WC, Frazier L, Rosner B, Tamimi RM, Rockett HRH, Colditz GA. Prospective study of adolescent alcohol consumption and risk of benign breast disease in young women. *Pediatrics.* 2010;125:e1081–1087

40. Linos E, Willett WC, Cho E, Colditz G, Frazier L. Adolescent diet in relation to breast cancer risk among premenopausal women. *Cancer Epidemiol Biomarkers Prev.* 2010;19:689–696

41. Linos E, Willett WC, Cho E, Colditz G, Frazier L. Red meat consumption during adolescence among premenopausal women and risk of breast cancer. *Cancer Epidemiol Biomarkers Prev.* 2008;17:2146–2151

42. Dorgan JF, Liu L, Klifa C, Hylton N, Shepherd JA, Stanczyk FZ, et al. Adolescent diet and subsequent serum hormones, breast density, and bone mineral density in young women: results of the

Dietary Intervention Study in Children follow-up study. *Cancer Epidemiol Biomarkers Prev.* 2010;19:1545–1556

43. Marchbanks PA, McDonald JA, Wilson HG, Folger SG, Mandel MG, Daling JR, et al. Oral contraceptives and the risk of breast cancer. *N Engl J Med.* 2002;346:2025–2032

44. American College of Obstetricians and Gynecologists. Use of hormonal contraception in women with coexisting medical conditions: Practice Bulletin No. 73. *Obstet Gynecol.* 2006;107:1453–1472

45. Qureshi S, Sultan N. Topical nonsteroidal anti-inflammatory drugs versus oil of evening primrose in the treatment of mastalgia. *Surgeon.* 2005;3:7–10

46. Loud KJ, Micheli LJ. Common athletic injuries in adolescent girls. *Curr Opin Pediatr.* 2001;13:317–322

47. Liu H, Yeh ML, Lin KJ, Huang CK, Hung CM, Chen YS. Bloody nipple discharge in an adolescent girl: unusual presentation of juvenile fibroadenoma. *Pediatr Neonatol.* 2010;51:190–192

48. Stricker T, Navratil F, Forster I, Hurlimann R, Sehhhauser FH. Nonpuerperal mastitis in adolescents. *J Pediatr.* 2006;148:278–281

49. Dabbas N, Chand M, Pallett A, Royle GT, Sainsbury R. Have the organisms that cause breast abscess changed with time?—Implications for appropriate antibiotic usage in primary and secondary care. *Breast J.* 2010;16:412–415

50. Braverman PK. Body art: piercing, tattooing, and scarification. *Adolesc Med Clin.* 2006;17:505–519

51. Jacobs VR, Golombeck K, Jonat W, Kiechle M. Mastitis nonpuerperalis after nipple piercing: time to act. *Int J Fertil Womens Med.* 2003;48:226–231

52. Mayers LB, Moriarty BW, Judelson DA, Rundell KW. Complications of body art. *Consultant.* 2002;42:1744–1752

53. Braithwaite RL, Stephens T, Sterk C, Braithwaite K. Risks associated with tattooing and body piercing. *J Public Health Policy.* 1999;20:459–470

54. Pugatch D, Mileno M, Rich JD. Possible transmission of human immunodeficiency virus type 1 from body piercing. *Clin Infect Dis.* 1998;26:767–768

55. Bengualid V, Singh V, Singh H, Berger J. Mycobacterium fortuitum and anaerobic breast abscess following nipple piercing: case presentation and review of the literature. *J Adolesc Health.* 2008;42:530–532

56. American College of Obstetricians and Gynecologists. Breast concerns in the adolescent: ACOG Committee Opinion No. 350. *Obstet Gynecol.* 2006;108:1329–1336

57. Koltz PF, Sbitany H, Myers RP, Shaw RB, Patel N, Girotto JA. Reduction mammoplasty in the adolescent female: the URMC experience. *Inter J Surg.* 2011;9:229–232

58. Neto MS, Dematte MF, Freire M, Garcia EB, Quaresma M, Ferreira LM. Self esteem and functional capacity outcomes following reduction mammoplasty. *Aesthetic Surge J.* 2008;28:417–420

59. McGrath MH, Schooler WG. Elective plastic surgical procedures in adolescence. *Adolesc Med Clin.* 2004;15:487–502

60. Aillet S, Watier E, Chevrier S, Pailheret JP, Grall JY. Breast feeding after reduction mammaplasty performed during adolescence. *Eur J Obstet Gynecol Reprod Biol.* 2002;101:79–82

61. American Society of Plastic Surgeons. Report of the 2010 Plastic Surgery Statistics. http://www.plasticsurgery.org/Documents/news-resources/statistics/2010-statisticss/Patient-Ages/2010-teen-cosmetic-surgery-minally-invasive-13-19.pdf. Accessed August 3, 2011

62. American Society of Plastic Surgeons. Plastic surgery for teenagers briefing paper. http://www.plasticsurgery.org/Media/Briefing_Papers/Plastic_Surgery_for_Teenagers.html. Accessed August 3, 2011

63. Michalopoulos K. The effects of breast augmentation surgery on future ability to lactate. *Breast J.* 2007;13:62–67

Adolesc Med 23 (2012) 53–72

Excessive Uterine Bleeding

Hina J. Talib, MD[a], Susan M. Coupey, MD[*b]

[a]Postdoctoral Fellow, Adolescent Medicine, Children's Hospital at Montefiore, Albert Einstein College of Medicine, Bronx, New York

[b]Chief, Adolescent Medicine, Professor of Pediatrics, Children's Hospital at Montefiore, Albert Einstein College of Medicine, Bronx, New York

INTRODUCTION

Adolescence is a time of great physical, psychological, cognitive, and social change. At the crossroads of this change in adolescent girls is the onset of menstruation. Perceived and actual disruptions in the normal menstrual cycle may be a cause of concern and anxiety for many girls and their families. In fact, menstrual disorders are one of the leading reasons for physician office visits by adolescent girls in the United States.[1] Excessive uterine bleeding resulting in anemia or hemodynamic instability may be especially disrupting in the lives of adolescent girls because it can lead to emergency room visits, hospitalizations, and consultations with adolescent medicine specialists, gynecologists, hematologists, or endocrinologists.[2] Of adolescents hospitalized with menorrhagia and severe anemia, an estimated 75% have anovulatory dysfunctional uterine bleeding and the remaining 25% have an identifiable structural, infectious, or hematological disorder.[3,4]

Terminology used to describe abnormal uterine bleeding can be confusing, and it is important to understand commonly used definitions. Menorrhagia is defined as heavy or prolonged uterine bleeding. Dysfunctional uterine bleeding (DUB) is defined as irregular, painless bleeding of endometrial origin that is prolonged, unpatterned, and excessive. DUB can range from spotting to heavy bleeding and is associated with physiologic (perimenarchal/perimenopausal) or pathologic (eg, polycystic ovary syndrome) causes of anovulation. DUB is a diagnosis of exclusion, and this article discusses etiology and management of

---

*Corresponding author.
E-mail address: scoupey@montefiore.org (S. M. Coupey).

hormonally mediated anovulatory bleeding, as well as excessive uterine bleeding secondary to local genital tract conditions (structural and infectious), hematologic, and other medical disorders that are clinically relevant in the adolescent age group.

MENSTRUAL CYCLES: DEFINING "NORMAL" IN ADOLESCENTS

In order to evaluate and manage excessive uterine bleeding in adolescents, one must first understand the characteristics of menstrual bleeding in this age group. Menarche is a hallmark event in pubertal development and most often occurs at a sexual maturity rating (SMR) of 3 or 4. Analysis of National Health and Nutrition Examination Survey (NHANES) Wave III data on a representative sample of adolescents in the United States shows that the median age at menarche for all girls is 12.43 years, with some notable ethnic differences: non-Hispanic white girls have a median age at menarche of 12.55 years; non-Hispanic black girls achieve menarche, on average, nearly 6 months earlier than white girls at 12.06 years; and Mexican-American girls are in the middle at 12.25 years.[5]

The American Academy of Pediatrics and the American College of Obstetricians and Gynecologists published a consensus report in 2006 entitled *Menstruation in Girls and Adolescents: Using the Menstrual Cycle as a Vital Sign.* This report describes the normal range for age at menarche as 11–14 years, normal menstrual cycle interval as 21–45 days, normal duration of bleeding as up to 7 days, and normal flow as requiring 3–6 menstrual pads or tampons per day.[6] In addition to knowledge of these normal ranges, an understanding of the physiology of the adolescent menstrual cycle and its regulatory mechanisms is key to appropriate diagnosis and management of excessive uterine bleeding.

Ovulatory menstrual cycles in both adolescent and adult women are characterized by an initial follicular phase where estrogen, secreted from a maturing ovarian follicle, stimulates growth of the endometrial lining of the uterus (proliferative endometrium) and a later luteal phase where progesterone, secreted from the corpus luteum, differentiates and stabilizes the endometrial lining (secretory endometrium). In an ovulatory cycle, a midcycle luteinizing hormone (LH) surge triggered by rising estrogen levels influences release of an ovum and subsequent development of a corpus luteum. During the next 14 days, the corpus luteum involutes, estrogen and progesterone levels fall, and the secretory endometrium sheds in a controlled fashion producing a menstrual period. Cycles that are regular, associated with breast tenderness, premenstrual symptoms, and/or dysmenorrhea are usually ovulatory.

Anovulatory menstrual cycles may also be normal in adolescents, especially at younger gynecologic ages. Gynecologic age is defined as chronological age minus age at menarche and is a good clinical measure of the maturity of the hypothalamic-pituitary-ovarian (HPO) axis. The spectrum of anovulatory cycles in adolescent girls ranges from primary or secondary amenorrhea to oligomenorrhea to DUB to regular menstrual periods. A World Health Organization 2-year prospective study of more than 600 early adolescent girls using menstrual calendars showed that 67% of menstrual cycles are regular (bleeding for less than 10 days and at intervals of 20–40 days) by 2 years after menarche.[7] Furthermore, this study shows that in the first 24 months after menarche, approximately 5% of bleeding episodes last longer than 7 days and less than 0.5% last longer than 10 days. Biochemical studies of the adolescent menstrual cycle demonstrate an absent progesterone peak indicating anovulation (no corpus luteum formation) in the majority of cycles, also up to the second gynecologic year.[8,9] Studies also show that older age at menarche is associated with a longer interval of maturation from anovulatory to ovulatory cycles.[10] These studies, however, cannot differentiate physiologic anovulation from other pathologic causes of anovulation that may be more relevant in the early adolescent girl presenting with excessive uterine bleeding.

For clinical diagnostic purposes, the HPO axis is generally considered to be mature at a gynecologic age of 3 years. Thus a girl who had menarche at age 10 should have a mature HPO axis by age 13, whereas a girl whose menarche occurred at age 13 may not have a mature axis until age 16. At gynecologic ages younger than 3 years, anovulatory cycles can be physiologic. In physiologic anovulation in adolescents with a young gynecologic age, the immature HPO axis does not respond to rising estrogen levels with an LH surge (lack of maturation of the positive feedback mechanism) and the endometrium continues to proliferate under the influence of estrogen secreted by the developing follicle without progesterone-mediated stabilization. Fortunately, even in the absence of ovulation, there is negative feedback of estrogen at the hypothalamus, which leads to a cyclic fall in estrogen levels and an estrogen withdrawal bleed. Thus, most anovulatory cycles due to HPO axis immaturity result in relatively regular bleeding episodes that are not excessive. Only rarely is HPO axis immaturity associated with irregular sloughing of the unstable endometrium resulting in dysfunctional uterine bleeding that is excessive, prolonged, or associated with symptomatic anemia.

ETIOLOGIES OF EXCESSIVE UTERINE BLEEDING IN THE ADOLESCENT

Pathologic causes of excessive uterine bleeding in the adolescent may be as common or more common as those due to physiologic anovulation. We believe that the diagnosis of pathologic conditions in adolescent girls may sometimes be delayed due to the incorrect assumption that the majority of menstrual disorders result from HPO axis immaturity. Here we review clinically significant causes of pathologic anovulation, as well as other important causes of excessive uterine bleeding in adolescent girls including pregnancy, local pathology, and coagulopathies, as well as other medical disorders. Early identification of the etiology of uterine bleeding is important for appropriate and timely management. Table 1 outlines the etiologies of excessive bleeding in the adolescent girl.

Pathologic Anovulation

The normal regulatory mechanisms of the HPO axis on the menstrual cycle are susceptible to disruption by several hormonally mediated processes. Chief among these in adolescent girls is functional ovarian hyperandrogenism or polycystic ovary syndrome (PCOS). PCOS is the most common endocrine disorder in women and affects up to 15% of the population. PCOS usually presents in the perimenarcheal period with menstrual disorders. Oligomenorrhea and secondary amenorrhea are the menstrual disorders most commonly associated with PCOS; however, girls with PCOS may also have excessive uterine bleeding due to anovulatory DUB.[11] Common clinical signs of androgen excess in adolescents with PCOS include moderate to severe acne and, often, relatively mild hirsutism. Many adolescents with PCOS also are obese and have insulin resistance.[12,13] The etiology of PCOS is multifactorial and includes ovarian overproduction of androgens stimulated by elevated LH levels and hyperinsulinemia leading to chronic anovulation. Peripheral conversion of dehydroepiandrosterone (DHEA) and androstenedione into estrogen and testosterone further contributes to the hyperandrogenic state. Please see the article "Adolescent Polycystic Ovary Syndrome" on page 164 in this journal for an in-depth update on PCOS and its associated endocrine dysfunctions.

Other hyperandrogenic states that similarly affect the menstrual cycle and should be considered as a cause of anovulation and DUB in adolescents include Cushing syndrome, late-onset congenital adrenal hyperplasia (CAH), and the rare androgen-secreting tumors. Unlike the multifactorial mechanisms causing hyperandrogenism and menstrual disorders in PCOS, it has been proposed that the mechanism underlying menstrual disorders in Cushing syndrome is secondary to cortisol inhibition at the level of the hypothalamus, causing chronic anovulation from hypogonadotropic hypogonadism.[14] Late-onset, or nonclassical, CAH usually presents in adolescence with menstrual irregularity and, usually, moderate to severe hirsutism and occasional clitoromegaly. Those with the most common enzyme deficiency, 21-hydroxylase deficiency, have elevated 17-hydroxy progesterone levels and an exaggerated response to adrenocorticotropic hormone (ACTH) stimulation tests. In late-onset CAH, this elevated 17-hydroxy progesterone, expression of 5-alpha reductase in the ovary, and a direct glucocorticoid effect all contribute to hormonal disruption of the HPO axis.[15]

Hyperprolactinemia causes inhibition of gonadotropin releasing hormone (GnRH) at the level of the hypothalamus and also leads to pathologic anovulation. Additionally, there is a decrease in sex hormone binding globulin (SHBG) and an increase in DHEA and testosterone levels that are associated with increased prolactin levels. Clinical signs of a prolactin secreting pituitary adenoma include

Table 1.
Etiologies of Excessive Uterine Bleeding in Adolescent Girls

Hormonally Mediated Dysfunctional Uterine Bleeding

- Physiologic anovulation
- Hyperandrogenic anovulation
  - Polycystic ovary syndrome
  - Congenital adrenal hyperplasia
  - Adrenal/ovarian tumor
- Hypothalamic anovulation
  - Stress
  - Weight loss
  - Exercise
  - Chronic illness
- Endocrine disorders
  - Thyroid dysfunction
  - Diabetes mellitus
- Primary ovarian insufficiency
- Hyperprolactinemia

Systemic Medical Disorders

- Bleeding disorders
  - Inherited (eg, von Willebrand disease)
  - Acquired (eg, thrombocytopenia, leukemia)
- Liver disease
- Kidney disease
- Autoimmune disease
  - Inflammatory bowel disease
  - Rheumatologic

Local Genital Tract Pathology

- Sexually transmitted infection
  - Endometritis
  - Pelvic inflammatory disease
- Trauma
  - High vaginal laceration
- Structural lesions
  - Neoplasm
  - Arteriovenous malformation

Pregnancy-related

- Spontaneous abortion
- Ectopic pregnancy

Iatrogenic

- Medications
  - Anticoagulants
  - Hormonal contraceptives
  - Chemotherapy

headaches, vision changes, and galactorrhea, in addition to the signs of excess androgens mentioned earlier. Most often hyperprolactinemia is associated with secondary amenorrhea, but it can also present with DUB. Other than primary pituitary tumors such as prolactinomas, certain psychiatric drugs, including risperidone, haloperidol, and phenothiazines, may also increase prolactin levels in adolescent girls.[16]

Thyroid dysfunction also interacts at the HPO axis causing menstrual irregularities and excessive uterine bleeding. Although both hyper- and hypothyroidism may cause menstrual disorders, menorrhagia is more commonly associated with hypothyroidism. In hypothyroidism, thyroid releasing hormone (TRH) is released by the hypothalamus, which signals the pituitary to make thyroid stimulating hormone (TSH) and prolactin. In addition to hyperprolactinemia, hypothyroidism is also associated with decreased SHBG, which results in decreased clearance of estrogens and androgens. Hypothyroidism can also result in decreased levels of factors VII, VIII, IX, and XI, which may further predispose an adolescent to develop symptomatic menorrhagia.[17]

Diabetes mellitus is a common chronic illness in adolescents and has been shown to be associated with menstrual abnormalities. Studies suggest that hyperglycemia directly suppresses the GnRH pulse generator, causing hypogonadotropic hypogonadism. Accordingly, poor glycemic control is associated with anovulation and DUB, specifically in girls with hemoglobin A1c levels greater than 12.8 mg/dL or serum glucose levels greater than 240 mg/dL. In those adolescents with type 2, insulin-resistant, diabetes mellitus, hyperinsulinism contributes to a hyperandrogenic state that causes anovulatory cycles.[18,19] With the obesity epidemic in full force among today's adolescents, many more are developing type 2 diabetes than in the past, and even those who do not have frank diabetes have marked insulin resistance. Many of these obese teens have anovulation, irregular menses, and DUB related to the accompanying metabolic derangements.

Anovulation may also be related to suppression of the HPO axis secondary to physical and emotional stress, eating disorders, weight loss from other causes such as inflammatory bowel disease, and excessive exercise. Although these anovulatory states most often present as primary or secondary amenorrhea and are frequently referred to as hypothalamic amenorrhea, DUB can also be a feature, especially at the onset and during recovery from the condition. In the early stages and during recovery of any cause of hypothalamic amenorrhea, oligo-ovulatory cycles may lead to persistently elevated estrogen and result in irregular sloughing of the endometrium. Stress and weight loss often accompany a variety of chronic illnesses and can contribute to menstrual disorders in adolescents with such illnesses.

Finally, premature ovarian insufficiency and/or ovarian failure may also be associated with DUB, although eventually this condition leads to amenorrhea. Many adolescent girls who have been treated for cancer have a temporary period of ovarian insufficiency with oligo-ovulation that often results in excessive uterine bleeding, especially if there are also hematologic abnormalities such as thrombocytopenia associated with the cancer treatment.

Pregnancy-Related Complications

When excessive uterine bleeding is associated with lower abdominal pain, the evaluation should pay special attention to pregnancy-related causes or those due to local pathology such as infection in the genital tract. In fact, pregnancy should always be an early consideration in the evaluation of excessive menstrual bleeding in an adolescent girl, regardless of a stated history of sexual activity and especially to rule out life-threatening complications. Given that adolescents may not acknowledge sexual activity and the United States has the highest teenage pregnancy rate among developed nations, a pregnancy test should always be done. Recent national estimates have shown a teenage birthrate in the United States in 2006 of 41.9 births per 1000 women and 19.3 abortions per 1000 women.[20] Like adults, adolescents have a risk of miscarriage and also have a 2% risk of ectopic pregnancy, both of which can present with excessive uterine bleeding and pain in an adolescent who has no idea that she is pregnant. Adolescents with ectopic pregnancy are more likely than adults to present with abdominal pain and a current gonorrhea or chlamydia infection.[21] Centers for Disease Control and Prevention (CDC) surveillance data show that mortality rates associated with ectopic pregnancies are highest in adolescents, further underscoring the importance of its consideration in a sexually active adolescent with uterine bleeding.[22]

Local Pathology: Infectious, Trauma, Structural Lesions, Tumors

Adolescents with menorrhagia should be evaluated for infectious etiologies, most often sexually transmitted, including endometritis or pelvic inflammatory disease (PID). Infectious endometritis, with or without salpingitis, often presents with painful heavy uterine bleeding. Obtaining a confidential history from an adolescent girl is essential for eliciting an accurate sexual history. In 2009, the CDC reported that the highest age specific rates of chlamydia and gonorrhea among sexually active females are among girls aged 15–19.[23] Given these high rates of infection, the risk of PID is much higher in adolescents than in adults. Adolescent girls are also biologically at increased risk of acquiring sexually transmitted infections (STIs) and PID as many have a cervical ectropion, exposing the columnar cells of the endocervix on the portio of the cervix where they are easily infected during sexual intercourse. Given this biological risk factor, as well as the high rates of STIs in adolescents, it is important to include infection in the differential diagnosis of heavy uterine bleeding in any sexually active girl, especially if presenting with lower abdominal pain.

Profuse bright red vaginal bleeding that requires a blood transfusion is suspicious for traumatic causes such as a deep vaginal laceration, which may result from voluntary or involuntary sexual intercourse.[24,25] An examination under anesthesia, to localize the source of the bleeding and repair the laceration, is often necessary. A deep vaginal laceration resulting from a high pressure insufflation injury (secondary to water slides, jet ski, or spa jets) presents similarly and also requires an examination under anesthesia and surgical repair.[26,27] Although rare, abrupt, bright red, heavy uterine bleeding may also be secondary to a congenital hemangioma or arteriovenous malformation.[28]

When excessive uterine bleeding is refractory to traditional hormonal treatment, one must consider structural lesions. Lesions such as uterine myomas (fibroids) and cervical or uterine polyps are much more common in adults but may occur in adolescents and can be associated with excessive or prolonged bleeding.[29,30] Malignant tumors of the lower genital tract are exceedingly rare in adolescents; however, rhabdomyosarcoma is seen more commonly in the adolescent age group. About 20% of rhabdomyosarcomas arise from the genitourinary tract and often cause vaginal bleeding that is refractory to hormonal treatment, with or without a visible or palpable mass.[31,32] Foreign bodies retained in the vagina usually present with purulent discharge that may be bloody but do not produce excessive bleeding. Similarly, partially obstructive congenital Müllerian anomalies can present with prolonged bleeding and pain but do not usually produce excessive bleeding.

Bleeding Disorders and Other Medical Conditions

Menorrhagia is often the first presenting symptom of inherited or acquired bleeding disorders in adolescents. With inherited bleeding disorders, menorrhagia usually begins at menarche or soon thereafter and is often associated with significant anemia requiring hospitalization. With acquired bleeding disorders, new-onset menorrhagia in a girl with previously normal menses may be the presenting symptom of leukemia or thrombocytopenia and also may require hospitalization and transfusion.

Bleeding disorders that affect adolescents can be divided into 2 main categories: coagulation factor abnormalities and acquired or inherited platelet disorders. Von Willebrand disease (vWD), a deficiency or abnormality in a clotting factor critical in platelet adhesion, is one of the most common inherited bleeding disorders found among women with menorrhagia.[33] Other coagulation factor abnormalities include factor deficiencies, hemophilia A or B, and fibrinogen disorders. Acquired platelet disorders include those associated with idiopathic thrombocytopenia purpura (ITP), autoimmune diseases, leukemia, aplastic anemia, hypersplenism, myelosuppression from chemotherapy or other drugs, and liver failure. Inherited platelet disorders, including Glanzmann thrombasthenia and Bernard-Soulier syndrome, are rare but are also associated with menorrhagia in adolescents.[34]

Small, single-center studies have shown that the prevalence of bleeding disorders among adolescents hospitalized with menorrhagia and severe anemia ranges from 5–28%. [2,35-38] These studies found that the most common bleeding disorder in hospitalized adolescents with menorrhagia is vWD, followed by thrombocytopenia and other platelet disorders, and finally, clotting factor deficiencies. Screening for the most common bleeding disorders should be considered when menorrhagia causes severe enough anemia to require hospitalization, presents at menarche, is associated with other signs of bleeding such as petechiae, or when there is a family history of bleeding disorders.

Adolescents with chronic renal disease or liver failure may also have excessive uterine bleeding. In chronic renal disease or failure, hypothalamic suppression due to rising azotemia and/or hyperprolactinemia resulting from decreased renal clearance can lead to oligo-ovulation and DUB. Anemia (due to decreased erythropoietin production), platelet dysfunction, and decreased fibrinogen levels (due to uremia) also contribute to excessive uterine bleeding in girls with chronic renal failure.[39] In chronic liver failure, the production of vitamin K dependent coagulation factors, protein C, protein S, fibrinogen levels, and the number and function of platelets are all decreased, resulting in an increased risk of menorrhagia. In liver failure, hypothalamic suppression from excess estrogen, in the setting of decreased SHBG produced in the liver, may result in anovulatory DUB.[40]

Menstrual abnormalities, including excessive uterine bleeding, have also been associated with other chronic conditions in adolescents including juvenile idiopathic arthritis, systemic lupus erythematosus, and inflammatory bowel disease.[41-43] Here the mechanisms are less clear; however, menstrual dysfunction is correlated with disease onset. Suggested mechanisms include hypothalamic suppression resulting from stress, poor nutrition, and side effects of medications used in the management of these conditions.[44]

Iatrogenic or Drug-Mediated

Taking a thorough medication history, especially in adolescents with chronic medical illnesses or in those who are sexually active and using hormonal contraception, is important when evaluating causes of excessive uterine bleeding. Drugs that alter clotting parameters, such as aspirin or warfarin, may increase susceptibility to heavy uterine bleeding. Chemotherapy and its associated myelosuppression may also lead to coagulation dysfunction. Some medications, such as valproic acid, are independently associated with PCOS and DUB in adolescents.[45,46]

Both combined and progesterone-only contraceptives may be associated with irregular uterine bleeding but are usually not associated with significant anemia or menorrhagia. Progesterone-only formulations, including depo-medroxyprogesterone acetate (DMPA), the levonorgestrel-releasing intrauterine system, and norethindrone oral contraceptive pills, are more likely to result in irregular bleeding than combined estrogen-progestin formulations and, over time, are more often associated with amenorrhea. With combined oral contraception (COC), break-through bleeding may result from missed pills, inconsistent timing of pills, or from medication interactions that decrease estrogen concentrations. A wide array of drug classes are known to increase the metabolism of estrogen, thus effectively lowering the estrogen dose and producing breakthrough bleeding in girls taking COCs. These include anticonvulsants, central nervous system stimulants (modafinil), selected antibiotics (rifampin, griseofulvin), and herbal supplements (St. John's wort, garlic).[47]

EVALUATION OF EXCESSIVE UTERINE BLEEDING IN ADOLESCENTS

The first priority in the evaluation of excessive uterine bleeding in an adolescent girl is to establish if they are hemodynamically stable and to perform a complete blood count. Pregnancy should also be an early consideration and should be ruled out with a urine or serum ß-human chorionic gonadotropin (HCG) level.

History

A careful and complete menstrual, medical, family, and psychosocial history must be elicited. For every girl who is evaluated for excessive uterine bleeding, no matter how young she is, a portion of this history should be obtained from the girl, herself, in private, without the mother or other family members present. It is crucial to elicit a private, confidential, sexual history from the adolescent, including a history of sexual abuse. Other essential components of the adolescent history, including body image and eating behaviors, mood and stress, and drug and alcohol use, are also best elicited in private.

For the menstrual history, obtaining a gynecologic age (in months if less than 3 years); quantifying blood loss, blood clots, and product use; and screening for missed school days and clothing accidents are all important to obtain, preferably from the adolescent rather than the mother. However, adolescent girls (and their mothers) frequently underestimate or overestimate amounts of blood loss and a hemoglobin level should always be obtained before planning management. Excessive uterine bleeding, by definition, falls outside the normal ranges of menstrual bleeding, which is greater than 7 days or 80 mL per cycle. As mentioned, obtaining an accurate estimate of blood loss may be challenging. One prospective tool to help quantify excessive blood loss is a pictorial bleeding assessment calendar (Figure 1).[48] Lightly stained products are scored with 1 point, moderately stained with 5 points, and soaked products with 10 points. Scoring greater than 100 points on this tool has been shown to be 89% sensitive and 86% specific for identifying heavy menstrual bleeding (> 80 mL) in adult women. Using such a pictorial tool or keeping a menstrual diary, either on paper (Figure 2) or using a smart phone application, may be especially helpful when evaluating bleeding in an adolescent. A thorough review of systems, especially noting any chronic or

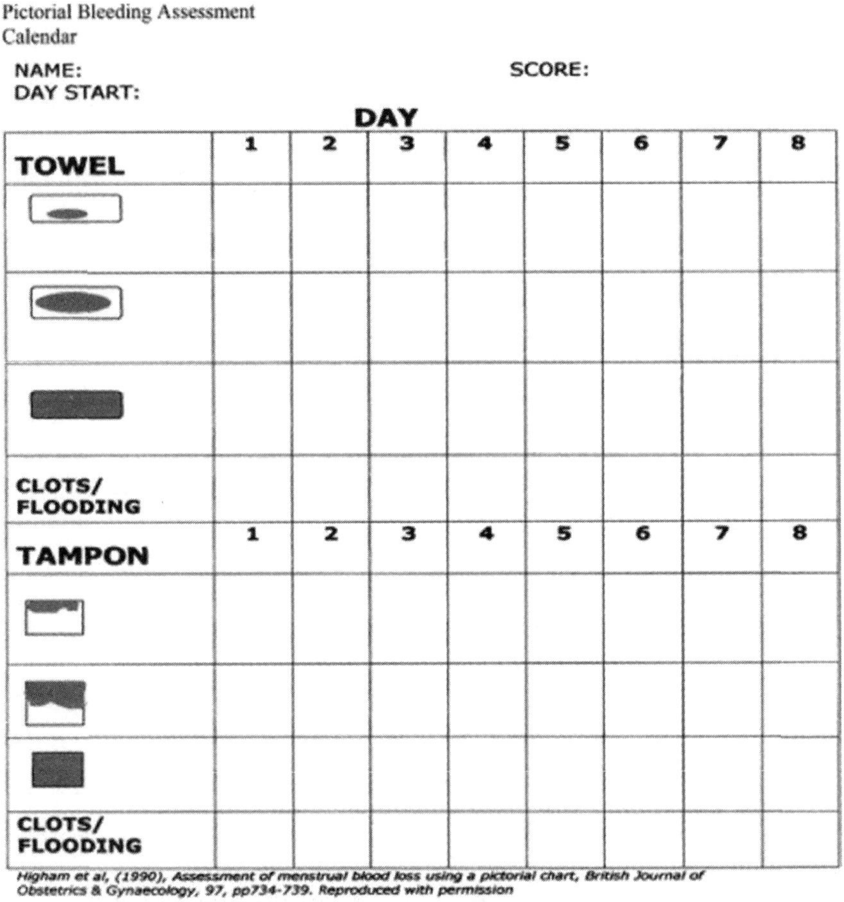

Pictorial Bleeding Assessment
Calendar

NAME: SCORE:
DAY START:

DAY

TOWEL	1	2	3	4	5	6	7	8
(light)								
(moderate)								
(heavy)								
CLOTS/ FLOODING								

TAMPON	1	2	3	4	5	6	7	8
(light)								
(moderate)								
(heavy)								
CLOTS/ FLOODING								

Higham et al, (1990), Assessment of menstrual blood loss using a pictorial chart, British Journal of Obstetrics & Gynaecology, 97, pp734-739. Reproduced with permission

Figure 1. Pictorial Bleeding Assessment Calendar: A Prospective Tool to Help Estimate Blood Loss (Source: Higham JM, O'Brien PM, Shaw RW. Assessment of menstrual blood loss using a pictorial chart. *Br J Obstet Gynecol.* 1990;97:734–739. Reprinted with permission from John Wiley & Sons, Inc.).

systemic illnesses, medications, recent weight changes, dieting and exercise behavior, stressors, and symptoms of systemic bleeding disorders, is warranted. A family history of infertility, menstrual disorders, and bleeding disorders may provide more clues toward the etiology.

Physical Examination

On physical examination, the clinician should pay particular attention to the skin examination looking for signs of bleeding (pallor, ecchymosis, petechiae), hyperandrogenism (acne, hirsutism, clitoromegaly), hyperinsulinemia (acanthosis nigricans), hyperprolactinemia (galactorrhea), and other endocrine dis-

Menstrual Calendar

Name_____Year_____

	Jan	Feb	Mar	Apr	May	Jun	Jul	Aug	Sep	Oct	Nov	Dec
1												
2												
3												
4												
5												
6												
7												
8												
9												
10												
11												
12												
13												
14												
15												
16												
17												
18												
19												
20												
21												
22												
23												
24												
25												
26												
27												
28												
29												
30												
31												
# of days between periods												

■ Exceptionally heavy flow

X Normal flow

L Exceptionally light flow

• Spotting

Figure 2. Sample Menstrual Calendar

eases (thyromegaly, striae). In order to achieve this, a complete examination with the adolescent undressed and gowned is required. SMR staging of breast and pubic hair should be performed to assess pubertal stage. An external genital examination with separation/traction of the labia majora in the lithotomy or frog-leg position, evaluating for vulvar lesions, masses, and anatomy and to document the source of the bleeding, is indicated in every adolescent presenting with bleeding. If the adolescent is sexually active, a complete pelvic examination, including a speculum examination and a bimanual vaginal examination, is indicated to further visualize the genital tract, localize the bleeding, palpate for tenderness and masses, and obtain samples for STI testing. In cases of vaginal trauma with profuse bleeding, an examination under anesthesia is usually needed to visualize and repair the source of bleeding.

Laboratory Tests

A complete blood count (with attention to both hemoglobin and platelet values) and a urine ß-HCG pregnancy test should ideally be done before the history and physical examination so that results are immediately available for decision making after the visit. A few other tests guided by the history and physical examination may be warranted. If hormonally mediated DUB is suspected, thyroid function tests, prolactin, and a workup for PCOS (LH, FSH, free and total testosterone, DHEAS) should be performed. Of note, gonadotropin and androgen levels are suppressed if the patient is taking COCs or other hormonal contraceptives, and one cannot accurately diagnose PCOS under these conditions.

If there is orthostasis, marked anemia, or physical signs or a family history of systemic bleeding disorders, screening tests for the most common coagulation disorders should be considered. These would include prothrombin time (PT), partial thromboplastin time (PTT), fibrinogen level, a vWD panel (vWF antigen, factor VIII, ristocetin cofactor activity), bleeding time, and liver function tests. vWF levels are lowest during menses, and therefore, it is best to screen for these abnormalities within the first 3 days of a menstrual bleed. Exogenous estrogen and thyroid hormone also interfere with this assay by elevating vWF and factor VIII levels, and ideally, this test should be performed before prescribing any hormonal treatment. In the emergent setting, it is important to note that all of these tests should be sent before any required blood transfusions or hormonal stabilization of the endometrium. However, in cases of severe bleeding, coagulation factors may be depleted and accurate testing may not be possible until the emergent event has resolved and effects of blood transfusion have dissipated. Thus, if there is a high index of suspicion for a bleeding disorder, testing should be repeated a few months later. When using combination contraceptive pills in the treatment of these patients, testing should be done during the placebo week to prevent false elevations of these factors as a result of estrogen.

In the sexually active adolescent girl, an infectious workup, including a gonorrhea and chlamydia test, as well as inflammatory markers such as white blood cell count, erythrocyte sedimentation rate, and C-reactive protein level, is important. If PID is diagnosed clinically by physical examination, a pelvic ultrasound to evaluate for a tubo-ovarian abscess may be considered. If the adolescent is pregnant, an ultrasound to locate, assess viability, and date the pregnancy is necessary.

In the rare cases when structural pathology is a concern, a pelvic ultrasound or magnetic resonance imaging (MRI) study may be indicated. Endometrial biopsy has little role in the evaluation of the adolescent.

MANAGEMENT OF EXCESSIVE UTERINE BLEEDING IN ADOLESCENTS

The goals of management for adolescent girls with excessive uterine bleeding in order of importance are (1) to correct hemodynamic imbalance; (2) to stabilize the endometrium and stop the bleeding; to prevent future uncontrolled blood loss; (3) to correct the anemia; (4) and to replenish iron stores. Management must be tailored to the severity and rate of the bleeding and the degree of anemia, as well as to the underlying etiology. Regardless of the etiology, however, if there is significant anemia, hormonal treatment to stabilize the endometrium and control future bleeding episodes is usually needed until the anemia resolves. Low dose COCs ($\leq$ 35 μg of ethinyl estradiol) are the mainstay of hormonal therapy for this age group. However, treatment with progestin-only preparations (eg, medroxyprogesterone acetate) may be suitable for some adolescents when estrogen is contraindicated. Antifibrinolytics (eg, tranexamic acid), alone or in combination with hormonal therapy, may also be helpful. Here we discuss the management of adolescents with bleeding secondary to hormonally mediated DUB, as well as systemic bleeding disorders (Figure 3). Bleeding secondary to pregnancy, local pathology, drugs, and other medical conditions require condition-specific management.

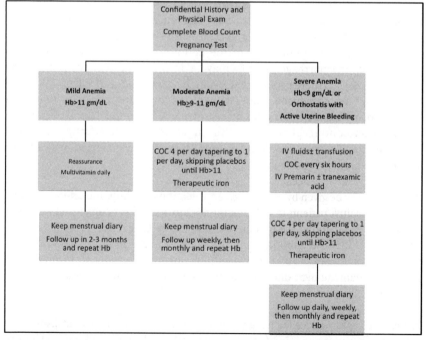

Figure 3. Sample Algorithm for the Management of Excessive Uterine Bleeding in Adolescents According to Severity. Used at Children's Hospital at Montefiore. Hb, hemoglobin; COC, combination oral contraceptive

Inpatient Management

Adolescents with active heavy uterine bleeding; hemodynamically unstable, symptomatic anemia; or a Hgb less than 9g/dL may need emergent intravenous fluids, blood transfusion, and hospitalization. In these patients, pregnancy, bleeding disorders, trauma, or other local pathology should be ruled out. Inpatient management of severely anemic adolescents with menorrhagia varies from institution to institution, and there is a lack of consensus and evidence as to the most efficacious approach. Initial management may include intravenous conjugated estrogens, 25 mg every 4 hours to a maximum of 4 doses or until the bleeding significantly slows. Most adolescents only require 1 or 2 doses. It is postulated that intravenous estrogen acts by rapidly constricting the spiral arteries in the endometrium and can be used to help stop uterine bleeding from any nonstructural cause.[49] Intravenous estrogen should not be used in those with estrogen contraindications or in those who, despite severe anemia, are not currently bleeding heavily. In our inpatient protocol, we begin a monophasic COC concurrent with the administration of intravenous estrogen or as a single therapeutic agent when intravenous dosing is not required at a dose of 4 pills a day (1 pill every 6 hours) for the first day or two, tapering down to 2 pills a day (1 pill every 12 hours) once the bleeding stops. Of note, this regimen may be associated with nausea and antiemetics should be provided prophylactically. An alternative regimen that is used in the United Kingdom and may be especially helpful in girls with bleeding disorders is to give tranexamic acid 1300 mg (two 650 mg tablets) by mouth 3 times daily (every 8 hours) with or without a COC taper as described earlier.[50] Tranexamic acid is an antifibrinolytic agent that was approved by the Food and Drug Administration (FDA) in the United States for use in menorrhagia in 2010.[51] It has fewer side effects than epsilon aminocaproic acid and is a more potent antifibrinolytic. Tranexamic acid blocks the action of plasmin, thereby reducing fibrin degradation, stabilizing clots, and reducing bleeding. It has no effect on standard blood coagulation parameters such as PT, PTT, or platelet count. However, in the United States, the package insert for tranexamic acid warns about the potential increased risk for thromboembolic events and cautions regarding use with COCs. If estrogen contraindications exist, medroxyprogesterone acetate 5–10 mg twice a day or norethindrone acetate 5 mg twice a day may be given by mouth with or without an antifibrinolytic. On discharge from the hospital, patients should continue to take 2, tapering to 1 COC per day continuously, discarding the placebo pills. Those who are estrogen intolerant may taper to 1 pill of progestin per day and then switch to a progestin-only contraceptive pill, 1 pill daily continuously. In addition, at hospital discharge, the adolescent should begin taking a therapeutic dose of iron such as ferrous gluconate 325 mg twice a day. Outpatient regimens for tapering of COCs or progestins in the management of excessive menstrual bleeding are highly variable and, as with inpatient management, there is a lack of evidence for differential efficacy of any regimen over another.

Adherence to and understanding the medication regimen after discharge from the hospital may be challenging for adolescent patients and their families, especially for young girls in the 10- to 14-year age group. The parents of young adolescents are understandably reluctant to keep their child on "contraceptive pills." We have found it helpful with our population to call them "hormone pills" and to explain that older girls and women use the same pills for contraception or birth control but that we are using them to stop the bleeding. Clear and concrete discharge instructions are needed. It is important to impress on the parent and the adolescent that if the girl stops taking the COC pill she will bleed again. Having the parent fill the COC prescription before discharge and showing them how to discard the placebo pills is helpful to ensure continuous hormonally active pill administration at home. Because the patient is not taking the placebo pills, she needs to start a new package of pills every 3 weeks rather than the usual 4 weeks used for contraception. Therefore, the prescription must be written for the pharmacist to dispense 2 packages of pills at each refill, giving 6 weeks of continuous use. Because of various insurance company and Medicaid regulations, we often have difficulty getting the pharmacy to dispense 2 packs at once and may have to call the pharmacy or the insurance company to facilitate dispensing. When the adolescent is still severely anemic on discharge from hospital (Hgb $\leq$ 8 gm/dL), close follow up within 2–3 days of discharge to address bleeding control and medication adherence is helpful. Surprisingly, we find clinically that many girls are reluctant to take the therapeutic iron supplement, and they require much counseling and support to correct their anemia. We prescribe ferrous gluconate rather than ferrous sulfate because it is less irritating to the stomach, and we prescribe it twice a day, with breakfast and dinner, rather than the usual 3 times a day, to facilitate adherence. We also prescribe 100 mg of docusate sodium to be taken twice a day with the iron pill, along with plenty of water, to prevent constipation.

Outpatient Management

Adolescents who present with mild (Hgb $\geq$ 11 g/dL) or moderate (Hgb = 9–11 g/dL) anemia as a result of excessive uterine bleeding may be managed in the outpatient setting, with close physician follow-up. For moderate anemia, depending on the amount and rate of bleeding, a COC taper (varying from 4 pills to 2 pills a day) tailored to the adolescent's presentation may be started. Continuous COCs, 1 pill a day and discarding the placebo pills, should be continued until the hemoglobin level is greater than or equal to 11 g/L. At this point, a withdrawal bleed should be allowed and the adolescent should then continue cycling with COCs, 1 pill a day including the placebo pills, to control menstrual bleeding for at least 3 months. During this time, they should continue taking the therapeutic iron supplement twice a day to replenish iron stores. By this time, results of tests investigating the etiology of the uterine bleeding will be available and treatment of the underlying cause should be considered. If the adolescent is sexually active and wants contraception or is found to have a hormonal cause of DUB that is managed by COCs, such as PCOS, the COCs may be continued indefinitely. If the patient has vWD or another bleeding disorder and does not want to continue on

COCs, she may be well controlled by taking tranexamic acid 1300 mg three times daily for the first 5 days of every menstrual period, or if she is sexually active, by a levonorgestrel-releasing intrauterine system.[52] Adolescents with a young gynecologic age, who are thought to have HPO axis immaturity, should be counseled to stop taking the COCs and keep a menstrual calendar.

Adolescents with mild excessive bleeding (Hgb ≥ 11) only need reassurance and outpatient follow-up for a repeat hemoglobin level in 2–3 months. Appropriate anticipatory guidance about early menstrual bleeding patterns has been shown to decrease young adolescents' anxiety about their bleeding.[53] Adolescents with mild excessive bleeding may be prescribed a daily multivitamin with iron, and if the bleeding causes anxiety or is associated with dysmenorrhea, nonsteroidal anti-inflammatory drugs (NSAIDS) such as naproxen sodium, 550 mg by mouth twice a day, help to decrease flow and menstrual cramps.[54,55]

SUMMARY

Menstrual bleeding that falls outside the range of normal in adolescents is often a cause of great concern for both girls and their families. Often, much of this anxiety can be alleviated with proper anticipatory guidance about menarche and early menstrual bleeding patterns. Eliciting a menstrual history from an adolescent girl is challenging, and the use of concrete methods to chart their patterns and flow, such as menstrual calendars and pictorial bleeding assessment calendar (PBAC) tools, may be helpful. The importance of obtaining a confidential history from the adolescent girl cannot be overestimated. A confidential sexual history is essential so that pregnancy and infectious causes of bleeding are addressed.

Not all menstrual bleeding in young girls is attributable to immaturity of the HPO axis. Anovulation and DUB from other clinically relevant conditions in adolescent girls must also be considered. Chief among these is PCOS, which should always be ruled out when a girl presents with excessive bleeding associated with clinical signs of hyperandrogenism, obesity, or insulin resistance. Attention must also be paid to signs or a family history of a bleeding disorder, as vWD is commonly associated with excessive uterine bleeding. Importantly, the laboratory testing for both PCOS and vWD is affected by therapies for the excessive bleeding, and it should be performed before hormonal interventions or blood products are administered or during the placebo phase if treatment has begun.

Management goals for excessive uterine bleeding include stabilizing the endometrium and stopping further blood loss, as well as preventing future uncontrolled blood loss. Hormonal stabilization of the endometrium is often helpful regardless of the cause of bleeding and especially in those with hormonally mediated anovulation. New antifibrinolytics, such as tranexamic acid, may also be helpful in the emergent setting and in adolescents with bleeding disorders.

References

1. Ziv A, Boulet JR, Slap GB. Utilization of physician offices by adolescents in the United States. *Pediatrics.* 1999;104:35–42
2. Iglesias EA, Coupey SM. Menstrual cycle abnormalities: diagnosis and management. *Adolesc Med.* 1999;10:255–273
3. Claessens EA, Cowell CA. Acute Adolescent Menorrhagia. *Am J Obstet Gynecol.* 1981;139:277–280
4. Smith YR, Quint EH, Hertzberg RB. Menorrhagia in adolescents requiring hospitalization. *J Pediatr Adolesc Gynecol.* 1998;11:13–15
5. Chumlea WC, Schubert CM, Roche AF, et al. Age at menarche and racial comparisons in US girls. *Pediatrics.* 2003;111:110–113
6. Diaz A, Laufer MR, Breech LL, American Academy of Pediatrics Committee on Adolescence, American College of Obstetrician and Gynecologists Committee on Adolescent Health Care. Menstruation in girls and adolescents: using the menstrual cycle as a vital sign. *Pediatrics.* 2006;118:2245–2250
7. World Health Organization multicenter study on menstrual and ovulatory patterns in adolescent girls. II. Longitudinal study of menstrual patterns in the early postmenarcheal period, duration of bleeding episodes and menstrual cycles. World Health Organization Task Force on Adolescent Reproductive Health. *J Adolesc Health Care.* 1986;7:236–244
8. Read GF, Wilson DW, Hughes IA, et al: The use of salivary progesterone assays in the assessment of ovarian function in postmenarchal girls. *J Endocrinol.* 1984;102:265–268
9. Apter D, Viinikka L, Vihko R. Hormonal patterns of adolescent menstrual cycles. *J Clin Endocrinol Metab.* 1978;47:944–954
10. Vikho R, Apter D. Endocrine characteristics of adolescent menstrual cycles: impact of early menarche. *J Steroid Biochem.* 1984;20:231–236
11. Azziz R, Woods KS, Reyna R, et al. The prevalence and features of the polycystic ovary syndrome in an unselected population. *J Clin Endocrinol Metab.* 2004;89:2745–2749
12. Rieder J, Santoro N, Cohen HW, Marantz P, Coupey SM. Body shape and size and insulin resistance as early clinical predictors of hyperandrogenic anovulation in ethnic minority adolescent girls. *J Adolesc Health.* 2008;43:115–124
13. Franks S, Gilling-Smith C, Watson H, et al. Insulin action in the normal and polycystic ovary. *Endocrinol Metab Clin North Am.* 1999;28:361–378
14. Lado-Abeal J, Rodriguez-Arnao J, Newell-Price JDC, et al. Menstrual abnormalities in women with Cushing's disease are correlated with hypercortisolism rather than raised circulating androgen levels. *Clin J Endocrinol Metab.* 1998;83:3083–3088
15. Witchel SF, Azziz R. Congenital adrenal hyperplasia. *J Pediatr Adolesc Gynecol.* 2011;24(3):116–126
16. Roke Y, van Harten PN, Boot AM, Buitelaar JK. Antipsychotic medication in children and adolescents: a descriptive review of the effects on prolactin level and associated side effects. *J Child Adolesc Psychopharmacol.* 2009;19(4):403–414
17. Krassas G. Thyroid disease and female reproduction. *Fertil Steril.* 2000;4:1063–1070
18. Schroeder B, Hertweck SP, Sanfilippo J, et al. Correlation between glycemic control and menstruation in diabetic adolescents. *J Reprod Med.* 2000;45:1–5
19. Strotmeyer E, Steenkiste A, Foley TP, et al. Menstrual cycle differences between women with type 1 diabetes and women without diabetes. *Diabetes Care.* 2003;26:1016–1021
20. Guttmacher Institute. U.S. teenage pregnancies, births and abortions: national and state trends and trends by race and ethnicity. January 2010. Available at: www.guttmacher.org/pubs/USTP-trends.pdf. Accessed June 26, 2011
21. Menon S, Sammel MD, Vichnin M, Barnhart KT. Risk factors for ectopic pregnancy: a comparison between adult and adolescent women. *J Pediatric Adolesc Gynecol.* 2007;20(3):181–185
22. Centers for Disease Control and Prevention. Surveillance for ectopic pregnancy—United States, 1970–1989. *MMWR.* 1993;42(SS-6):73–85
23. Centers for Disease Control and Prevention. *Sexually Transmitted Disease Surveillance 2009.* Atlanta: U.S. Department of Health and Human Services; 2010

24. Frioux SM, Blinman T, Christian CW. Vaginal lacerations from consensual intercourse in adolescents. *Child Abuse Negl.* 2011;35(1):69–73
25. Perlman SE, McDanald M, Templeman C. Unrecognized coital laceration in a series of nonvirginal adolescent girls. *J Pediatr Adolesc Gynecol.* 2001;14(3):149–155
26. Merritt DF. Genital trauma in children and adolescents. *Clinical Obstet Gynecol.* 2008;51:237–248
27. Lacy J, Brennand E, Ornstein M, Allen L. Vaginal laceration from high-pressure water jet in a prepubescent girl. *Pediatr Emerg Care.* 2007;23(2):112–114
28. Wang S, Lang JH, Zhou HM. Venous malformations of the female lower genital tract. *Eur J Obstet Gynecol Reprod Biol.* 2009;145(2):205–208
29. Fields KR, Neinstein LS. Uterine myomas in adolescents: case reports and a review of the literature. *J Pediatr Adolesc Gynecol.* 1996;9:195–198
30. Noorhasan DJ, Weiss G. Perimenarchal menorrhagia: evaluation and management. *J Pediatr.* 2010;158:162
31. Ortner A, Weiser G, Haas HM, Resch R, Dapunt O. Embryonal rhabdomyosarcoma (botryoid type) of the cervix: a case report and review. *Gynecol Oncol.* 1982;13:115–119
32. Ghaemmaghami F, Zarchi M, Ghasemi M. Lower genital tract rhabdomyosarcoma: case series and literature review. *Arch Gynecol Obstet.* 2008;278(1):65–69
33. Kadir RA, Economides DL, Sabin CA, Owens D, Lee CA. Frequency of inherited bleeding disorders in women with menorrhagia. *Lancet.* 1998;351(9101):485–489
34. Philipp CS. Platelet disorders in adolescents. *J Pediatr Adolesc Gynecol.* 2010;23:S11–14
35. Smith YR, Quint EH, Hertzberg RB. Menorrhagia in adolescents requiring hospitalization. *J Pediatr Adolesc Gynecol.* 1988;11:13–15
36. Oral E, Cagdas A, Gezer A, et al. Hematological abnormalities in adolescent menorrhagia. *Arch Gynecol Obstet.* 2002;266:72–74
37. Bevan JA, Maloney KW, Hillery CA, et al. Bleeding disorders: a common cause of menorrhagia in adolescents. *J Pediatr.* 2001;138:856–61
38. Jayasinghe Y, Moore P, Donath S, et al. Bleeding disorders in teenagers presenting with menorrhagia. *Aust N Z J Obstet Gynaecol.* 2005;45:439–443
39. Cochrane R, Regan L. Undetected gynaecological disorders in women with renal disease. *Human Reprod.* 1997;12:667–670
40. Mass K, Quint E, Punch M, et al. Gynecological and reproductive function after liver transplantation. *Transplantation.* 1996;62:476–479
41. Ostensen M, Almberg K, Koksvik H. Sex, reproduction, and gynecological disease in young adults with a history of juvenile chronic arthritis. *J Rheumatol.* 2000;27:1783–1787
42. Pasto SG, Mendonca BB, Bonfa E. Menstrual disturbances in patients with systemic lupus erythematosus without alkylating therapy: clinical, hormonal and therapeutic associations. *Lupus.* 2002;11:175–180
43. Weber AM, Belinson JL. Inflammatory bowel disease a complicating factor in gynecologic disorders. *Medscape Gen Med.* 1999;2:4
44. LaCour DE, Long DN, Perlman SE. Mini-review: dysfunctional uterine bleeding in adolescent females associated with endocrine causes and medical conditions. *J Pediatr Adolesc Gynecol.* 2010;23:62–70
45. Morrell MJ, Hayes FJ, Sluss PM, et al. Hyperandrogenism, Ovulatory dysfunction and polycystic ovary syndrome with valproate versus lamotrigine. *Ann Neurol.* 2008;64:200–211
46. Isojarvi JI, Laatikainen TJ, Pakarinen AJ, et al. Polycystic ovaries and hyperandrogenism in women taking valproate for epilepsy. *N Engl J Med.* 1993;329:1383–1388
47. Tom WC. Oral contraceptive (OC) drug interactions. *Pharmacist's Letter/Prescriber's Letter.* 2005;21:210903
48. Higham JM, O'Brien PM, Shaw RW. Assessment of menstrual blood loss using a pictorial chart. *Br J Obstet Gynecol.* 1990;97:734–739
49. DeVore GR, Owens O, Kase NL. Use of intravenous premarin in the treatment of dysfunctional uterine bleeding: a double blind randomized control study. *Obstet Gynecol.* 1982;59:285–291

50. Chi C, Pollard D, Tuddenham E, Kadir RA. Menorrhagia in adolescents with inherited bleeding disorders. *J Pediatr Adolesc Gynecol.* 2010:23;215–222
51. Lukes AS, Moore KA, Muse KN, et al. Tranexamic acid treatment for heavy menstrual bleeding: a randomized control trial. *Obstet and Gynecol.* 2010;116(4):865–875
52. Chi C, Huq FY, Kadir RA. Levonorgestrel-releasing intrauterine system for the management of heavy menstrual bleeding in women with inherited bleeding disorders: long-term follow-up. *Contraception.* 2011; 83(3):247–257
53. Frank D, Williams T. Attitudes about menstruation among fifth- sixth-, and seventh-grade pre- and post-menarcheal girls. *J Sch Nurs.* 1999;15:25–31
54. Hall P, Maclachlan N, Thorn N et al. Control of menorrhagia by the cyclo-oxygenase inhibitors naproxen sodium and mefenamic acid. *Brit J of Obstet Gynecol.* 1987;94:554–558
55. Lethaby A, Augwood C, Duckitt K et al. Nonsteroidal anti-inflammatory drugs for heavy menstrual bleeding. *Cochrane Database Syst Rev.* 2008;1:CD000400

Adolesc Med 23 (2012) 73–94

Overview of Sexually Transmitted Infections in Adolescents

Fareeda Haamid, DO[a]*,
Cynthia Holland-Hall, MD, MPH[b]

[a]*Section of Adolescent Medicine, Department of Pediatrics, Assistant Professor of Clinical Pediatrics, The Ohio State University College of Medicine, Nationwide Children's Hospital, Columbus, Ohio*

[b]*Associate Professor of Clinical Pediatrics, The Ohio State University College of Medicine, Columbus, Ohio*

THE SCOPE OF THE ISSUE

The Youth Risk Behavior Surveillance System (YRBSS) describes self-reported health risk behaviors among a nationally representative sample of in-school youth.[1] It is implemented by the Centers for Disease Control and Prevention (CDC) in conjunction with local and state education and health entities. In 2009, 31.6% of high school freshmen reported ever having sexual intercourse. The percentage nearly doubles to a rate of 62.3% in twelfth graders. The YRBSS sample population is smaller for middle school students.[2] In 2005, 11% of sixth graders and approximately 18% of eighth graders stated they had ever had sexual intercourse.

Healthy People 2010 (HP 2010) included the objective of increasing to 56% the percentage of ninth to twelfth graders who either abstain from sexual intercourse or use condoms if they are currently sexually active.[3] In 1999, HP 2010 reported that 50% of ninth graders stated they had never been sexually active. In 2009 this number had increased to 54%. Additionally, HP 2010 included an objective to reduce the proportion of adolescents and young adults with chlamydia infection. Data from 2009 indicate that among females aged 15–24 years attending STD clinics, 16.4% tested positive for chlamydia; the HP 2010 target was 3%.

The CDC's 2009 Sexually Transmitted Disease (STD) Surveillance Data indicate that adolescent females aged 15–19 years have the highest rates of chlamydia and

*Corresponding author.
E-mail address:* fareeda.haamid@nationwidechildrens.org (F. Haamid).

gonorrhea infection among all age and gender groups, with a rate of 3329 cases and 569 cases (respectively) per 100,000 population[4] (Figure 1). Young women 20–24 years old have similarly high rates of infection. This rate has risen annually, in part due to improved diagnostic techniques. Among 15–19-year-old males, the rates of diagnosis with chlamydia and gonorrhea are 735 cases and 250 cases (respectively) per 100,000 population. Rates of both infections are significantly higher in 20–24-year-old men.

Adolescent females have a higher risk than adult women of acquiring a sexually transmitted infection (STI).[5] There are a multitude of influential factors. Biological factors include cervical ectopy, a common finding in which columnar epithelial cells, typically found in the endocervix of a mature woman, are located on the ectocervix. This may predispose adolescent females to STIs, especially those pathogens that preferentially infect the columnar epithelial cells, such as *C. trachomatis* and *N. gonorrhoeae,* and those that affect cells undergoing squamous metaplasia, such as human papillomavirus (HPV).[6,7,8] Psychosocial factors that influence STI acquisition among adolescents include inconsistent and improper condom use,[9,10] concurrent partnerships,[11] complex romantic/sexual networks,[12] and poor decision-making skills. Early initiation of sexual activity has also been to shown to correlate with STIs in adolescents.[13]

SCREENING GUIDELINES

All sexually active adolescents should be screened for STIs (Table 1). The United States Preventive Services Task Force (USPSTF) provides evidence based clinical guidelines regarding screening for myriad conditions, including STIs. In its most recent publication, *The Guide to Clinical Preventive Services 2010–2011,* clinicians can find evidence-based recommendations concerning the care of adolescents.[14] The CDC and many medical professional societies also publish recommendations for screening, or may issue statements endorsing USPSTF or other existing

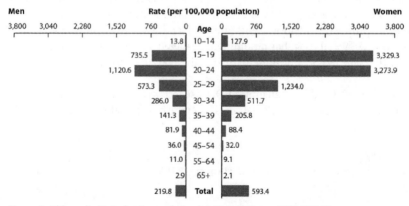

Figure 1. Chlamydia Rates by Age and Gender, United States, 2009 (CDC)

Table 1.
Screening Recommendations for Sexually Active Adolescents

	Chlamydia trachomatis	Neisseria gonorrhoeae	Trichomonas vaginalis	HIV	HPV	Hepatitis B Virus	HSV-2	Syphilis
Females (all sexually active)	Annual screening recommended*	Annual screening recommended*	Consider annual screening*	Screening recommended	Begin testing at 21 years of age	Screen based on personal risk factors; immunize	Routine screening not recommended	Screen based on epidemiology and personal risk factors
Males (female partners only)	Consider screening high-risk individuals†	Consider screening high-risk individuals	Routine screening not recommended	Screening recommended	Routine screening not recommended	Screen based on personal risk factors; immunize	Routine screening not recommended	Screen based on epidemiology and personal risk factors
MSM	Annual screening recommended*‡	Annual screening recommended*‡	Routine screening not recommended	Annual screening recommended*	Routine screening not recommended	Screen based on personal risk factors; immunize	Routine screening not recommended	Annual screening recommended*
Preferred test for screening	Nucleic acid amplification test; culture§	Nucleic acid amplification test; culture§	Light microscopy, culture, or rapid antigen detection	Serology	Papanicolaou smear	Serology	Type-specific (G2) serology	Serology (RPR or VDRL)

Abbreviations: MSM: males who have sex with males; HIV: human immunodeficiency virus; HPV: human papillomavirus; HSV: herpes simplex virus; RPR: rapid plasma reagin; VDRL: Venereal Disease Research Laboratory
*Consider more frequent screening in high-risk individuals
†Males attending sexually transmitted disease clinics; males entering the military or National Job Training Program; males in juvenile detention facilities, adolescent medicine clinics, emergency departments, and high school based health centers serving high risk communities
‡Site(s) of testing based on individual sexual practices
§NAAT is not currently FDA approved for pharyngeal or rectal specimens
From Holland-Hall C. Sexually transmitted infections. In Berlan EB, Bravender T (Eds). Adolescent Medicine Today: A Guide to Caring for the Adolescent Patient. World Scientific

guidelines. In June 2011 the World Health Organization (WHO) published *The Prevention and Treatment of HIV and Other Sexually Transmitted Infections Among Men Who Have Sex with Men and Transgender People,* representing the first-ever global public health guidelines focusing on these populations.[15]

Chlamydia and Gonorrhea

All sexually active adolescent females should receive annual screening for chlamydia and gonorrhea. High risk adolescents, including those previously diagnosed with an STI, may be screened more frequently due to rapid rates of reinfection in this population.[16,17] Currently, the evidence has not demonstrated cost-effectiveness of routine screening in males. However, a recent longitudinal cohort study of adolescent females indicated that reinfection by male partners contributes greatly to repeated chlamydial infections, highlighting the potential utility of screening at-risk adolescent males.[18] Clinicians should therefore consider individual risk factors, as well as epidemiologic data of the populations they serve. Nucleic acid amplification testing (NAAT) using urine, vaginal, cervical, or urethral specimens are the preferred screening tools, given their high sensitivity and specificity.

Syphilis

Routine screening of youth for syphilis is not recommended.[14] Adolescents at increased risk for acquiring syphilis, as determined by epidemiologic data and personal risk behaviors, should be screened. Populations such as men who have sex with men (MSM), persons in correctional facilities, and those who exchange sex for money or drugs have an elevated risk for infection with syphilis. The WHO strongly recommends MSM and transgender people receive periodic serologic screening for asymptomatic infection.[15] Additionally, the revised USP-STF recommendations indicate that all pregnant women should be screened. Screening may be done using a nontreponemal test such as the Venereal Disease Research Laboratory (VDRL) or rapid plasma reagin (RPR) test.

Genital Herpes

Routine screening for herpes simplex virus (HSV) in asymptomatic adolescents is not recommended. Where clinically indicated, for example, in patients with infected sexual partners who wish to know their serostatus, or as part of an evaluation of genital lesions, patients may receive type-specific serological testing for HSV-2.

HIV

The CDC states that more than half of all HIV-infected adolescents are believed not to have been tested and therefore are unaware of their HIV status.[19,20] HIV screening should be discussed with all adolescents and encouraged for those who are sexually active to reduce HIV associated morbidity and mortality. Moreover, HIV education, including information about modes of transmission, infection, and testing should be included as part of the primary care services rendered to all adolescents. The CDC recommends routine "opt-out" HIV screening for all persons older than the age of 13 years and further advises that all patients who request treatment for an STI receive HIV testing, regardless of whether they have specific behavioral risks for HIV infection. The USPSTF strongly recommends screening for HIV in adolescents who are at increased risk for this infection but makes no recommendation for or against screening adolescents who are not at increased risk. One should keep in mind, however, that adolescents may belong to many of the high-risk groups for HIV acquisition, including those who have unprotected intercourse with multiple partners, those who are treated for an STI, and those who receive care in high-risk settings such as STD clinics or adolescent health clinics where the STI prevalence is high.

Other Infections

There are currently no indications for screening immunocompetent adolescents for human papillomavirus (HPV). Cervical cancer screening using a Pap smear should be initiated at 21 years of age. The USPSTF recommends against screening for hepatitis B and C viruses in the general population of adolescents and adults who do not have symptoms or risk factors for these infections. Adolescents who have not been immunized against HPV or hepatitis B virus should be vaccinated.

No published guidelines recommend screening for infection with *Trichomonas vaginalis*. However, many adolescent health providers routinely test for this infection due to its high prevalence in adolescents and its association with increased risk for HIV transmission and adverse pregnancy outcomes.

MANAGEMENT PRINCIPLES

Directly observed therapy is regarded as the standard of care for the treatment of gonorrhea, chlamydia, nongonococcal urethritis, and trichomoniasis.[21] Single dose antibiotic regimens are preferred to increase adherence when possible.[22] Patient adherence with multiple-dose regimens has been shown to be less than ideal.[23] Partner notification and treatment is critical, and adolescents may need counseling regarding how to approach this challenge.[24] Expedited partner therapy (EPT), in which a sexual partner of an infected individual can be provided with therapy without being seen by a clinician, is legal in some states and is a viable option in certain populations.[25,26] Retesting at 3 months for repeat infections is advised following a diagnosis of chlamydia or gonorrhea.[22] The CDC maintains up-to-date treatment guidelines, as well as state-specific information about EPT, at www.cdc.gov/std.[22]

Diseases with Vaginal Discharge

Bacterial Vaginosis

Epidemiology Bacterial vaginosis (BV) is the most common cause of vaginal discharge among sexually active females.[27] Risk factors include sexual activity and douching.[28,29] Those who are not sexually active may acquire BV as well. Black females are at higher risk than other ethnicities.[30] BV is not sexually transmitted, but it may place those who have it at greater risk for acquiring other STIs such as *N. gonorrhoeae, C. trachomatis,* and HIV.[30,31] BV has also been associated with an increased risk of pregnancy complications, such as preterm labor and birth and chorioamnionitis.[32,33]

Etiology BV is a clinical syndrome characterized by a shift in the normal vaginal flora in which hydrogen peroxide–producing lactobacilli no longer predominate; instead there is a proliferation of anaerobic and facultative anaerobic bacteria. These may include *Gardnerella vaginalis, Prevotella, Mobiluncus, Ureaplasma,* and *Mycoplasma* species. The cause of these changes in the vaginal ecosystem is not well understood.

Clinical Manifestations BV is often asymptomatic, but it may cause significant vulvovaginal symptoms. One of the cardinal features of BV is vaginal discharge that is often malodorous. The discharge typically has a homogeneous gray or milky appearance with a fishy odor.

Diagnosis The diagnosis of BV is often made clinically, but the use of specific criteria is encouraged to improve diagnostic accuracy. Physical examination often reveals a thin, white, homogenous discharge that may smell fishy. Diagnostic tools include evaluation of vaginal fluid using light microscopy and pH testing. Amsel's criteria include 4 elements, of which at least 3 must be present to diagnose BV: (1) vaginal discharge that is thin, white, and homogeneous; (2) vaginal fluid (ideally collected from the lateral vaginal wall) pH > 4.5; (3) a predominance of clue cells (> 20% of epithelial cells) on microscopy: and (4) a positive "whiff test," which occurs when vaginal discharge has a fishy odor (due to the presence of amines) before or after the addition of 10% potassium hydroxide. The OSOM® BVBLUE® Test (Sekisui Diagnostics) is a rapid "point of care" assay that tests for enzymatic activity of many of the common BV pathogens. The sensitivity of this test is comparable to that of Amsel's criteria, and the specificity is greater than 90%, making it a viable diagnostic tool.[34,35] Furthermore, this rapid test eliminates the need for microscopy and provides results at the time of the patient encounter. BV may be reported as an incidental finding on Pap smear reports, but sensitivity of this method for diagnosing BV is low.

Treatment BV is treated with antibiotics that eradicate vaginal anaerobes. Recommended treatment is with metronidazole 500 mg orally twice daily for 7 days, or a 5-day course of intravaginal clindamycin or metronidazole. Alternative oral regimens include tinidazole 2 g daily for 2 days or clindamycin 300 mg twice daily for 7 days. Pregnant women may be treated with oral metronidazole or clindamycin. Women may be counseled to avoid douching because it may cause an imbalance in the normal vaginal flora that favors overgrowth of anaerobic organisms. There is no evidence to support treatment of sexual contacts.

Trichomonas vaginalis

Epidemiology Trichomonas vaginalis is a flagellated protozoan that is transmitted via sexual intercourse and is a common cause of vaginal discharge among sexually active females. Trichomoniasis may also cause nongonococcal urethritis (NGU) in males. Fomite transmission is postulated but is rare.[36] The overall prevalence among reproductive aged women is 3.1% based on National Health and Nutrition Examination Survey (NHANES) data from 2001–2004, with comparable rates reported in adolescents.[5,37] Laga et al[38] report increased HIV seroconversion in females with *Trichomonas* infections.

Clinical Manifestations Trichomoniasis presents with vaginal discharge that is often copious. Discharge is commonly yellow-green, frothy, and may be malodorous. Patients may also complain of vulvovaginal irritation. Both female and male patients can be asymptomatic. On physical examination, the cervix may have a classic "strawberry" appearance due to development of punctate hemorrhages caused by *T. vaginalis* infection. Although this finding is often absent, its presence is virtually pathognomonic for *T. vaginalis* infection.[39]

Diagnosis The index of suspicion for *T. vaginalis* should be high when clinicians obtain a history of vaginal discharge in a sexually active female or urethral symptoms in a male. Traditionally, vaginal microscopy has been used as a common method of diagnosis, requiring visualization of motile trichomonads. Its sensitivity is approximately 50–70% and specificity is high.[40] This diagnostic method is dependent on the examiner's skill and the availability of materials needed for microscopy. Vaginal pH greater than 4.5 is consistent with this diagnosis, but is nonspecific. *Trichomonas vaginalis* infection may be confirmed by obtaining a culture of the vaginal discharge. Culture methods boast higher sensitivity than microscopy, and easy-to-use "pouch" culture media are available.

In April 2011, the FDA approved the APTIMA® *Trichomonas vaginalis* Assay (Gen-Probe). This is the first NAAT specifically approved for the diagnosis of *T. vaginalis* in females. The advantage of this test is that it can be used on the same vaginal, cervical, or urine samples collected from females for detection of chlamydia and gonorrhea, and it offers superior sensitivity to other diagnostic methods.[41,42] Rapid testing (OSOM® Trichomonas Rapid Test; Sekisui Diagnostics) is also available and has a higher sensitivity than microscopy.[43]

Treatment The recommended treatment for trichomoniasis is metronidazole or tinidazole 2 grams orally in a single dose. Alternatively, metronidazole 500 mg orally twice daily for 7 days may be used. This may be a preferred regimen in a patient who has a concomitant diagnosis of BV. Intravaginal metronidazole is not effective in eradicating *T. vaginalis.*

Infected individuals are advised to use condoms and notify their partners, who must be treated to prevent reinfection.

Urethritis

Epidemiology Infectious urethritis is a clinical syndrome that involves inflammation of the urethra that may result in urethral discharge and dysuria. Urethritis is caused by a host of pathogens, most of which are bacterial. Both males and females may be affected. In females, some of the organisms that cause urethritis also cause cervicitis, such as *C. trachomatis.*

Etiology Urethritis in males is classified as either gonococcal or nongonococcal urethritis (NGU). *Chlamydia trachomatis* is the most common pathogen identified in NGU.[44] Other causes of NGU include *Mycoplasma genitalium, Ureaplasma urealyticum, T. vaginalis,* HSV, and adenovirus.[45]

Clinical Manifestations Dysuria is typically the presenting symptom, with or without a urethral discharge. However, no clinical features reliably differentiate between gonococcal urethritis and NGU.

Diagnosis Diagnosis is made based on the presence of mucopurulent or purulent discharge, and/or evidence of white blood cells (WBCs) in the urine. Diagnosis should not be based solely on the presence of dysuria without objective evidence of inflammation. Inflammation may be documented by urethral fluid containing greater than 5 WBCs per oil immersion field on a Gram stain, a first-void urine specimen containing greater than 10 WBCs per high-powered field, or positive leukocyte esterase testing of a first-void urine. Etiology should be investigated using a nucleic acid amplification test for gonorrhea and chlamydia on a first-catch urine specimen. Alternatively, culture for these organisms may be performed on a urethral specimen. If Gram staining of urethral fluid is available, it may be useful for the diagnosis of gonococcal urethritis, in which gram-negative intracellular diplococci may be visualized in WBCs. Tests for other NGU pathogens often are not widely available and are not recommended for use in initial evaluation. They may be appropriate in cases of persistent or recurrent urethritis.

Treatment Empiric treatment is reasonable for persons with objective evidence of urethritis. Recommended treatment for NGU includes single dose azithromycin 1 g orally, or doxycycline 100 mg orally twice daily for 7 days. The preferred treatment of all gonococcal infections is ceftriaxone 250 mg IM as a single dose, plus azithromycin 1 g orally, or doxycycline 100 mg orally twice daily for 7 days. For nonresponsive urethritis with persistent, objective evidence of infection, the clinician may consider treatment for possible *T. vaginalis* infection with metronidazole 2 g, or for *M. genitalium* with moxifloxacin 400 mg daily for 7 days.

Cervicitis

Cervicitis is the clinical syndrome of cervical inflammation, manifesting as a mucopurulent or purulent cervical discharge. The inflamed cervix is more susceptible to bleeding when touched. Patients with cervicitis may have one or both of these findings. However, most girls and women with cervical infections are asymptomatic.

Etiology The two pathogens most often isolated in women with cervicitis are *N. gonorrhoeae* and *C. trachomatis.*[46] However, in most women with clinical cervicitis, no pathogen is isolated.[47] Conversely, most women who screen positive for gonorrhea or chlamydia at the cervix do not have clinical signs of cervicitis, underscoring the poorly understood nature of this condition. HSV, *T. vaginalis,* and *M. genitalium* are potential pathogens as well.

Clinical Manifestations Most cervical infections are asymptomatic; even patients with objective signs of cervicitis on speculum examination may not report symptoms. Symptomatic patients may report vaginal discharge or abnormal vaginal bleeding, such as intermenstrual "spotting" or bleeding after intercourse.

Diagnosis All patients with signs of cervicitis should have cervical NAAT testing for *C. trachomatis* and *N. gonorrhoeae*. If clinically indicated, testing for other causes of cervicitis such as *T. vaginalis* or HSV may be considered. The presence of WBCs on microscopic evaluation of cervical exudate is supportive of a bacterial infection. It is imperative to evaluate for evidence of ascending genital tract infection (ie, pelvic inflammatory disease) to avoid complications and sequelae such as tubo-ovarian abscess and infertility.

Treatment Adolescents are high risk for STI based on their age, potential for unprotected sexual encounters, and possible inability to appropriately follow-up. Clinicians should therefore have a low threshold for treating empirically for gonorrhea and chlamydia infections in adolescents with clinical cervicitis, while awaiting test results. Azithromycin 1 g orally in a single dose or doxycycline 100 mg orally twice daily for 7 days should be given for coverage of chlamydial infections. Where gonorrhea is prevalent, as is the case in many adolescent health settings, patients should be treated for this as well, with ceftriaxone 250 mg IM. Oral regimens for the treatment of gonorrhea include cefixime 400 mg as a single dose or cefuroxime axetil 1 g as a single dose; however, these regimens are less effective than parenteral ceftriaxone at eradicating gonococcal infections, particularly in persons with known or suspected pharyngeal infections. The CDC recommends that all persons with gonococcal infections receive dual treatment with azithromycin or doxycycline (in addition to the cephalosporin) to discourage the development of cephalosporin-resistant *N. gonorrhoeae*.

Pelvic Inflammatory Disease

Pelvic inflammatory disease (PID) is an upper genital tract infection involving the endometrium, fallopian tubes, and/or ovaries. It is a serious consequence of untreated STI in females, potentially leading to infertility, ectopic pregnancy, and chronic pelvic pain.

Epidemiology The incidence of PID is unclear; it is not a reportable condition, and clinical diagnostic criteria have limited sensitivity and specificity. The CDC estimates that approximately 750,000 women are affected annually.[48] Sexually active adolescents and young women are at highest risk of PID. Other risk factors include multiple sexual partners, history of STI, and failure to use contraception.[49,50]

Etiology *Neisseria gonorrhoeae* and *C. trachomatis* are the most commonly isolated organisms in adolescents with PID and are isolated in approximately one half of all cases.[51,52] PID is often a polymicrobial infection; anaerobic organisms, including *Bacteroides* spp., *Prevotella*, *G. vaginalis*, and others may be isolated from intraoperative cultures, although it is not clear what role they play in pathogenesis.[53] *Mycoplasma genitalium* has been detected in a disproportionate number of women with PID in a research setting, and it is postulated to be a causative organism.[54,55] In many cases of PID diagnosed clinically, no organism is identified. It is presumed that PID is caused by spread of sexually transmitted organisms along mucosal surfaces from the cervix to the upper genital tract.

Clinical Manifestations PID typically presents with lower abdominal or pelvic pain, which may vary from mild to severe and debilitating. Patients may report pain with intercourse, vaginal discharge, or irregular vaginal bleeding. Patients with more severe disease may have fever, vomiting, or pain with ambulation. Research supports the existence of asymptomatic PID as well, demonstrating antibodies to *C. trachomatis* in women with tubal scarring but no history of clinical disease.[56] On examination, lower abdominal tenderness is present. Cervicitis or vaginal discharge may be seen on speculum examination. Bimanual examination may reveal uterine, adnexal, or cervical motion tenderness. Gonococcal PID is more likely to present with acute, severe symptomatology than chlamydial PID.[57]

Clinical complications of PID include the development of a tubo-ovarian complex, an inflammatory mass of the adnexa. This requires prolonged treatment with broad-spectrum parenteral antibiotics and, in some cases, surgical intervention. Fitz-Hugh-Curtis syndrome is a perihepatic inflammation that causes painful adhesions to form between the liver capsule and the diaphragm or anterior abdominal wall. Patients may present with acute right upper quadrant pain. Treatment for Fitz-Hugh-Curtis syndrome is the same as for uncomplicated PID. Long-term sequelae of PID include chronic pelvic pain, which can occur in up to 40% of adolescents.[52] The risk of infertility from tubal scarring is about 10% following a single episode of PID; the risk increases to nearly 50% following

3 episodes of PID.[58] Tubal scarring also increases a woman's risk of ectopic pregnancy by 3- to 10-fold.[59]

Diagnosis Laparoscopy is the traditional gold standard for the diagnosis of PID, demonstrating visible inflammation of the adnexal structures. In practice, however, PID is diagnosed clinically, using less costly and invasive means. Clinicians must consider this diagnosis in all sexually active adolescent females with abdominal pain and should have a low threshold for performing a pelvic examination in these patients. Minimum clinical criteria endorsed by the CDC for the diagnosis of PID include the presence of adnexal tenderness, uterine tenderness, *or* cervical motion tenderness on a bimanual examination.[22] Additional findings that enhance the specificity of these minimal criteria include fever, cervical or vaginal discharge, the presence of WBCs in the vaginal fluid, and an elevated erythrocyte sedimentation rate (ESR) or C-reactive protein (CRP). Endocervical testing for *N. gonorrhoeae* and *C. trachomatis* should be performed; their presence also supports the diagnosis. In patients with no evidence of lower genital tract infection, PID is less likely, and other causes of pain should be considered. Pelvic ultrasound may be considered to evaluate for tubo-ovarian complex, but it is often normal in mild to moderate PID. Patients with PID should be tested for HIV and other STIs as well.

Treatment Patients who meet the minimal clinical criteria for PID with no other explanation for their symptoms should be treated. Mild to moderate PID is treated in the outpatient setting; there is no evidence that adolescents or adults have better outcomes when treated as inpatients.[60] Outpatient treatment is with ceftriaxone 250 mg IM in a single dose, in combination with doxycycline 100 mg twice daily for 14 days. Clinicians may consider adding metronidazole 500 mg twice per day to enhance anaerobic coverage.[22] Alternative regimens include cefoxitin 2 g intramuscularly (with probenecid 1 g orally) and doxycycline, or other parenteral third-generation cephalosporins with doxycycline. Oral regimens using quinolones are no longer recommended for the treatment of PID, due to unacceptably high rates of antimicrobial resistance. Patients should be reevaluated in 48–72 hours for clinical improvement.

Hospitalization may be indicated in patients with more severe disease, pregnant patients, patients who do not respond to outpatient therapy or cannot tolerate oral therapies (eg, due to excessive vomiting), patients with tubo-ovarian abscess, and patients in whom surgical emergencies such as appendicitis cannot be ruled out. Parenteral antibiotic regimens include (1) cefoxitin 2 g IV every 6 hours, with doxycycline 100 mg by mouth or intravenously every 12 hours, or (2) clindamycin 900 mg IV every 8 hours, with gentamicin 2 mg/kg loading dose, followed by 1.5 mg/kg every 8 hours. Single daily dosing of gentamicin (3–5 mg/kg) may be substituted. Patients should continue to receive parenteral treatment for 24 hours after clinical improvement and should then complete the remainder of a 14-day course of oral doxycycline, with or without additional anaerobic coverage using metronidazole.

Ulcerative Lesions

In North America, HSV is by far the most common cause of genital ulcerations. Syphilis remains prevalent in the United States but is relatively uncommon among heterosexual adolescents. Chancroid and lymphogranuloma venereum are less commonly encountered in North America, though some speculate that chancroid is underdiagnosed.

Herpes Simplex Virus

Epidemiology HSV is a common cause of ulcerative anogenital lesions in sexually active individuals.[61] In 2009, 306,000 initial visits to physicians' offices were reported for genital herpes.[62] National trend data from 2005–2008 indicate that the seroprevalence of HSV type 2 (HSV-2) among those aged 14–49 has declined as compared with previous years, and blacks have higher rates of infection than whites.[63] The prevalence of HSV-2 in sexually experienced 14–19-year-old females in the NHANES 2003–2004 survey was 3.4%.[5]

HSV is an enveloped, double-stranded DNA virus belonging to the *Herpesviridae* family and alpha-herpesvirus subfamily. HSV infection is most commonly acquired via direct contact with infected lesions or genital secretions. The incubation interval in the non-neonatal populations is 2–14 days. Following the primary infection, the virus remains in a latent state, most commonly in the sacral dorsal root ganglia, throughout the lifespan of the infected individual. This period of latency may be followed by recurrent symptomatic episodes, caused by reactivation of the virus. Thus genital herpes is a chronic infection. Transmission of HSV can occur via sexual contact with asymptomatic or symptomatic hosts in any stage of infection, although the degree of viral shedding is higher when lesions are present. Primary, symptomatic infection is associated with the greatest degree of viral shedding, which may persist for several weeks. Compared with HSV-1, HSV-2 is more commonly associated with asymptomatic viral shedding, especially in the first year following the primary infection.

Although HSV-2 infections most commonly affect the genitalia, both HSV-1 and HSV-2 can cause both oral and genital lesions. The belief that HSV-1 is found only in lesions above the waist and genital lesions are exclusively caused by HSV-2 is now outdated. In fact, there has been an increase in the identification of HSV-1 in primary genital infections. Episodic recurrences of genital herpes, however, are more commonly caused by HSV-2 than HSV-1, the latter being associated with less frequent outbreaks.[64,65]

Clinical Manifestations The primary infection may go unnoticed and remain undiagnosed; subclinical infections are common. Alternatively, primary infection may be characterized by a painful and protracted course with systemic viral symptoms. Genital lesions may vary in appearance. Classic lesions progress from vesicular to ulcerative stages and are often symmetrical, but more subtle skin changes such as fissures or excoriations may be present. HSV-2 is associated with more frequent outbreaks than HSV-1, but the manifestations of the individual outbreaks, either primary or secondary, are clinically indistinguishable. Infected persons may experience a prodromal phase before a recurrence that can present as pruritus, tingling, or burning at the site. HSV-2 infections can be complicated by aseptic meningitis, which may be associated with a nonprotracted course with mild symptoms.

Diagnosis Clinicians must maintain a high level of suspicion for HSV upon obtaining a history of painful genital lesions. However, not all patients have this classic presentation. The CDC recommends that viral culture (or NAAT) and type-specific serology be utilized whenever available because clinical diagnosis has limited sensitivity and specificity. Distinguishing HSV-2 from HSV-1 is useful for providing appropriate STI counseling. Tzanck smears have unacceptably low sensitivity and specificity. Differential diagnosis includes other causes of genital ulcers including syphilis, chancroid, lymphogranuloma venereum, and granuloma inguinale. The latter two are very uncommonly diagnosed in adolescents in North America and can often be effectively ruled out based on this low prevalence. Other uncommon causes of vulvar ulcers may include cytomegalovirus, Epstein-Barr virus, or idiopathic aphthous vulvitis.

The virologic diagnostic modalities of choice are cell culture and polymerase chain reaction (PCR) for lesions affecting the anogenital or oral areas. HSV grows quickly in culture, but the yield is dependent on the quality of the specimen sent, and sensitivity declines the longer the lesion has been present. PCR testing of cerebrospinal fluid is the mainstay of confirming the diagnosis of central nervous system infection and may be used as a more sensitive method of diagnosing genital lesions as well.

HSV antibodies appear within weeks following primary infection. The FDA has approved type-specific serologic assays that utilize the HSV-1 and HSV-2 glycoproteins. Providers now have access to laboratory-based and point-of-care testing. The sensitivity of the HSV-specific glycoprotein G2 (for HSV-2) assays approaches 98% and specificities are excellent.[66,67] The CDC delineates circumstances in which type-specific serologic assays might be valuable, such as (1) recurrent genital symptoms or atypical symptoms with negative HSV cultures; (2) a clinical diagnosis of genital herpes without laboratory confirmation; or (3) a patient whose partner has genital herpes, who wishes to know his/her own serostatus.

Treatment There is no effective medication to eliminate latent HSV. Moreover, antiviral agents have not been shown to influence recurrences following cessation of these medications. However, antivirals remain the basis of genital herpes treatment because they have been shown to shorten the viral shedding period and abate symptoms. The optimal time of treatment for episodic recurrences is early in the course of the outbreak—ideally within the first 24 hours of symptoms. Acyclovir, valacyclovir, or famciclovir may be given orally. Dosing varies, depending on whether one is treating primary infection, recurrence, or providing daily suppressive therapy, or if the patient is HIV-positive or otherwise immunocompromised (Table 2). Clinicians may offer daily suppressive courses of therapy for those with frequent or severe outbreaks, or in persons who wish to decrease viral shedding and the risk of transmission to seronegative partners. The role of supportive care to ameliorate the discomfort caused by the lesions is important and often neglected. Supportive care may include sitz baths, oral analgesics, and soothing topical medications such as viscous lidocaine jelly. The role of topical antivirals has not been substantiated.

Management Research has consistently demonstrated that there is recurrent, intermittent viral shedding even in the absence of visible lesions. The viral load required to transmit infection during times when no lesions are apparent is unknown. Patients must be counseled to inform sexual partners of their infection, to avoid sexual contact when lesions are present, and to use latex condoms during all sexual encounters. Providers should ensure that patients have access to episodic treatment in a timely manner. Women should inform their obstetricians of their history of HSV given the implications for method of delivery if lesions are present.

Table 2.
Recommended Regimens for Treatment of Genital Herpes[*][1]

	Acyclovir	Valacyclovir	Famciclovir
First clinical episode	400 mg po 3×/day for 7–10 days[2] 200 mg po 5×/day for 7–10 days[2]	1 gram po 2×/day for 7–10 days[2]	250 mg po 3×/day for 7–10 days[2]
Episodic therapy for recurrences	400 mg po 3×/day for 5 days 800 mg po 2×/day for 5 days 800 mg po 3×/day for 2 days	500 mg po 2×/day for 3 days 1 gram po 1×/day for 5 days	125 mg po 2×/day for 5 days 1000 mg po 2×/day for 1 day 500 mg po once, then 250 mg 2×/day for 2 days
Suppressive therapy[3] for recurrences	400 mg po 2×/day	500 mg po 1×/day 1 gram po 1×/day	250 mg po 2×/day
Severe disease[4]	5–10 mg/kg IV every 8 hrs for 2–7 days, until improved, then oral treatment for a total of a minimum of 10 days of therapy		

*Adapted from CDC MMWR *Sexually Transmitted Diseases Treatment Guidelines, 2010*
[1]Specific regimens exist for persons with HIV
[2]May extend treatment course beyond 10 days if inadequate healing is present
[3]May discontinue treatment after one year and reassess frequency of recurrences
[4]CNS complications, disseminated infection, pneumonitis, hepatitis

Syphilis

Epidemiology Syphilis is a sexually transmitted infection caused by *Treponema pallidum,* a bacterial spirochete. Syphilis varies in presentation based on the stage of illness. For the purpose of this article, tertiary syphilis is not discussed, as it is extremely uncommon among adolescents and should only be managed by experienced clinicians. According to CDC's 2009 STD surveillance data, primary and secondary syphilis rates among women aged 15–19 years have risen every year since 2004 to a current rate of 3.3 per 100,000 population.[4] Among women, those aged 20–24 years account for the highest rates of infection. Adolescent males aged 15–19 years also experienced an increase in rates to 6.0 per 100,000 population in 2009, although older males still have significantly higher rates.

Clinical Manifestations Primary syphilis is characterized by the presence of a single or multiple painless ulcers (chancres) at the site of infection that is commonly unnoticed by the patient. Although the chancre resolves spontaneously, inadequately treated primary syphilis will become latent and may subsequently develop into secondary syphilis, which is typified by constitutional symptoms; dermatologic signs, including rashes, alopecia, and condyloma lata; and cardiac manifestations, among others. Neurosyphilis may be present at any stage.

Diagnosis Syphilis is definitively diagnosed when *T. pallidum* is visualized using darkfield microscopy or direct fluorescent antibody tests are performed on syphilitic lesions or tissue. Nontreponemal serologic screening tests include the rapid plasma reagin (RPR) and the Venereal Disease Research Laboratory (VDRL) tests. Nontreponemal tests have limited sensitivity during primary or latent syphilis and can yield false positive results in those with pregnancy, viral illnesses, connective tissue diseases, and other systemic diseases. Positive nontreponemal screening tests require confirmation with a treponemal serologic test such as the fluorescent treponemal antibody absorption (FTA-ABS) test or the *T. pallidum* passive particle agglutination (TP-PA) assay. Treponemal antibody tests may remain reactive for life, whereas nontreponemal titers should resolve with adequate treatment. HIV testing is recommended in those infected with syphilis due to the increase risk of HIV transmission associated with this infection.

Treatment Parenteral penicillin G is the treatment of choice for all stages of syphilis. Specific dosing regimens depend on the stage of treatment and can be readily accessed at www.cdc.gov/std. Nontreponemal tests are used to monitor treatment responses, as titers should decrease following therapy. Doxycycline or tetracycline can be used for treatment of nonpregnant patients with penicillin allergies. Pregnant patients with penicillin allergies should be desensitized so that penicillin may be safely administered.

Chancroid

Epidemiology Chancroid is a condition marked by painful genital ulcers caused by *Haemophilus ducreyi*, a gram-negative coccobacillus. Prevalence data worldwide indicate that there are a decreasing number of cases. Twenty-eight cases (20 from non-STD clinics) were reported by state health departments in the United States in 2009; this reflects a decrease from 110 cases in 1999.[4] Twenty-eight percent of cases were reported in Texas, followed by North Carolina and Wisconsin with 6 cases each. True prevalence is difficult to determine because *H. ducreyi* is not easily isolated by widely available culture methods. Infection with chancroid is a known risk factor for transmission of HIV.

Clinical Manifestations Chancroid is characterized by a painful ulcerative lesion that may begin as an erythematous papule that progresses into a pustule, which erodes to form an ulcer. A bubo refers to the resultant unilateral inguinal lymph nodes that are painful and often suppurative.

Diagnosis The diagnosis is made by culture of fluid from the lesions; it requires special media that are not widely available. Clinical diagnosis may be considered in the presence of solitary or multiple ulcers that are painful, localized lymphadenopathy, and when testing of the ulcer confirms the absence of both syphilis and genital HSV. Regional prevalence should also be considered.

Treatment
Eradication of chancroid may be accomplished with antibiotic therapy. Single-dose treatment with either oral azithromycin 1 g or ceftriaxone 250 mg given intramuscularly is recommended. Other effective treatments include ciprofloxacin for 3 days or erythromycin for 1 week.

Lymphogranuloma Venereum

Epidemiology Lymphogranuloma venereum (LGV) is caused by *C. trachomatis* serovars L1-L3. LGV is not common in the United States, although outbreaks have been recently reported in other countries. There is a concern for a possible increase in diagnosis in this country, particularly in MSM.

Diagnosis Lesions from genitalia and lymph node aspirates can be sent for culture, direct immunofluorescence, or NAAT where available. Chlamydia serology may also be used to support the clinical diagnosis. Clinicians may need to rely on clinical manifestations if appropriate testing is not available.

Clinical Manifestations LGV can present as a painless genital ulcer followed by tender inguinal lymphadenopathy that is usually unilateral. The adenopathy may be a more notable clinical finding than the ulcer, which typically resolves spontaneously. Proctocolitis can occur in patients engaged in receptive anal intercourse.

Treatment Doxycycline 100 mg orally twice daily for 21 days is the preferred treatment in nonpregnant patients. Effective treatment is curative and prevents progression to systemic involvement.

Human Papillomavirus

Epidemiology Human papillomavirus (HPV) is a DNA virus that causes a range of clinical manifestations including condyloma acuminata (anogenital warts), cervical dysplasia, cervical cancer, and certain vulvar, vaginal, anal, and oropharyngeal cancers.[68] HPV is the most common STI, ubiquitous among sexually active persons. Infections are frequently cleared or suppressed by an intact immune response. Cervical dysplasia is the result of persistence of HPV in the cervical mucosa. More than 100 types of HPV have been identified. Oncogenic types include 16, 18, 31, and 33, the first two being responsible for 70% of all cervical cancers.[69,70,71] Low-risk types may be associated with genital warts; types 6 and 11 are responsible for 90% of cases.[72,73,74] In a longitudinal study of at-risk adolescent females followed for approximately 2 years, the cumulative prevalence of genital HPV infection was 81.7%, with several different HPV types identified.[75] There is a high prevalence of genital HPV among males as well.[76,77]

Clinical Manifestations Genital warts present with various morphologies including condyloma acuminata and keratotic or papular warts. They may be found on the vulva and in the vaginal introitus or on the penis, urethral meatus, scrotum, or perianal areas. Genital warts are often asymptomatic and may be found incidentally by clinicians during routine inspection of the external genitalia. Subclinical infections are common. Symptomatic patients may describe burning, pruritus, or local irritation, based on the location or number of warts. The natural history of genital warts that do not undergo treatment is varied; some fully resolve, others increase in size or remain unchanged.

Diagnosis Genital warts are diagnosed clinically based on their appearance. Applying 3–5% acetic acid to HPV infected areas produces a characteristic whitening of the area but lacks specificity. Biopsy may be used to confirm the diagnosis in questionable cases but is not typically necessary. Current CDC recommendations do not advocate HPV DNA testing in the evaluation of genital warts.

Treatment Patients who wish to eradicate symptomatic or unsightly lesions have a choice of patient-applied or provider-administered treatments. Clearance rates of 23–94% were reported in one critical appraisal of genital wart treatments.[78] Currently there are 3 patient-applied methods available in the United States, which are podofilox 0.5% solution or gel;[79] imiquimod 5% cream;[80] and sinecatechins 15%, a newly approved regimen that is a green-tea extract ointment applied 3 times daily for a maximum of 16 weeks.[81,22] There has been no determination of the safety of the patient-applied methods during pregnancy, and all 3 may cause local skin irritation. The risk-benefit ratio does not appear to favor treatment of subclinical infections.[82,83]

Provider-administered treatment options include trichloroacetic acid (TCA) or bichloracetic acid (BCA) 80–90%; cryotherapy; podophyllin resin 10–25%; laser therapy; or surgical removal, which often requires 1 treatment only via excision or electrosurgery.[84] TCA is commonly used and can be reapplied weekly. It is corrosive to the wart and adjacent tissues, thus care should be taken to apply it sparingly and with caution, particularly near mucosal surfaces. The use of cryotherapy and surgical modalities require provider training. Urethral, rectal, and intravaginal warts are best treated by an experienced clinician.

SUMMARY

STIs are very common among adolescents, thus routine screening is warranted. Recognition of common clinical syndromes can aid in timely diagnosis and treatment. Preventive measures, including vaccines, may significantly impact the disease burden in this vulnerable population.

References

1. Centers for Disease Control and Prevention. Youth Risk Behavior Surveillance: United States. *MMWR Surveill Summ.* 2010;59:1–142
2. Shanklin SL, Brener N, McManus T, Kinchen S, Kann L. *2005 Middle School Youth Risk Behavior Survey.* Atlanta, GA: U.S. Department of Health and Human Services, Centers for Disease Control and Prevention; 2007
3. U.S. Department of Health and Human Services. *Healthy People 2010: Understanding and Improving Health.* 2nd ed. Washington, DC: U.S. Government Printing Office; November 2000
4. Centers for Disease Control and Prevention. *Sexually Transmitted Disease Surveillance 2009.* Atlanta, GA: U.S. Department of Health and Human Services; 2010
5. Forhan SE, Gottlieb SL, Sternberg MR, et al. Prevalence of sexually transmitted infections among female adolescents aged 14 to 19 in the United States. *Pediatrics.* 2009;124:1505–1512
6. Stergachis A, Scholes D, Heidrich FE, Sherer DM, Holmes KK, Stamm WE. Selective screening for *Chlamydia trachomatis* infection in a primary care population of women. *Am J Epidemiol.* 1993;138:143–153
7. Moss GB, Clemetson D, D'Costa L, et al. Association of cervical ectopy with heterosexual transmission of human immunodeficiency virus: results of a study of couples in Nairobi, Kenya. *J Infect Dis.* 1991;164:588–591
8. Monroy OL, Aguilar C, Lizano M, Cruz-Talonia F, Cruz RM, Rocha-Zavaleta L. Prevalence of human papillomavirus genotypes, and mucosal IgA anti-viral responses in women with cervical ectopy. *J Clin Virol.* 2010;47(1):43–48
9. Abma JC, Martinez GM, Copen CE. Teenagers in the United States: sexual activity, contraceptive use, and childbearing, national survey of family growth 2006–2008. *Vital Health Stat 23.* 2010;(30):1–47
10. Paz-Bailey G, Koumans EH, Sternberg M, et al. The effect of correct and consistent condom use on chlamydial and gonococcal infection among urban adolescents. *Arch Pediatr Adolesc Med.* 2005;159:536–542
11. Kretzschmar M, Morris M. Measures of concurrency in networks and the spread of infectious disease. *Math Biosci.* 1996;133:165–195

12. Bearman PS, Moody J, Stovel K. Chains of affection: the structure of adolescent romantic and sexual networks. *Am J Sociol.* 2004;110:44–91

13. Tu W, Batteiger BE, Wiehe S, et al. Time from first intercourse to first sexually transmitted infection diagnosis among adolescent women. *Arch Pediatr Adolesc Med.* 2009;163:1106–1111

14. U.S. Preventive Services Task Force. December 2010. *The Guide to Clinical Preventive Services 2010–2011.* http://www.uspreventiveservicestaskforce.org/about.htm. Accessed July 13, 2011

15. World Health Organization. Prevention and treatment of HIV and other sexually transmitted infections among men who have sex with men and transgender people. http://whqlibdoc.who.int/publications/2011/9789241501750_eng.pdf. Accessed July 13, 2011

16. Burstein GR, Gaydos CA, Diener-West M, et al. Incident *Chlamydia trachomatis* infections among inner-city adolescent females. *JAMA.* 1998;280:521–526

17. Orr DP, Johnston K, Brizendine E, et al. Subsequent sexually transmitted infection in urban adolescents and young adults. *Arch Pediatr Adolesc Med.* 2001;155:947–953

18. Batteiger BE, Tu W, Ofner S, et al. Repeated *Chlamydia trachomatis* genital infections in adolescent women. *J Infect Dis.* 2010;201(1):42–51

19. Rotheram-Borus MJ, Futterman D. Promoting early detection of human immunodeficiency virus infection among adolescents. *Arch Pediatr Adolesc Med.* 2000;154:435–439

20. National Institutes of Health, Office of AIDS Research. *Report of the working group to review the NIH perinatal, pediatric, and adolescent HIV research priorities.* Bethesda, MD: National Institutes of Health; 1999

21. World Health Organization. *Sexually Transmitted and Other Reproductive Tract Infections: A Guide to Essential Practice.* Geneva, Switzerland: World Health Organization; 2005. Available at: http://www.who.int/reproductivehealth/publications/rtis/9241592656/en/index.html. Accessed July 13, 2011

22. Centers for Disease Control and Prevention. Sexually transmitted diseases treatment guidelines, 2010. *MMWR.* 2010;59:1–95. Available at: http://www.cdc.gov/std/treatment/2010. Accessed July 13, 2011

23. Brookoff D. Compliance with doxycycline therapy for outpatient treatment of pelvic inflammatory disease. *South Med J.* 1994;87;1088–1091

24. Trelle S, Shang A, Nartey L, et al. Improved effectiveness of partner notification for patients with sexually transmitted infections: systematic review. *BMJ.* 2007;334(7589):354

25. Hodge JG Jr, Pulver A, Hogben M, et al. Expedited partner therapy for sexually transmitted diseases: assessing the legal environment. *Am J Public Health.* 2008;98:238–243

26. Schillinger JA, Kissinger P, Calvet H, et al. Patient-delivered partner treatment with azithromycin to prevent repeated *Chlamydia trachomatis* infection among women: a randomized, controlled trial. *Sex Transm Dis.* 2003;30:49–56

27. Spiegel CA. Bacterial vaginosis. *Clin Microbio Rev.* 1991;4(4):485–502

28. Amsel R, Totten PA, Spiegel CA, et al. Nonspecific vaginitis: diagnostic criteria and microbial and epidemiological associations. *Am J Med.* 1983;74:14–22

29. Ness RB, Kip KE, Soper DE, et al. Douching in relation to bacterial vaginosis, lactobacilli, and facultative bacteria in the vagina. *Obstet Gynecol.* 2002;100:765

30. Royce RA, Jackson TP, Thorp JM Jr, et al. Race/ethnicity, vaginal flora patterns and pH during pregnancy. *Sex Transm Dis.* 1999;26:96–102

31. Taha TE, Hoover DR, DAllabeta GA, et al. Bacterial vaginosis and disturbances of vaginal flora: association with increased acquisition of HIV. *AIDS.* 1998;12(13):1699–1706

32. Hillier SL, Nugent RP, Eschenbach DA, et al. Association between bacterial vaginosis and preterm delivery of a low birth infant. *N Engl J Med.* 1995;333:1737–1742

33. Meis PJ, Goldenberh RL, Mercer B, et al. The preterm prediction study: significance of vaginal infection. *Am J Obstet Gynecol.* 1995;173:1231–1235

34. Myziuk L, Romanowski B, Johnson SC. BVBlue test for diagnosis of bacterial vaginosis. *J Clin Microbiol.* 2003;41:1925–1928

35. Bradshaw CS, Morton AN, Garland SM, Hovarth LB, Kuzeveska I, Fairley CK. Evaluation of a point-of-care test, BVBlue, and clinical and laboratory criteria for diagnosis of bacterial vaginosis. *J Clin Microbiol.* 2005;43:1304–1308

36. Fotus AC, Kraus SJ. *Trichomonas vaginalis:* reevaluation of its clinical presentation and laboratory diagnosis. *J Infect Dis.* 1980;141:137–143
37. Sutton M, Sternberg M, Koumans EH, McQuillan G, Berman, S, Markowitz LE. The prevalence of *Trichomonas vaginalis* infection among reproductive-age women in the United States, 2001–2004. *Clin Infect Dis.* 2007;45(10):1319–1326
38. Laga M, Manoka A, Kivuvu M, Malele B, Tuliza M, Nzila N. Nonulcerative sexually transmitted diseases as risk factors for HIV-1 transmission in women: results from a cohort study. *AIDS.* 1993;7(1):95–102
39. Sonnex C. Colpitis macularis and macular vaginitis unrelated to *Trichomonas vaginalis* infection. *Int J STD AIDS.* 1997;8:589–591
40. Krieger JN, Alderete JF. *Trichomonas vaginalis* and trichomoniasis. In: Holmes KK, Sparling PF, Mardh P, et al., eds. *Sexually Transmitted Diseases.* 3rd ed. New York, NY: McGraw-Hill; 2000: 587
41. Hollman D, Coupey SM, Fox AS, Herold BC. Screening for *Trichomonas vaginalis* in high-risk adolescent females with a new transcription-mediated nucleic acid amplification test (NAAT): associations with ethnicity, symptoms, and prior and current STIs. *J Pediatr Adolesc Gynecol.* 2010;23(5):312–316
42. Andrea SB, Chapin KC. Comparison of Aptima *Trichomonas vaginalis* transcription-mediated amplification assay and BD affirm VPIII for detection of *T. vaginalis* in symptomatic women: performance parameters and epidemiological implications. *J Clin Microbiol.* 2011;49(3):866–869
43. Campbell L, Woods V, Lloyd T, Elsayed S, Church DL. Evaluation of the OSOM *Trichomonas* Rapid Test versus Wet Preparation Examination for Detection of *Trichomonas vaginalis* Vaginitis in Specimens from Women with a Low Prevalence of Infection. *J Clin Microbiol.* 2008;46(10):3467–3469
44. Tait IA, Hart CA. *Chlamydia trachomatis* in non-gonococcal urethritis patients and their heterosexual partners: routine testing by polymerase chain reaction. *Sex Transm Infect.* 2002;78(4):286–288
45. Maeda S, Deguchi T, Ishiko H, et al. Detection of *Mycoplasma genitalium, Mycoplasma hominis, Ureaplama parvum* (biovar 1), and *Ureaplasma urealyticum* (biovar 2) in patients with non-gonococcal urethritis using polymerase chain reaction-microtiter plate hybridization. *Int J Urol.* 2004;11(9):750–754
46. Paavonen J, Critchlow CW, DeRouen T, et al. Etiology of cervical inflammation. *Am J Obstet Gynecol.* 1986;154(3):556–564
47. Manhart LE, Critchlow CW, Holmes KK, et al. Mucopurulent cervicitis and *Mycoplasma genitalium.* *J Infect Dis.* 2003;187:650–657
48. Sutton MY, Sternberg M, Zaidi A, et al. Trends in pelvic inflammatory disease hospital discharges and ambulatory visits, United States, 1985–2001. *Sex Transm Dis.* 2005;32:778–784
49. Simms I, Stephenson JM, Mallinson H, et al. Risk factors associated with pelvic inflammatory disease. *Sex Transm Infect.* 2006;82:452–457
50. Jossens MO, Eskenazi B, Schachter J, Sweet RL. Risk factors for pelvic inflammatory disease. A case control study. *Sex Transm Dis.* 1996;23:239–247
51. Wasserheit JN, Bell TA, Kiviat NB, et al. Microbial causes of proven pelvic inflammatory disease and efficacy of clindamycin and tobramycin. *Ann Intern Med.* 1986;104:187–193
52. Trent M, Haggerty CL, Jennings JM, et al. Adverse adolescent reproductive health outcomes after pelvic inflammatory disease. *Arch Pediatr Adolesc Med.* 2011;165:49–54
53. Saini S, Gupta N, Aparna, et al. Role of anaerobes in acute pelvic inflammatory disease. *Indian J Med Microbiol.* 2003;21:189–192
54. Simms I, Eastick K, Mallinson H, et al. Associations between *Mycoplasma genitalium, Chlamydia trachomatis* and pelvic inflammatory disease. *J Clin Pathol.* 2003;56:616–618
55. Haggerty CL. Evidence for a role of *Mycoplasma genitalium* in pelvic inflammatory disease. *Curr Opin Infect Dis.* 2008;21:65–69
56. World Health Organization Task Force on the Prevention and Management of Infertility. Tubal infertility: serologic relationship to post chlamydial and gonococcal infection. *Sex Transm Dis.* 1995;33:747–752

57. Short VL, Totten PA, Ness RB, et al. Clinical presentation of *Mycoplasma genitalium* infection versus *Neisseria gonorrhoeae* infection among women with pelvic inflammatory disease. *Clin Infect Dis.* 2009;48:41–47

58. Weström L, Joesoef R, Reynolds G, et al. Pelvic inflammatory disease and fertility. A cohort study of 1,844 women with laparoscopically verified disease and 657 control women with normal laparoscopic results. *Sex Transm Dis.*1992;19(4):185–192

59. Buchan H, Vessey M, Goldacre M, Fairweather J. Morbidity following pelvic inflammatory disease. *Br J Obstet Gynecol.* 1993;100:558–562

60. Ness RB, Hillier SL, Kip KE, et al. Effectiveness of inpatient and outpatient treatment strategies for women with pelvic inflammatory disease: results from the Pelvic Inflammatory Disease Evaluation and Clinical Health (PEACH) randomized trial. *Am J Obstet Gynecol.* 2002;186:929–937

61. Mertz KJ, Trees D, Levine WC, et al. Etiology of genital ulcers and prevalence of human immunodeficiency virus coinfection in 10 US cities. The Genital Ulcer Disease Surveillance Group. *J Infect Dis.* 1998;178(6):1795–1798

62. Centers for Disease Control and Prevention. The 2009 Sexually Transmitted Diseases Surveillance page. Selected STDs and Complications—Initial Visits to Physicians' Offices, National Disease and Therapeutic Index, United States, 1966–2009. http://www.cdc.gov/std/stats09/tables/43.htm. Accessed July 13, 2011

63. Centers for Disease Control and Prevention. Seroprevalence of herpes simplex virus type 2 among persons aged 14–49 years—United States, 2005-2008. *MMWR.* 2010;59(15):456–459

64. Benedetti JK, Corey L, Ashley R. Recurrence rates in genital herpes after symptomatic first-episode infection. *Ann Intern Med.* 1994;121:847–854

65. Engelberg, R, Carrel D, Krantz E, Corey L, Wald A. Natural history of genital herpes simplex virus type 1 infection. *Sex Transm Dis.* 2003;30(2):174–177

66. Whittington WL, Celum CL, Cent A, Ashley RL. Use of a glycoprotein G-based type-specific assay to detect antibodies to herpes simplex virus type 2 among persons attending sexually transmitted disease clinics. *Sex Transm Dis.* 2001;28(2):99–104

67. Prince HE, Ernst CE, Hogrefe WR. Evaluation of an enzyme immunoassay system for measuring herpes simplex virus (HSV) type 1-specific and HSV type 2-specific IgG antibodies. *J Clin Lab Anal.* 2000;14(1):13–16

68. Cogliano V, Baan R, Straif K, et al. Carcinogenicity of human papillomaviruses. *Lancet Oncol.* 2005;6:204

69. Clifford GM, Smith JS, Plummer M, Münoz N, Franceschi S. Human papillomavirus types in invasive cervical cancer worldwide: a metaanalysis. *Br J Cancer.* 2003;88:63–73

70. Walboomers JM, Jacobs MV, Manos MM, et al. Human papillomavirus is a necessary cause of invasive cervical cancer worldwide. *J Pathol.* 1999;189(1):12–19

71. Smith JS, Lindsay L, Hoots B, et al. Human papillomavirus type distribution in invasive cervical cancer and high-grade cervical lesions: a meta-analysis update. *Int J Cancer.* 2007;121(3);621–632

72. Brown DR, Schroeder JM, Bryan JT, Stoler MH, Fife KH. Detection of multiple human papillomavirus types in *Condylomata acuminata* lesions from otherwise healthy and immunosuppressed patients. *J Clin Microbiol.* 1999;37(10):3316–3322

73. Greer CE, Wheeler CM, Ladner MB, et al. Human papillomavirus (HPV) type distribution and serological response to HPV type 6 virus-like particles in patients with genital warts. *J Clin Microbiol.* 1995;33(8):2058–2063

74. Garland SM, Steben M, Sings HL, et al. Natural history of genital warts: analysis of the placebo arm of 2 randomized phase III trials of a quadrivalent human papillomavirus (types 6, 11, 16, and 18) vaccine. *J Infect Dis.* 2009;199(6):805–814

75. Brown DR, Shew ML, Qadadri B, et al. A longitudinal study of genital human papillomavirus infection in a cohort of closely followed adolescent women. *J Infect Dis.* 2005;191:182–192

76. Dunne E, Nielson C, Stone K, Markowitz L, Giuliano A. Prevalence of HPV infection among men: a systematic review of the literature. *J Infect Dis.* 2006;194:1044–1057

77. Revzina N, Diclemente R. Prevalence and incidence of human papillomavirus infection in women in the USA: a systematic review. *Int J STD AIDS.* 2005;16:528–537

78. Maw R. Critical appraisal of commonly used treatment for genital warts. *Int J STD AIDS.* 2004;15(6):357–364
79. Wiley DJ. Genital warts. *Clin Evid.* 2002;(8):1620–1632
80. Edwards L, Ferenczy A, Eron L, et al. Self-administered topical 5% imiquimod cream for external anogenital warts. HPV Study Group. Human Papilloma Virus. *Arch Dermatol.* 1998;134(1):25–30
81. Tatti S, Swinehart JM, Thielert C, Tawfik H, Mescheder A, Beutner KR. Sinecatechins, a defined green tea extract, in the treatment of external anogenital warts: a randomized controlled trial. *Obstet Gynecol.* 2008;111(6):1371–1379
82. Reid R. The management of genital condyloma, intraepithelial neoplasia, and vulvodynia. *Obstet Gynecol Clin North Am.* 1996;23(4):917–991
83. Beutner KR, Conant MA, Friedman-Kien AE, et al. Patient-applied podofilox for treatment of genital warts. *Lancet.* 1989;1(8642):831–834
84. Wiley DJ, Douglas J, Beutner K, et al. External genital warts: diagnosis, treatment, and prevention. *Clin Infect Dis.* 2002;35(Suppl 2):S210–224

Adolesc Med 23 (2012) 95–110

Contraception for Primary Care Providers

Shon Patrick Rowan, MD[a], Jean Someshwar, MD[b], Pamela Murray, MD, MHP[b]*

[a]*West Virginia University Department of Obstetrics and Gynecology, Morgantown, West Virginia*

[b]*West Virginia University Department of Pediatrics, Morgantown, West Virginia*

INTRODUCTION

Adolescence is a time of growth, both physical and mental, bringing many changes and challenges. During this period, teens take on increasing responsibilities and autonomy as they prepare themselves for independence. Education plays a key role, not only for academic achievement, but also in social and life skills development. Beginning in early adolescence, anticipatory guidance may begin with water and bicycle safety and progress to driving safety as teens continue to develop new skills and take on added responsibilities (Table 1). Sexual safety and literacy are particularly important objectives, with almost half of male and female high school age students in the United States (US) being sexually experienced according to the 2009 National Youth Risk Behavior Survey conducted by the Centers for Disease Control and Prevention (CDC).[1] Although the US teen pregnancy rate has decreased over the past 2 decades, the US teen birth rate remains the highest in the industrialized world.[2] Sexually active female adolescents who do not use contraception have an 85–90% chance of pregnancy within 1 year.[3] Primary care providers can address this issue by educating patients about condoms, emergency contraception, and selection of contraceptive methods. Discussion of risks, benefits, and limitations of the various modalities of contraception should aim to maximize effectiveness, minimize discontinuation, and avoid contraceptive failure. We offer a review of current contraceptive options and offer suggestions for the primary care provider.

---

*Corresponding author.
E-mail address: pmurray@hsc.wvu.edu (P. Murray).

Table 1.
Early Adolescent Skill Development Checklist

Water safety—swim and float
Bicycle safety—ride and wear helmet
Illness safety—swallow pills and read labels
Motor vehicle safety—seatbelts, speed limits, eliminate distractions
Sexual safety—condoms and emergency contraception

REPRODUCTIVE HEALTH CARE

Providers can alleviate anxiety in the initiation of hormonal contraceptives by communicating with their patients that neither a Pap smear (ie, speculum examination) nor simple pelvic examination is required before beginning contraceptive use. Ideally, an inspection of the external genitalia, an evaluation for vaginitis, and testing for STIs is recommended, but some patients prefer to have this done after initiating contraception or sexual activity. In a patient without symptoms of genitourinary disease, this can be performed at a subsequent visit with increased patient comfort, if not done initially. A follow-up visit 1–3 months after initiation of contraception is recommended to see if there are complications from the contraceptive choice or interim discontinuation of the method. A focused gynecologic examination would be indicated in a patient experiencing symptoms suggestive of STI at any time but is not tied specifically to the initiation of hormonal contraceptives. A provider would be prudent to examine the external genitalia for any evidence of lesions or discharge and may consider vaginal self-swabs or urine testing for chlamydia and gonorrhea. Vaginal swabs allow for evaluation for vaginitis, and a bimanual examination is critical if an evaluation for possible pelvic inflammatory disease is needed. A speculum examination may only be required for the collection of Pap smear specimens or when inspection of the cervix and vaginal walls is clinically indicated, as in the evaluation of undiagnosed vaginal or uterine bleeding, pain, or trauma.[4] Pap smears are now recommended to begin at age 21 in all immunocompetent females regardless of their sexual history[5]; sexually experienced patients with immunocompromise, including HIV-infected individuals, should initiate Pap smears earlier as a part of comprehensive reproductive health care. Patients should be reminded which contraceptives prevent pregnancy but do not protect against STIs and that condom use is always recommended.

SEXUAL SAFETY

Dual protection should be reinforced with all adolescents. Condoms alone have a typical pregnancy failure rate of 15%[6] (Table 2) but provide protection against many STIs, whereas hormonal contraceptives do not substantially protect against STIs. Discussion of proper condom placement and strategies to ensure effective and consistent use is important and can be found online at http://www.

Table 2.
Effectiveness of Contraceptive Methods

Method	Failure Rate (Typical use)	Failure Rate (Perfect use)	Women Continuing Use at 1 Year
No method	85%	85%	
Spermicide	28%	18%	42%
Withdrawal	22%	4%	46%
Fertility awareness-based methods	24%	3–5%	47%
Female condom	21%	5%	41%
Male condom	18%	2%	43%
Hormonal pills	9% (26% teens)	0.3%	67%
Depo-Provera	6%	0.2%	56%
IUD, progesterone	0.2%	0.2%	80%
Implanon	0.05%	0.05%	84%
Female sterilization	0.5%	0.5%	100%

Adapted from Hatcher RA, Trussell J, Nelson AL, Cates W, Kowal D, Policar MS. *Contraceptive Technology.* 20th revised ed. New York, NY: Ardent Media; 2011.

cdc.gov/mmwr/preview/mmwrhtml/00001053.htm. Adolescents should be offered condoms while in the office or clinic and given locations where they can be obtained at low or no cost. Nonlatex condoms are available for people with a latex allergy but have an increased slippage and breakage rate.[7] Female condoms also offer protection against STIs and are made of a polyurethane sheath with 2 polyurethane rings. They are expensive, cumbersome, have a high rate of slippage, are less effective than male condoms, and have more reported problems.[8] They have not received wide acceptance among adolescent women.

EMERGENCY CONTRACEPTION

Emergency contraceptive pills (ECPs) provide high dose progestin to prevent pregnancy up to 5 days after unprotected intercourse and are most effective when taken closer to the event. ECP use may be associated with mild nausea and occasional vomiting and may also cause menstrual irregularity and short-term headache, fatigue, and mastalgia. Different emergency contraceptive regimens can be used. The most commonly used contains levonorgestrel 0.75 mg, which can be taken 1 tab 12 hours apart or 2 tablets at once with similar efficacy.[9] One time dosing is more practical for teenagers. A combined hormonal method, but with more gastrointestinal side effects and less efficacy than levonorgestrel alone, can also be used.[9] This is known as the Yuzpe method, which contains 100 mcg ethinyl estradiol combined with a progestin, either levonorgestrel 0.50 mg, norgestrel 1.0 mg, or norethindrone 2.0 mg.[9] Even with the Yuzpe method, the progestin dose is most critical to ECP effectiveness. The Yuzpe regimens are less effective and have more side effects than the progestin only regimen. Emergency contraceptives became available over-the-counter in the United States for women 17 years and older in August 2006.[10] There are variations from state to state in access to emergency contraceptives through pharmacists.[11] Ullipristal acetate is marketed in the United States and received Food and Drug Administration (FDA) approval in August 2010. It works as a selective progesterone receptor modulator.[12] It can be used up to 5 days following intercourse, with a pregnancy rate of 1.8% compared to 2.6% for 1.5 mg of levonorgestrel.[13]

Emergency contraception has traditionally been associated with conflict and controversy because of its perceived associations with promiscuity and pregnancy termination. In fact, emergency contraceptive pills are not abortifacients but work primarily by preventing ovulation.[14] If a pregnancy were to occur with their use, the ECP, as with all hormonal contraceptives, is not teratogenic and does not interrupt an established pregnancy. Advance provision of emergency contraception has not been shown to increase risky sexual behaviors.[15]

HORMONAL CONTRACEPTIVES

Combination Hormonal Contraceptives

The most common method of contraception chosen by adolescents is oral combination pills (OCPs) [16,17] (Table 3). Many formulations of the combination pill are marketed; almost all include the estrogen ethinyl estradiol (EE) and a progestin. In 2010, a pill containing the estrogen estradiol valerate was approved by the FDA. The combination pills work in large part by suppression of the luteinizing hormone (LH) surge, thus inhibiting ovulation. Also, cervical mucous is thickened due to a progestin effect, which inhibits sperm motility and could aid in prevention of STIs.

The estrogen component is dosed in variable increments, with most pills containing 35 mcg or less of EE, which is considered low-dose estrogen. Available formulations range from 10–50 mcg of EE per pill. Table 4 lists common hormonal side effects. The most serious side effect and risk of estrogen administration is thrombosis and stroke. This risk is very low in healthy adolescents with-

Table 3.
Contraceptive Method Use at First Sex and Last Sex (Sexually Active Adolescent Females)

	First Sex	1995 (last sex)	2002 (last sex)	2008 (last sex)
Condoms	70	38	54	55
Pills	15	25	34	31
Injections		7	10	
Withdrawal		7	12	
Dual methods		8	20	21
No methods		29	17	17

Adapted from Abma JC, Martinez GM, Copen CE. Teenagers in the United States: Sexual activity, contraceptive use, and childbearing, National Survey of Family Growth 2006–2008. National Center for Health Statistics. *Vital Health Stat.* 2010;23(30).

out a personal or family history of thromboembolic events, approximately 1–10 per 100,000 healthy adolescents.[18] Some medical conditions, including migraine with aura, complicated valvular heart disease, or surgery leading to prolonged immobility, increase this risk. Other medical conditions in which the combination pill is contraindicated include diabetes with end-organ damage, breast cancer, and liver disease or dysfunction, which are all relatively uncommon in adolescents. Tobacco use prevention and cessation is encouraged, but smoking is not a specific contraindication to OCP use in adolescents. Higher doses of estrogen may lead to nausea and vomiting, which may be decreased if the patient takes the pill at night. Birth control pills are not a gastric irritant, but the systemic effects of hormones may cause nausea. This side effect often is most problematic in the first pill cycle, when both endogenous and exogenous hormones contribute to hormonally influenced nuisance side effects. In subsequent cycles, when endogenous hormone production is suppressed by the effect of OCPs on pituitary production of gonadotropins, these symptoms abate. If side effects of estrogen are significant, one of the lower dose estrogen options can be used. However, when using lower doses of estrogen, amenorrhea or irregular bleeding can occur due to thinning of the endometrium. Concerns about decreased bone mineral density in young women on the lowest estrogen dosing have been raised, but long-term clinical significance is not established.[19]

Many different progestins are used in combination pill formulations and may be broadly categorized into first, second, and third generation progestins (Table 5). Estranes, which are first generation progestins, have a half-life of approximately 8 hours. Gonanes, second and third generation progestins, have a longer half-life, approximately 16 hours. Combination pills containing gonanes may have less breakthrough bleeding because of the longer half-life. A fourth generation progestin, drosperidone, has some spironolactone-like, antiandrogenic, and diuretic (mineralocorticoid) activity, theoretically enhancing the improvement in acne and hirsutism seen with most OCPs and decreasing premenstrual fluid retention. However, concerns have been raised regarding the increased thrombotic risk in pills containing some third and fourth generation progestins. Published articles addressing this question have had conflicting conclusions. However, 2 recent studies published in the *British Medical Journal* found a 2–3 fold

Table 4.
Common Hormonal Side Effects

Estrogen	Progesterone
Nausea	Breast size increase
Headache	Appetite increase
Mastalgia	Mood changes
Leukorrhea	Decreased libido
Fluid retention	Acne
Thrombosis	Pruritus
Telangiectasia	Headache

Table 5.
Choosing a Progestin

Estranes

First generation
Norethindrone, norethindrone acetate, ethynodiol diacetate
half-life = 8 hours

Gonanes

Second generation
Norgestrel, levonorgestrel
half-life = 11–16 hours; better cycle control
Third generation*
Desogestrel, norgestimate, gestodene
half-life = 11–16 hours; better cycle control

Spironolactone analog

Fourth generation*
drospirenone (Yasmin*)
may cause potassium retention
modest increased risk of thromboembolism

*increased thrombotic risk

higher risk of venous thromboembolism in patients taking drospirenone compared to levonorgestrel.[20,21] Similar concerns have been raised about desogestrel, with several epidemiologic studies supporting an increased risk of thromboembolic events.[22] The FDA issued a safety warning in June 2011 advising caution in prescribing drospirenone.[23]

The benefits of OCPs, beyond pregnancy prevention, include menstrual regulation; improvement in dysmenorrhea and menorrhagia; prevention of ovarian cysts; and a decreased risk for colorectal, ovarian, and endometrial cancer.[24] Combination OCPs also provide treatment of polycystic ovary syndrome (PCOS), including improvements in acne and hirsutism, and are helpful in treating endometriosis.[24] Extended cycling, a regimen of oral contraceptives that includes an increased duration of active hormone days can be used in adolescents preferring less frequent menses. It is particularly useful for those with certain medical conditions, including bleeding disorders, menorrhagia with iron deficiency or secondary anemia, severe dysmenorrhea or endometriosis, premenstrual syndrome, menstrual migraines, or other cyclical conditions exacerbated by menses. Extended cycling can be instituted using packaged regimens with 84 hormone and 7 placebo days or can be designed by skipping the placebo week after any number of packs of combination pills. Flexibility can be allowed for making a limited extended cycling regimen to avoid menses during special events, such as performances, sporting activities, and vacations. Extended cycling improves contraceptive effectiveness but may be associated with increased frequency of unscheduled irregular bleeding,[25] which is a poorly tolerated side effect for many women.[26] Many teens prefer to plan their withdrawal bleed, and some choose to extend their hormone pills continuously until bleeding starts. With spontaneous bleeding, stopping hormones for 3–4 days allows a withdrawal bleed.

Initiating CHCs can be handled in several ways, including using a "Sunday start," a "first day start," or a "quick start" (Table 6). The Sunday start entails asking patients to begin the CHC on the Sunday associated with the start of their menses. This has been the most traditional starting regimen, popular with patients because it usually results in menses-free weekends. The first day of menses start instructs patients to begin the first pill pack on the first day of the next menses. The quick start method allows patients to begin their CHC pack on the day of their visit; it can be used in those patients who have not had unprotected sex in the 2 weeks before their visit and have a negative urine pregnancy test. Patients using the quick start method should be counseled that they should consider themselves unprotected from pregnancy for 2 weeks after starting the pill and should use a backup method of contraception. Information on condoms and ECPs should be provided, as with all contraceptive starts. A repeat pregnancy test can be performed in 2 weeks to confirm that the patient is not pregnant. Prescribers should become familiar with several brands of pills with varying doses of estrogen and various progesterone components, as well as with insurance coverage in their locale. This makes prescribing oral contraceptives simpler for the clinician and the patient. A complete and up-to-date list of oral contraceptives can be found at websites such as http://www.nlm.nih.gov/medlineplus/druginfo/meds/a601050.html. Key resources for clinical care and patient education can be found on websites

Table 6.
Quick Start Checklist

Condoms—education and samples
ECP—education and prescribing
Pregnancy test—βhCG (urine)
Sexual health evaluation (as indicated)
Wet prep or point-of-care testing for vaginitis (vaginal swab)
NAAT for gonorrhea and chlamydia (vaginal swab or urine)
HIV and syphilis (blood work)
Contraceptive choice
Quick start OCPs on day of appointment
LARC options education
DMPA if βhCG negative and no risk of pregnancy
If LARC initiation delayed—use OCPs or abstinence as bridging contraception
Follow-up appointment

ECP = emergency contraception; βhCG = human chorionic gonadotropin; NAAT = nucleic acid amplification testing; HIV = human immunodeficiency virus; LARC = long acting reversible contraception; DMPA = depo medroxyprogesterone acetate (Depo-Provera); OCPs = oral contraceptive pills

such as bedsider.org, http://www.cdc.gov/mmwr/preview/mmwrhtml/mm6026a3
.htm#tab1, and www.thenationalcampaign.org.

Another combination hormone method is the vaginal contraceptive ring, which
delivers 120 mcg etonogestrel and 15 mcg of ethinyl estradiol directly into the
vaginal wall from a soft flexible ring that is inserted into the vagina. The ring
stays in place for 21 days, although it can be removed intermittently for up to
3 hours, for example during intercourse, and still remain effective.[27] Advantages
of this method include its privacy and comfort. In a study of women and their
partners, the majority of participants reported no undesirable effects even when
the ring remained in place during coitus.[27] Drawbacks to the use of the vaginal
ring in adolescents might include a reticence in those who express discomfort
with the self-touching needed for insertion and removal of the device.

Another hormonal method, similar in hormonal composition to the OCP, the
transdermal patch, may be a good alternative method for those patients who
have difficulty complying with a daily regimen. The patch contains 6 mg of
norelgestromin and 0.75 mg of ethinyl estradiol, releasing 159 mcg of the progestin and 20 mcg of the estrogen component daily. The patch is a thin, beige, 20
cm square that is applied to fleshy parts of the body except for breast tissue. It
should be left in place for 1 week, then changed weekly to complete 3 patches,
followed by a patch-free week in which menses occurs. If replacing a patch is
inadvertently delayed, there is a "grace period" giving the adolescent patient up
to 48 hours to apply the second or third patch in a cycle without an increased
risk of pregnancy.[28] The transdermal patch has a similar side effect profile to that
of OCPs, with the addition that adolescents may have difficulty with the adhe-
sive on the patch and skin discoloration.[29] This was shown in a 3-month study of
adolescents in which more than one-third of participants experienced complete
or partial detachment of at least 1 patch.[30,31] The transdermal patch may be less
effective in women weighing more than 90 kg, according to one study.[32] Further,
concerns have been raised regarding the possibility of higher thrombotic risk
using the transdermal patch because of the continuous administration of estrogen resulting in a larger "area under the curve" of estrogen exposure. One study
by Cole et al[33] suggested that patients using the transdermal patch may have a
2-fold risk of venous thromboembolism compared to patients using the OCP.
Because of these findings, the FDA instituted new labeling requirements for the
patch in 2006, cautioning prescribers and patients.

Progesterone-Only Contraceptives

Progesterone-only contraceptive pills are typically reserved for women with
contraindications or intolerance to estrogen as listed previously. Progesterone-
only contraceptive package inserts list the same contraindications as those for
estrogen-containing contraceptives but are believed to be safe in most patients.
Progesterone-only contraceptive pills contain 0.35 mg of norethindrone and

have both a lower dose of progesterone and no hormone-free period as in combination contraceptive pills. Ovulation is not consistently inhibited by these pills, as approximately 40% of patients ovulate normally. Rather, progesterone-only pills work by thickening cervical mucus and creating an atrophic endometrium.[34] Progesterone-only pills need to be taken at the same time every day, as the effect of cervical mucus thickening diminishes in 22 hours, with complete resolution by 24 hours. Intercourse is contraindicated in the 3 hours before and after pill ingestion because of diminished efficacy. Minimal effects on lipid and carbohydrate metabolism are seen with these pills.[35] However, a 3-fold increase in developing diabetes mellitus in women with recent gestational diabetes and progestin-only contraceptive use compared to nonhormonal or combination contraception has been reported.[36] The most common reason for discontinuation is irregular menses.[37] Functional ovarian cysts are also associated with progestin-only contraceptive use.[38]

Injections

Depo medroxyprogesterone acetate (DMPA) is a good option for many adolescents, as it is a very effective long-acting contraceptive. It is an injection given every 3 months and it can be given intramuscularly with a 150 mg dose or subcutaneously with a newer 104 mg dose. The lower dose formulation allows a lower hormone dose while providing a slower and more sustained absorption.[39] The 150 mg formulation is generic, making it available at lower cost in many settings.

DMPA thickens cervical mucus and alters the endometrium, as do other progesterone-only contraceptives. However, it also suppresses ovulation by blocking the LH surge.[40] Return to fertility is variable after DMPA use. Irregular menses, weight gain, and headaches lead to a discontinuation rate of 33–75% after 1 year.[41,42,43]

Bone mineral density (BMD) loss has been documented with DMPA use, leading to an FDA black box warning cautioning against use for more than 2 years. However, although BMD does decrease in adolescents using DMPA, the loss appears to slow down after 1 year of use,[44] and after discontinuation of use, the BMD partially or fully recovers at the spine and partially recovers at the hip.[45] The American College of Obstetricians and Gynecologists (ACOG) states, however, that concerns about possible BMD loss should not prevent prescribing DMPA or limit its use. They state that other long-acting reversible contraception (LARC) options, including implants and IUDs, which do not have a documented effect on BMD, should be considered as first-line options in adolescents.[46]

DMPA has long been considered a safe alternative to estrogen-containing contraceptives for patients with a history of venous thromboembolism (VTE). A recent study showed a 3.6-fold increase in VTE in DMPA users compared to nonhormonal users. However, this study was performed in a homogenous population in the Netherlands and therefore may not be generalizable; other studies have not shown an increased risk.[47]

Implants

The first implantable contraceptive device approved by the FDA was the 6-rod levonorgestrel Norplant system, but it was taken off the market in 2002 due to concerns regarding a greater than expected pregnancy rate. Implanon is a subdermal rod system that has been available in the United States since 2006. It consists of a single rod containing the progestin etonogestrel and measures 40 mm in length and 2 mm in diameter. Sixty-eight mg of etonogestrel is released at an initial rate of 60 to 70 mcg/day, decreasing to 35 to 45 mcg/day at the end of the first year, 30 to 40 mcg/day at the end of the second year, and 25 to 30 mcg/day at the end of the third year.[48] It works primarily by inhibiting ovulation.[49] It can be inserted and removed in the office or clinic by clinicians who have undergone a 3-hour training session. The insertion and removal procedures can be accomplished in less than 5 minutes. Approximately 3% of patients complain of pain at the insertion site. Removal complications have been reported in 1.7% of patients; these include implant breakage, inability to palpate the implant, difficult removal secondary to deep insertion, the implant being fixed by fibrous tissue, too much implant flexibility for easy removal, implant adherence to underlying tissue, and difficulty locating the implant. Drug-related adverse effects are similar to other progestin-only contraceptives, including headache, weight gain, acne, breast pain, emotional instability, and abdominal pain. In one review, 35% of patients discontinued implant use early, with adverse effects and bleeding irregularities being the most common reasons.[50]

Intrauterine Devices

Intrauterine devices (IUDs) provide a highly effective, cost-efficient, and relatively easy to reverse method that requires little compliance. It is the most widely used method of reversible contraception in the world, accounting for as much as 50% of contraceptive use in some countries, but only accounting for 2% of contraceptive use in the United States.[51] Concerns about increased rates of pelvic inflammatory disease (PID) and effects on future fertility have not been substantiated, making the IUD an appropriate contraceptive for some adolescents. The risk of PID is only increased at the time of insertion.[52] Patients often present for a visit to discuss contraception before IUD placement. This visit is a good time to collect sensitive and specific tests for gonorrhea and chlamydia, thus allowing time to receive results and implement treatment before insertion. In instances where IUD insertion is desired at the initial visit, it is acceptable to proceed, but the tests for gonorrhea and chlamydia should be performed and treatment should be provided as needed while the IUD is in place. Treatment of positive cultures decreases the risk of PID. In fact, the risk of acquiring PID during the time that the IUD is in place may actually be decreased with the levonorgestrel-releasing intrauterine device because it thickens cervical mucus and thins the endometrium. Infertility is not increased in IUD users after removal, and fecundity has been shown to quickly return after removal.[53] Discomfort with IUD insertion occurs in many patients. The use of misoprostol to soften the cervix and the use of anti-inflammatory medications may decrease discomfort.

There are 2 available devices in the United States: the copper IUD and the levonorgestrel-releasing intrauterine system (IUS). The IUS is a 32 mm, T-shaped, polyethylene frame that contains 52 mg of levonorgestrel and releases 20 mcg per day initially, decreasing to 11 mcg per day by 5 years. This device is associated with decreased uterine bleeding and is approved to remain in place for 5 years, making it a good option for adolescents. Fertility after removal of the system is similar to that for reproductive age women without prior IUS placement, with more than 70% of patients wanting to conceive becoming pregnant within 24 months.[54] Irregular menstrual bleeding may occur, mostly during the first 3–6 months. Fifty percent of women become amenorrheic after 1 year of use.[55] Side effects include headache, acne, and breast tenderness.[56] The copper IUD is a 36 mm long, T-shaped, polyethylene device with a 68.7 mg copper sleeve on each of its transverse arms and a 176 mg copper wire wrapped around its vertical axis. As with the IUS, it contains barium sulfate to make it radiopaque. It is approved for 10 years of effective contraception and intrauterine placement. After 5 years for the IUS or 10 years for the copper IUD, it should be removed and a new IUD may be placed immediately if desired.

Although rarely used, the copper IUD has been studied and found to be effective for emergency contraception.[57] The IUS has not been studied for this indication.

Postpartum Contraception

With an adolescent birth rate of 41.5 per 1000 teenagers, postpartum contraception in the adolescent must be considered.[2] Progesterone-only methods can be started immediately postpartum. Combined oral contraceptives have been typically started 3 weeks postpartum, due to the increased risk of peripartum thrombotic events, but the latest recommendations are to wait 6 weeks postpartum before starting OCPs.[58] This method has been shown to decrease milk supply in breastfeeding mothers, but infant growth is likely not affected.[59] IUDs can be placed immediately after delivery, but this comes with an expulsion rate of 24% compared to 4.4% when waiting 6–8 weeks postpartum.[60] Adolescents who choose DMPA over OCPs or the patch for postpartum contraception are much less likely to become pregnant within 1 year.[61]

Withdrawal

More than 50% of women report having ever used withdrawal as a method of birth control, with 12% of adolescents reporting withdrawal as their contraceptive method at last sex.[17] Withdrawal has the advantages of being free of cost, devices, and chemicals, but it has high failure rates and does not provide protection from STIs.

Barrier Devices

Barrier devices other than the condom that are available but rarely used by adolescents include the cervical cap, the diaphragm, and the sponge. Spermicides can be used with a condom or other barrier device. Nonoxynol-9 (N-9) damages the sperm cell membrane and is contained in nearly all spermicides available in the United States.[62] The dose ranges from 52.5–150 mg depending on the product and can be used in the form of gels, creams, foams, suppositories, and films. Suppositories and films must be placed 10–15 minutes before intercourse, making them a less than ideal contraceptive for adolescents. N-9 users may experience vaginal burning or irritation, which can lead to ulceration.[63] Although N-9 has been shown to inactivate some sexually transmitted pathogens in vitro, it does not appear to decrease the rate of infection compared to condom use alone.[61] Spermicides should not be used in HIV infected individuals or those at high risk of acquisition of HIV infection because of concerns with increased HIV transmission.

Male Contraception

Male contraception options in the United States currently include only condoms and vasectomy. The future of male contraception is worth noting. There are several forms in various stages of development, including hormonal methods, contraceptive vaccines, and easily reversed surgical occlusive procedures. The availability of additional male contraception methods in the future will allow male adolescents to have a greater role in preventing unintended pregnancies. Clinicians caring for male adolescents will then be able to expand contraceptive options beyond abstinence and condoms.

Special Needs

Adolescents with disabilities are as likely to be sexually active as those without disabilities and more likely to be sexually abused.[64] Menstruation for adolescents with severe disabilities may have a significant impact on hygiene. Therefore, contraception and menstrual management in the disabled adolescent needs consideration. Contraceptive options for this population need to be carefully chosen depending on the goals and specific conditions of the adolescent. Combination contraceptives remain an option. Chewable combined OCPs are available and can be given to patients with G-tubes or those unable to swallow pills. However, immobility and thromboembolic risks must be considered. Inadvertent removal of patches may be an issue in some adolescents. Contraceptive rings require insertion by the adolescent or a caregiver, limiting their use in some adolescents with disabilities. In patients with fear of blood or hygiene issues, irregular bleeding with progesterone-only pills and implants may pose a problem. DMPA is a good option for many disabled adolescents due to its efficacy, extended interval, and high rate of amenorrhea. The effect of long-term use on bone density needs to be considered, especially in young women with other risks for decreased BMD, such as those with immobility, malnutrition, or taking certain medications. Weight gain in this setting may also limit its use in these populations. IUDs also provide long-term effective contraception, with lighter menses or amenorrhea in most patients. IUD placement may be difficult in some patients but with appropriate technique it can be safely accomplished.

Surgical Methods of Contraception

These methods are not typically considered an option for adolescents. If menstrual elimination for hygiene reasons is a primary goal, then surgical options may become part of the informed discussion and could lead to permanent sterilization. Primary care physicians in the medical home are often asked their opinion about more permanent surgical procedures. Surgical methods for contraception short of hysterectomy do not play a role in hygiene. Hysterectomy may be an option for some adolescents with disabilities but is beyond the scope of this article. Laws concerning sterilization in adolescents vary by state.

INTERNATIONAL CONSIDERATIONS

As international travel for adolescents is not uncommon, clinicians may encounter contraceptives different from those available in the United States. Oral contraceptives may be marketed under different names, but the inserts usually have the estrogen and progesterone components noted in English. Although all progesterone-only pills in the United States contain norethindrone, pills containing only desogestrel are available in other countries. An implantable device similar to the etonogestrel rod has been approved by the FDA but is not yet marketed in the United States. Many different IUDs are available throughout the world. Patients with IUDs placed in other countries need further evaluation of the device, as some may not have strings and can be challenging to remove.

CONCLUSIONS

Knowledge of contraceptives and gynecologic care are standard components of well adolescent care. Use of dual methods is strongly encouraged to optimize pregnancy and STI prevention. Combination hormonal contraception is available in several delivery mechanisms and is safe and effective in most adolescents. Progesterone-only pills are an option for patients with contraindications to estrogen containing methods. The CDC and ACOG endorse broader use of long-acting reversible contraceptives in adolescents to decrease the teen pregnancy rate in the United States, and this would certainly be true in other nations as well.

ACKNOWLEDGMENTS

The authors want to thank Alexandra Carey and Sylvia Choi for their thoughtful reading and feedback on the manuscript, and Rhea Seddon for reinforcing the value of checklists in medical care.

References

1. Centers for Disease Control. Youth Risk Behavioral Surveillance-United States 2009. http://www. cdc.gov/mmwr/pdf/ss/ss5905.pdf. Accessed June 29, 2011
2. Centers for Disease Control. National Center for Health Statistics. http://www.cdc.gov/NCHS. Accessed June 5, 2011
3. Harlap S, Kosi K, Forrest JD. *Preventing Pregnancy, Protecting Health: A New Look at Birth Control Choices in the United States.* New York, NY: AGI; 1991
4. American Academy of Pediatrics. http://www.aap.org/sections/adolescenthealth/pdf. Accessed June 10, 2011
5. ACOG guidelines 2009. http://www.acog.org. Accessed June 5, 2011
6. Hatcher RA, Trussel J, Nelson AL, Cates W, Stewart FH, Kowal D. *Contraceptive Technology.* 19th ed. New York, NY:Ardent Media, Inc.; 2008
7. Freziers RG, Walsh TL, Nelson AL, et al. Breakage and acceptability of a polyurethane condom: a randomized, controlled study. *Fam Plann Perspect.* 1998;30(2):73–78
8. Galvão LW, Oliveira LC, Díaz J, et al. Effectiveness of female and male condoms in preventing exposure to semen during vaginal intercourse: a randomized trial. *Contraception.* 2005;71(2):130–136
9. Cheng L, Gülmezoglu AM, Piaggio G, Ezcurra E, Van Look PF. Interventions for emergency contraception. *Cochrane Database Syst Rev.* 2008;16(2):CD001324
10. Plan B (0.75mg levonorgestrel) and Plan B One-Step (1.5 mg levonorgestrel) Tablets information. http://www.fda.gov/drugs/drugsafety/postmarketdrugsafetyinformationforpatientsandproviders/UCM109775. Accessed June 5, 2011
11. The Emergency Contraception Website. http://ec.princeton.edu/emergency-contraception.html. Accessed June 10, 2011
12. Chabbert-Buffet N, Meduri G, Bouchard P, Spitz I. Selective progesterone receptor modulators and progesterone antagonists: mechanisms of action and clinical applications. *Hum Reprod Update.* 2005;11:293–307
13. Glasier A, Cameron S, Fine P, et al. Ulipristal acetate versus levonorgestrel for emergency contraception: a randomized non-inferiority trial and meta-analysis. *Lancet.* 2010;375:555–562
14. Gemzell-Danielsson K. Mechanism of action of emergency contraception. *Contraception.* 2010;82(5):404–409
15. Meyer JL, Gold MA, Haggerty CL. Advance provision of emergency contraception among adolescent and young adult women: a systematic review of literature. *J Pediatr Adolesc Gynecol.* 2011;24(1):2–9
16. Mosher WD, Martinez GM, Chandra A, Abma JC, Wilson SJ. Use of contraception and use of family planning services in the United States: 1982–2002. *Adv Data.* 2004;(350):1–36
17. Abma JC, Martinez GM, Copen CE. Teenagers in the United States: Sexual activity, contraception use, and childbearing, National Survey of Family Growth 2006–2008. National Center for Health Statistics. *Vital Health Stat.* 2010;23(30):1–47
18. Trenor CC, Chung RJ, Michelson AD, et al. Hormonal contraception and thrombotic risk: a multidisciplinary approach. *Pediatrics.* 2011;127:347–357
19. Scholes D, Ichikawa L, LaCroix AZ, et al. Oral contraceptive use and bone density in adolescent and young adult women. *Contraception.* 2010;81(1):35–40
20. Parkin L, Sharples K, Hernandez RK, Jick SS. Risk of venous thromboembolism in users of oral contraceptives containing drospirenone or levonorgestrel: nested case-control study based on UK General Practice Research Database. *BMJ.* 2011;342:d2139
21. Jick SS, Hernandez RK. Risk of non-fatal venous thromboembolism in women using oral contraceptives containing drospirenone compared with women using oral contraceptives containing levonorgestrel: case-control study using United States claims data. *BMJ.* 2011;342:d2151
22. Hannaford PC. Epidemiology of the contraceptive pill and venous thromboembolism. *Tromb Res.* 2011;127:Suppl3:S30–34

23. Medical product safety information. http://www.fda.gov/safety/medwatch/safetyinformation. Accessed June 5, 2011
24. Jensen JT, Speroff L. Health benefits of oral contraceptives. *Obstet Gynecol Clin North Am.* 2000;27:705–772
25. Gold MA, Duffy K. Extended cycling or continuous use of hormonal contraceptives for female adolescents. *Curr Opin Obstet Gynecol.* 2009;21(5):407–411
26. den Tonkelaar I, Oddens BJ. Preferred frequency and characteristics of menstrual bleeding in relation to reproductive status, oral contraceptive use, and hormone replacement therapy use. *Contraception.* 1999;59:357–362
27. Wieder DR, Pattimakiel L. Examining the efficacy, safety, and patient acceptability of the combined contraceptive vaginal ring (NuvaRing). *Int J Womens Health.* 2010;2:401–409
28. New Product Review (September 2003). Norelgestromin/ethinyl oestradiol transdermal contraceptive system (evra). *J Fam Plann Reprod Health Care.* 2004;30(1):43–45
29. Sucato GS, Land SR, Murray PJ, Cecchini R, Gold MA. Adolescents' experiences using the contraceptive patch versus pills. *J Pediatr Adolesc Gynecol.* 2011: epub ahead of print
30. Harel Z, Riggs S, Vaz R, Flanagan P, Dunn K, Harel D. Adolescents' experience with the combined estrogen and progestin transdermal contraceptive method Ortho Evra. *J Pediatr Adol Gynecol.* 2005;18(2):85–90
31. Rubinstein ML, Halpern-Felsher BL, Irwin CE Jr. An evaluation of the use of the transdermal contraceptive patch in adolescents. *J Adolesc Health.* 2004;34(5)395–401
32. Zieman M, Guillebaud J, Weisberg E, Shangold GA, Fisher AC, Creasy GW. Contraceptive efficacy and cycle control with the Ortho Evra/Evra transdermal system: the analysis of pooled data. *Fertil Steril.* 2002;77(2 Suppl 2):S13–18
33. Cole JA, Norman H, Doherty M, Walker AM. Venous thromboembolism, myocardial infarction, and stroke among transdermal contraceptive system users. *Obstet Gynecol.* 2007;109(2):339–346
34. Moghissi KA, Syner FN, McBride LC. Contraceptive mechanism of microdose norethindrone. *Obstet Gynecol.* 1971;4:585.
35. Godsland IF, Crook D, Simpson R, et al. The effects of different formulations of oral contraceptive agents on lipid and carbohydrate metabolism. *N Engl J Med.* 1990;15;323(20):1375–1381
36. Kjos SL, Peters RK, Xiang A, Thomas D, Schaefer U, Buchanan TA. Contraception and the risk of type 2 diabetes mellitus in Latina women with prior gestational diabetes mellitus. *JAMA.* 1998;280(6):533–538
37. Broome M, Fotherby K. Clinical experience with the progestogen-only pill. *Contraception.* 1990;42(5):489–495
38. Tayob Y, Adams J, Jacobs HS, Guillebaud J. Ultrasound demonstration of increased frequency of functional ovarian cysts in women using progestogen-only oral contraception. *Br J Obstet Gynaecol.* 1985;92(10):1003–1009
39. Jain J, Jakimiuk AJ, Bode FR, Ross D, Kaunitz AM. Contraceptive efficacy and safety of DMPA-SC. *Contraception.* 2004;70(4):269–275
40. Bassol S, Garza-Flores J, Cravioto MC, et al. Ovarian function following a single administration of depo-medroxyprogesterone acetate (DMPA) at different doses. *Fertil Steril.* 1984;42(2):216–222
41. Smith RD, Cromer BA, Hayes JR, et al., Medroxyprogesterone acetate (Depo-Provera) use in adolescents: uterine bleeding and blood pressure patterns, patient satisfaction, and continuation rates. *Adolesc Pediatr Gynecol.* 1995;8:24
42. Polaneczky M, Liblanc M. Long-term depot medroxyprogesterone acetate (Depo-Provera) use in inner-city adolescents. *J Adolesc Health.* 1998;23(2):81–88
43. Harel Z, Biro FM, Kollar LM, Rauh JL. Adolescents' reasons for and experience after discontinuation of the long-acting contraceptives Depo-Provera and Norplant. *J Adolesc Health.* 1996;19(2):118–123
44. Cromer BA, Bonny AE, Stager M, et al. Bone mineral density in adolescent females using injectable or oral contraceptives: a 24-month prospective study. *Fertil Steril.* 2008;90(6):2060–2067

45. Kaunitz AM, Miller PD, Rice VM, Ross D, McClung MR. Bone mineral density in women aged 25–35 years receiving depot medroxyprogesterone acetate: recovery following discontinuation. *Contraception.* 2006;74(2):90–99

46. Depot medroxyprogesterone acetate and bone effects. ACOG Committee Opinion No 415. American College of Obstetricians and Gynecologists. *Obstet Gynecol.* 2008;112:727–730

47. van Hylckama Vlieg A, Helmerhorst FM, Rosendaal FR. The risk of deep venous thrombosis associated with injectable depot-medroxyprogesterone acetate contraceptives or a levonorgestrel intrauterine device. *Arterioscler Thromb Vasc Biol.* 2010;30(11):2297–2300

48. Wenzl R, van Beek A, Schnabel P, Huber J. Pharmacokinetics of etonogestrel released from the contraceptive implant Implanon. *Contraception.* 1998;58(5):283–288

49. Mäkäräinen L, van Beek A, Tuomivaara L, Asplund B, Coelingh Bennink H. Ovarian function during the use of a single contraceptive implant: Implanon compared with Norplant. *Fertil Steril.* 1998;69(4):714–721

50. Darney P, Patel A, Rosen K, Shapiro LS, Kaunitz AM. Safety and efficacy of a single-rod etonogestrel implant (Implanon): results from 11 international clinical trials. *Fertil Steril.* 2009;91(5):1646–1653

51. MacIsaac L, Espey E. Intrauterine contraception: the pendulum swings back. *Obstet Gynecol Clin North Am.* 2007;34(1):91–111

52. Farley TM, Rosenberg MJ, Rowe PJ, Chen JH, Meirik O. Intrauterine devices and pelvic inflammatory disease: an international perspective. *Lancet.* 1992;339(8796):785–788

53. Intrauterine device and adolescents. ACOG Committee Opinion No. 392. American College of Obstetricians and Gynecologists. *Obstet Gynecol.* 2007;110:1493–1495

54. Andersson K, Batar I, Rybo G. Return to fertility after removal of a levonorgestrel-releasing intrauterine device and Nova-T. *Contraception.* 1992;46(6):575–584

55. Hidalgo M, Bahamondes L, Perrotti M, Diaz J, Dantas-Monteiro C, Petta C. Bleeding patterns and clinical performance of the levonorgestrel-releasing intrauterine system (Mirena) up to two years. *Contraception.* 2002;65(2):129–132

56. Andersson K, Odlind V, Rybo G. Levonorgestrel-releasing and copper-releasing (Nova T) IUDs during five years of use: a randomized comparative trial. *Contraception.* 1994;49(1):56–72

57. Zhou L, Xiao B. Emergency contraception with Multiload Cu-375 SL IUD: a multicenter clinical trial. *Contraception.* 2001;64(2):107–112

58. CDC. U.S. medical eligibility criteria for contraceptive use, adapted from the World Health Organization medical eligibility criteria for contraceptive use, 4th edition. *MMWR.* 2010; 59(No. RR-4)

59. Tankeyoon M, Dusitsin N, Chalapati S, et al. Effects of hormonal contraceptives on milk volume and infant growth. WHO Special Programme of Research, Development and Research Training in Human Reproduction Task force on oral contraceptives. *Contraception.* 1984;30(6):505

60. Chen BA, Reeves MF, Hayes JL, Hohmann HL, Perriera LK, Creinin MD. Postplacental or delayed insertion of the levonorgestrel intrauterine device after vaginal delivery: a randomized controlled trial. *Obstet Gynecol.* 2010;116(5):1079–1087

61. Thurman AR, Hammond N, Brown HE, Roddy ME. Preventing repeat teen pregnancy: postpartum depot medroxyprogesterone acetate, oral contraceptive pills, or the patch? *J Pediatr Adolesc Gynecol.* 2007;20(2):61–65

62. Nakajima ST. *Contemporary Guide to Contraception.* 3rd ed. Newtown, PA: Handbooks in Health Care; 2007

63. Roddy RE, Zekeng L, Ryan KA, Tamoufé U, Weir SS, Wong EL. A controlled trial of nonoxynol 9 film to reduce male-to-female transmission of sexually transmitted diseases. *N Engl J Med.* 1998;339(8):504–510

64. Surís JC, Resnick MD, Cassuto N, Blum RW. Sexual behavior of adolescents with chronic disease and disability. *J Adolesc Health.* 1996;19(2):124–131

Adolesc Med 23 (2012) 111–122

Fertility Preservation for Adolescent Women with Cancer

Jonathan D. Fish, MD*

Section Head, Survivors Facing Forward Program, Hematology/Oncology and Stem Cell Transplantation, Steven and Alexandra Cohen Children's Medical Center of New York, New Hyde Park, New York, 11040

INTRODUCTION

The past 4 decades have transformed outcomes for children with cancer, thereby completely altering the field of pediatric oncology itself. Although overall survival for a child diagnosed with cancer in 2011 is approaching 80%, the prospect of curing large numbers of children was only becoming reality in the 1970s. It was thus truly remarkable that in 1975 Dr. Giulio D'Angio presciently declared that "a parallel effort is required in oncology so that the children of today don't become the chronically ill adults of tomorrow."[1] With the prevalence of childhood cancer survivors in America now approaching 1 in 450 young adults,[2] recent publications have revealed that 62% of current survivors have developed at least one chronic health condition, 27% a severe or life-threatening condition, and 18% have died within 30 years of diagnosis.[3,4] These data have made survivorship, a focus on the long-term health and well-being of survivors of childhood cancer, a specialized field in its own right. The long-term, therapy-related complications faced by survivors can be multisystem and complex, requiring extensive, intricate follow-up to maintain survivors' health and quality of life.[5-7] It is thus imperative that primary care physicians and specialists develop a level of comfort both in understanding and managing the unique health challenges faced by survivors of adolescent cancer.[8]

The survival gains achieved in children with cancer have come as a result of improvements in surgical technique, supportive care, changes in dosing and scheduling of chemotherapeutic agents, and refinement in the modalities of radiation therapy. Although the improvement in survival has been truly remark-

*Corresponding author.
E-mail address: JFish1@NSHS.EDU (J. D. Fish).

able, even the most modern approaches to treating cancer can lead to life-altering, long-term morbidities. For many young women treated for cancer, ovarian dysfunction is one of those morbidities. Approximately 6% of female childhood cancer survivors experience acute ovarian failure (AOF), defined as permanent loss of ovarian function within 5 years of diagnosis.[9,10] An additional 15% experience premature ovarian insufficiency (POI), defined as loss of ovarian function before age 40.[10] The actual, or even potential, loss of fertility can have a profound impact on the well-being of childhood cancer survivors.[11-13]

Adolescent boys typically have the option of sperm banking before therapy to preserve fertility.[14] There is no analogous modality available to adolescent women. Embryo cryopreservation remains the only standard-of-care method for fertility preservation available to adolescent women. This modality involves ovarian stimulation, invasive harvest of oocytes, in vitro fertilization, frozen storage of the resulting embryos, and ultimately transfer back into the uterus. This sequence presents numerous, often insurmountable, barriers to adolescents, including the need to harvest oocytes before treatment and the need to identify a male to serve as the father of future children. Thus, although embryo cryopreservation is an option in the rare case, it is not an ideal approach to fertility preservation for most adolescent women. Several detailed reviews have been published on fertility preservation options for the young cancer patient.[15-17] The focus of this article is on the developing modalities of fertility preservation for adolescent women diagnosed with cancer. The topic is covered in three sections: (1) identifying those at risk for infertility; (2) methods of a priori risk reduction for infertility; and (3) oocyte and ovarian cryopreservation.

IDENTIFYING THOSE AT RISK FOR INFERTILITY

In a simplistic but reasonably accurate conception, cancers occur when a cell incurs functional changes that abrogate both its ability to undergo normal differentiation and its ability to undergo apoptosis, or programmed cell death.[18] Despite the many advances in cancer treatment over the past several decades, the general principle of most cancer therapies is to selectively damage and kill those cells undergoing uncontrolled division. Although this approach effectively targets cancerous cells, normal "bystander" tissues, including mucosal, hair, and gonadal tissue, are often affected by the toxins commonly used.

Although there has been a recent suggestion that ovarian germ cells may be able to expand after birth, most theories hold that women are born with a finite number of ovarian follicles.[19] As they age, women lose primordial follicles through maturation and atresia in an accelerating manner until a threshold is reached, at which point ovarian function ceases and menopause ensues. The size of the oocyte pool for a given age in an otherwise healthy woman can be predicted by mathematical models, such as the Faddy-Gosden model.[20,21] Injury to the ovaries caused by anticancer therapies, including chemotherapy or radiation, decreases the size of the remaining oocyte pool. The degree of oocyte depletion, in turn, affects the age at which a girl or woman treated with anticancer agents experiences ovarian failure and menopause.

The study of long-term childhood cancer survivors has taught us that the risk of late effects, including ovarian dysfunction, can be predicted based on the exposures a patient received as part of cancer treatment. The risk-based approach to providing an appropriate screening regimen for a given cancer survivor has been codified in a standardized set of guidelines developed by the Late Effects Committee and Nursing Discipline of the Children's Oncology Group[22] (available at www.survivorshipguidelines.org). Although there are no absolute predictive models of which female cancer patients will experience ovarian failure or when they may experience it, the past 40 years have provided a picture of the relative ovarian toxicities of various anticancer agents and regimens. In particular, radiation to the ovaries and high cumulative doses of alkylating agents carry the highest risks of significant ovarian damage. Models have been developed to predict the effective sterilizing doses of radiation based on the age of the patient at the time of treatment,[23] but even lower doses of direct radiation to the ovary as part of whole-abdomen, pelvic, or total body irradiation have a profound impact on ovarian reserves.[9,24,25] Likewise, higher cumulative doses of alkylating agents, a class of drugs including cyclophosphamide, ifosfamide, busulfan, melphalan, mechlorethamine, and procarbazine, can negatively affect ovarian function.[26-28] A recent study of survivors of Hodgkin lymphoma diagnosed at a young age (14–40 years) found that the alkylating agents had the strongest association with POI in a dose-dependent manner.[29] In the population of children with cancer, pelvic radiation and alkylating agents are commonly used as part of therapy for higher stage Hodgkin lymphoma, solid tumors such as rhabdomyosarcoma, Ewing sarcoma, or neuroblastoma and as part of conditioning regimens for hematopoietic stem cell transplantation for high-risk or relapsed leukemias. This is particularly relevant to the adolescent population as Hodgkin lymphoma and Ewing sarcoma predominantly occur in this age group. When assessing the risk for ovarian dysfunction and formulating a reproductive plan for adolescent cancer survivors, it is therefore imperative to have access to a total treatment summary and cumulative doses of alkylators and radiation in particular.

METHODS OF *A PRIORI* RISK REDUCTION FOR INFERTILITY

Reduction of Therapy

The best way to preserve fertility in adolescent women diagnosed with cancer is to reduce the risk of infertility by delivering less gonadal-toxic treatment. As the field of pediatric oncology has evolved to have a greater focus on the late effects of therapy, this has translated into a new paradigm of protocol development stressing the reduction of therapy whenever possible. This paradigm is perhaps best exemplified by the protocols being developed for the treatment of Hodgkin lymphoma. Hodgkin lymphoma is one of the more common cancers diagnosed in adolescence and is among the most curable.[30] Although the disease-free survival from Hodgkin lymphoma is outstanding, the modalities used to treat it have resulted in some of the highest rates of late effects.[31] Earlier treatment regimens involved substantial exposure to alkylators, and often pelvic radiation, resulting in high rates of reduced ovarian function.[26,27] Based on data showing that a group of patients with Hodgkin lymphoma may not benefit from radiation therapy,[32] the most recent protocols for Hodgkin lymphoma developed by the Children's Oncology Group have not only substantially reduced the exposure to alkylators but are also exploring the safety of eliminating radiation for a subset of patients. These modifications will hopefully result in improved fertility outcomes for these patients at high risk for ovarian dysfunction. Despite this change in focus, there are still many adolescent women for whom pelvic radiation will remain a mainstay of therapy for the foreseeable future. Modern techniques for delivering radiation, such as intensity-modulated radiotherapy, may minimize the exposure of the ovary to radiation used for the treatment of pelvic tumors.[33] Nonetheless, not all patients can benefit from these techniques, and for these patients, alternative means of reducing the risk of infertility require exploration.

Oophoropexy

Oophoropexy is a surgical procedure undertaken in women scheduled to receive focal pelvic radiation in which the ovaries are transposed within the pelvic cavity to a site outside of the radiation field. Although there is no benefit to oophoropexy in children receiving total body irradiation, partial pelvic radiation is commonly part of therapy for Hodgkin lymphoma and pelvic solid tumors, whereas total spinal radiation may be used for certain central nervous system tumors. For those patients in whom the elimination of pelvic radiation would substantially reduce their chance of cure, oophoropexy may help preserve ovarian function. The first report describing the use of oophoropexy to preserve fertility was in 1968, when it was performed in young women being treated for Hodgkin lymphoma.[34] This report described 8 live births from 6 patients who had undergone oophoropexy before radiation; it demonstrated a 60% pregnancy rate. Since that time, multiple studies have confirmed the utility of oophoropexy in young women who require pelvic radiation, including total spinal radiation.[35-38] Although oophoropexy was originally abandoned because it interfered with surgical staging and radiation fields, surgical staging for Hodgkin disease is no longer performed, and radiation fields have become much more precise. Additionally, surgical techniques have improved, and oophoropexy can now be performed laparoscopically in a minimally invasive manner.[38,39] Despite the apparent benefit for a subset of patients, there have been no large, randomized trials in young women undergoing pelvic radiation comparing the rate of fertility preservation in those who undergo oophoropexy before radiation with those who do not. There are additional concerns that impact the effectiveness of this technique. First, it would provide little benefit for those receiving higher doses of alkylators along with radiation. Second, women receiving pelvic radiation may also have their uterus radiated, thereby reducing the chance of a successful pregnancy.[40] Finally, the potential exists for oophoropexy to interfere with oocyte retrieval for in vitro fertilization, should it be needed by the patient in the future.

Ovarian Suppression

Historically, it was noted that younger girls had lower rates of ovarian failure than older girls and women when exposed to gonadal toxic chemotherapies.[41] It is now generally accepted that younger girls retain ovarian function for a period of time after therapy because they have a larger pool of primordial follicles at the time of treatment, not that the chemotherapy is less toxic to the ovary. Although these younger girls may retain ovarian function for a period of time, they remain at risk for POI.[10] Nonetheless, this historical observation helped lead to the hypothesis that ovarian suppression in the adolescent or young adult would mimic the pre-pubertal state and thereby offer ovarian protection from cancer treatment. This, in turn, has resulted in the postulate that gonadotropin releasing hormone (GnRH) analogs can act as an ovarian protector during the treatment of adolescents and young women with cancer. GnRH analogs impact pituitary function, reversibly decreasing the production of folliclular stimulating hormone (FSH) and luteinizing hormone (LH). As primordial follicles have not been demonstrated to express GnRH receptors, and the early phases of follicular maturation are thought to be FSH independent,[42,43] the mechanism through which GnRH analogs would offer protection to the oocyte pool remains unclear. Most studies examining the use of GnRH analogs for fertility preservation in cancer patients have been nonrandomized, retrospective trials and have examined disparate patient groups and disparate treatment regimens, thus rendering any conclusions questionable.[44,45] There have been a few prospective randomized trials examining this question, but these, too, have had conflicting results.[46,47] A recent meta-analysis of the available literature has done little to resolve the question.[48] This study found a protective effect for GnRH analogs on ovarian function when proxy outcomes were measured, such as the resumption of menses or FSH levels. When actual pregnancy rates were examined, they found higher success rates in the GnRH analog-treated patients when analyzing observational trials, but lower success rates than in the controls in randomized controlled trials.

In summary, the use of GnRH analogs for fertility preservation in adolescent women being treated for cancer has not been demonstrated to be efficacious. However, the data are less than conclusive, and prospective, randomized trials are desperately needed to answer this important question.

Oocyte and Ovarian Cryopreservation

Despite the methods described in the previous section for risk-reduction of infertility in adolescent women being treated for cancer, many still face the prospect of reduced fertility following treatment. For these women, fertility preservation presently hinges on the capacity to harvest and store the currency of fertility before the delivery of gonadal-toxic therapies; namely embryos, oocytes, or ovarian tissue. Although embryo cryopreservation has been extensively developed since the first pregnancy achieved from a cryopreserved embryo in 1983[49] and the first successful birth from a frozen embryo in 1984,[50] it is only rarely a viable option for the adolescent with cancer. Although the time and methodologies needed to achieve oocyte harvest are certainly barriers to the use of this modality, the most substantial barrier to embryo cryopreservation in this population is the need to identify a desirable sperm donor. Recognizing that many young women receiving treatment for cancer do not have a partner with whom they would wish to create embryos, for the past 2 decades fertility preservation science has been focused on cryopreservation of the oocyte and ovarian tissue.

Oocyte Cryopreservation

The first success at freezing, thawing, and fertilizing a human oocyte was reported in 1986.[51] Over the past $2^1/_2$ decades, the science of oocyte cryopreservation has experienced remarkable advances, with each year bringing improvements. The first successful live birth from an oocyte cryopreserved from a young woman with cancer was reported in 2007. The oocyte was harvested from a young woman with Hodgkin lymphoma, and the child was delivered through a surrogate gestational carrier.[52] The first case of a cancer survivor delivering her own child fertilized from a cryopreserved oocyte obtained before her cancer treatment was reported in 2008.[53] A meta-analysis published in 2006 on the effectiveness of oocyte cryopreservation based on reports in the literature found that the rate of live births per oocyte thawed was approximately 2%, and the live-birth rate per injected oocyte was 2.4% for cryopreserved oocytes, as compared to 6.6% for unfrozen oocytes.[54] Although this suggested that the efficiency of in vitro fertilization with unfrozen oocytes was substantially better than with frozen oocytes, oocyte cryopreservation reached a level of success such that it could become a viable fertility preservation option for adolescent girls with newly diagnosed cancer. With newer freezing techniques, including vitrification technology, the success of oocyte cryopreservation will likely continue to improve, although the data remain limited.[55] As the number of live births from cryopreserved oocytes has increased, the rates of chromosomal abnormalities and birth defects have remained reassuring.[56,57] To address the pressing need for more information on the efficiency and safety of oocyte cryopreservation, a 5-year national study, the Human Oocyte Preservation Registry, has been recently developed to monitor the long-term risk of this technique.[58] As oocyte cryopreservation for the adolescent with cancer is still considered experimental, it should be undertaken in the context of an Institutional Review Board (IRB)-approved clinical trial at a center with experience with the technique.

The process of oocyte cryopreservation typically involves gonadotropin administration for 10–14 days with close monitoring through transabdominal ultrasound and hormone levels, followed by a transvaginal oocyte harvest under sedation. In order to benefit from oocyte cryopreservation, adolescent women newly diagnosed with cancer must be informed of their risk for infertility; must regard fertility preservation as a high priority; and the patient, the family, and the oncologist must believe that fertility is likely to be best preserved through oocyte cryopreservation. Should the decision be made to pursue oocyte cryopreservation, a center must be identified with the capacity to undertake oocyte harvest and storage in an adolescent population, and the harvest must be able to proceed without substantial delay, as oocyte harvesting necessitates some delay in initiating treatment of the cancer. Many of these steps present significant barriers to undertaking this fertility preservation technique. Additionally, this technique is only applicable to adolescent patients who have experienced menarche. For those in whom oocyte cryopreservation is not an option, fertility researchers have begun to focus on ovarian harvest and cryopreservation.

Ovarian Cryopreservation

For premenarchal adolescent girls facing the risk of infertility from cancer treatment, or for those in whom the time required to perform an oocyte harvest would present an unacceptable delay in treatment, the ability to collect, preserve, and then reimplant ovarian tissue becomes the only option for fertility preservation. This has been accomplished by surgically collecting ovarian strips, either during a discrete laparoscopic procedure, or concomitantly with another planned procedure to minimize the number of episodes of general anesthesia. The advantages to this technique include the ability to perform it on any female, prepubertal or pubertal, and the lack of any significant delay in therapy as a consequence of the procedure.

Following several decades of progressively more intricate animal models,[59-61] researchers began to study human ovarian tissue autografting for women with cancer in the 1990s.[62,63] These groups faced many questions, including how best to cryopreserve the ovarian tissue and where to reimplant it. Conceptually, there are two possible re-implantation options—orthotopically into the decorticated remaining ovary or the pelvic peritoneum or heterotopically to other sites including the forearm, abdominal wall, or chest wall. The advantages to heterotopic sites include the ease of performing the reimplantation and the theoretical ease of later harvesting oocytes for in vitro fertilization. By the early 2000s one group reported a series of women who had had ovarian cortical autologous transplants.[64] Hormonal recovery was documented, several oocytes were aspirated, and 1 embryo was produced, but no pregnancies ensued from the transplants. They postulated that orthotopically placed ovarian tissue alters the quality of recovered oocytes. The first report of a live birth following autologous transplantation of ovarian tissue was recorded in 2004 for a woman who was menopausal following treatment for Hodgkin lymphoma.[65] Since then, a number of live births have been reported, including a child born to a woman who underwent a bone marrow transplant for sickle cell disease.[66] She was menopausal for 2.5 years after having received conditioning with high doses of alkylating agents. Following an autologous, orthotopic transplant of ovarian cortical tissue she conceived during a natural menstrual cycle and ultimately delivered a healthy child approximately 1 year after the ovarian transplant.

Although these successes demonstrate exciting potential for this method of fertility preservation, the feasibility and effectiveness of ovarian cryopreservation and reimplantation for large numbers of young women with cancer have not been adequately tested. Aside from the lack of comprehensive data, there remain many concerns. These include the concern that the removal of healthy ovarian tissue before treatment could negatively impact the fertility potential for a woman who could have otherwise experienced a period of ovarian functional recovery post-treatment; concern that the invasive nature of ovarian harvest may carry finite anesthetic or surgical risks; and concern that the reimplantation of autologous tissue harvested from a patient with cancer before any antineoplastic therapy could result in a reintroduction of the cancer. In addressing the latter question, one group examined 26 ovarian specimens from women with Hodgkin lymphoma before cancer treatment and found no evidence of disease.[67] Although the true risk of transmitting malignancy through ovarian autografting remains unknown, some groups are addressing the theoretical risk by harvesting ovarian tissue after the first cycle of chemotherapy,[63] or by examining the tissue with sensitive techniques to detect minimal residual disease.[68]

Although ovarian transplantation may represent an excellent option in the future for preserving fertility in the adolescent with cancer, much work remains to confirm its safety and feasibility on a larger scale. Given the potential risks, this method of fertility preservation for adolescents should only be undertaken at a center with experience harvesting and preserving ovarian tissue and should only be undertaken in the setting of an IRB-approved protocol.

CONCLUSION

As more and more adolescent and young adult women are surviving cancer, the focus on their reproductive potential has intensified. Although the optimal approach to fertility preservation in this patient group is to minimize the risk of infertility a priori, some patients are still at risk for infertility or a reduced fertility window with even the most modern therapies. To address the reproductive needs of these patients, techniques such as oocyte or ovarian tissue cryopreservation are undergoing substantial clinical investigation and will likely become standard-of-care fertility preservation options in the near future. Future avenues of research have included the ex vivo maturation of primordial follicles[69] and organ culture with the capacity to retain the organization structure of the ovarian tissue.[70]

For the individual adolescent woman with cancer, the best approach is for the physicians responsible for her care to assess the potential risk for infertility based on the treatments she is scheduled to receive and to carefully explain to the patient and her family the fertility preservation options that are available. Although this may be a very challenging conversation at the time that a young woman has just been given a diagnosis of cancer, it ensures that she and her family are able to make an informed decision about how they would like to approach her reproductive future.

ACKNOWLEDGEMENTS

The author receives funding as a St. Baldrick's Foundation Scholar. We thank Joel Brochstein, MD, for his critical appraisal of the manuscript.

References

1. D'Angio GJ. Pediatric cancer in perspective: cure is not enough. *Cancer.* 1975;35(3 suppl):866–870
2. Bhatia S, Yasui Y, Robison LL, Birch JM, Bogue MK, Diller L, et al. High risk of subsequent neoplasms continues with extended follow-up of childhood Hodgkin's disease: report from the Late Effects Study Group. *J Clin Oncol.* 2003;21(23):4386–4394
3. Armstrong GT, Liu Q, Yasui Y, Neglia JP, Leisenring W, Robison LL, et al. Late mortality among 5-year survivors of childhood cancer: a summary from the Childhood Cancer Survivor Study. *J Clin Oncol.* 2009;27(14):2328–2338
4. Oeffinger KC, Mertens AC, Sklar CA, Kawashima T, Hudson MM, Meadows AT, et al. Chronic health conditions in adult survivors of childhood cancer. *N Engl J Med.* 2006;355(15):1572–1582
5. Dickerman JD. The late effects of childhood cancer therapy. *Pediatrics.* 2007;119(3):554–568
6. Hudson MM. Survivors of childhood cancer: coming of age. *Hematol Oncol Clin North Am.* 2008;22(2):211–231, v–vi
7. Robison LL. Treatment-associated subsequent neoplasms among long-term survivors of childhood cancer: the experience of the Childhood Cancer Survivor Study. *Pediatr Radiol.* 2009;39 Suppl 1:S32–37
8. Oeffinger KC, Tonorezos ES. The cancer is over, now what?: understanding risk, changing outcomes. *Cancer.* 2011;117(10 Suppl):2250–2257
9. Chemaitilly W, Mertens AC, Mitby P, Whitton J, Stovall M, Yasui Y, et al. Acute ovarian failure in the childhood cancer survivor study. *J Clin Endocrinol Metab.* 2006;91(5):1723–1728
10. Sklar CA, Mertens AC, Mitby P, Whitton J, Stovall M, Kasper C, et al. Premature menopause in survivors of childhood cancer: a report from the childhood cancer survivor study. *J Natl Cancer Inst.* 2006;98(13):890–896
11. Schover LR. Psychosocial aspects of infertility and decisions about reproduction in young cancer survivors: a review. *Med Pediatr Oncol.* 1999;33(1):53–59
12. Wenzel L, Dogan-Ates A, Habbal R, Berkowitz R, Goldstein DP, Bernstein M, et al. Defining and measuring reproductive concerns of female cancer survivors. *J Natl Cancer Inst Monogr.* 2005(34):94–98
13. Schover LR. Patient attitudes toward fertility preservation. *Pediatr Blood Cancer.* 2009;53(2):281–284
14. Tournaye H, Goossens E, Verheyen G, Frederickx V, De Block G, Devroey P, et al. Preserving the reproductive potential of men and boys with cancer: current concepts and future prospects. *Hum Reprod Update.* 2004;10(6):525–532

15. Levine J, Canada A, Stern CJ. Fertility preservation in adolescents and young adults with cancer. *J Clin Oncol.* 2010;28(32):4831–4841

16. Oktay K, Oktem O. Fertility preservation medicine: a new field in the care of young cancer survivors. *Pediatr Blood Cancer.* 2009;53(2):267–273

17. Wallace WH, Anderson RA, Irvine DS. Fertility preservation for young patients with cancer: who is at risk and what can be offered? *Lancet Oncol.* 2005;6(4):209–218

18. Hanahan D, Weinberg RA. Hallmarks of cancer: the next generation. *Cell.* 2011;144(5):646–674

19. Johnson J, Canning J, Kaneko T, Pru JK, Tilly JL. Germline stem cells and follicular renewal in the postnatal mammalian ovary. *Nature.* 2004;428(6979):145–150

20. Faddy MJ, Gosden RG. A model conforming the decline in follicle numbers to the age of menopause in women. *Hum Reprod.* 1996;11(7):1484–1486

21. Faddy MJ, Gosden RG, Gougeon A, Richardson SJ, Nelson JF. Accelerated disappearance of ovarian follicles in mid-life: implications for forecasting menopause. *Hum Reprod.* 1992;7(10):1342–1346

22. Landier W, Bhatia S, Eshelman DA, Forte KJ, Sweeney T, Hester AL, et al. Development of risk-based guidelines for pediatric cancer survivors: the Children's Oncology Group Long-Term Follow-Up Guidelines from the Children's Oncology Group Late Effects Committee and Nursing Discipline. *J Clin Oncol.* 2004;22(24):4979–4990

23. Wallace WH, Thomson AB, Saran F, Kelsey TW. Predicting age of ovarian failure after radiation to a field that includes the ovaries. *Int J Radiat Oncol Biol Phys.* 2005;62(3):738–744

24. Bath LE, Wallace WH, Shaw MP, Fitzpatrick C, Anderson RA. Depletion of ovarian reserve in young women after treatment for cancer in childhood: detection by anti-Mullerian hormone, inhibin B and ovarian ultrasound. *Hum Reprod.* 2003;18(11):2368–2374

25. Wallace WH, Thomson AB, Kelsey TW. The radiosensitivity of the human oocyte. *Hum Reprod.* 2003;18(1):117–121

26. Byrne J, Mulvihill JJ, Myers MH, Connelly RR, Naughton MD, Krauss MR, et al. Effects of treatment on fertility in long-term survivors of childhood or adolescent cancer. *N Engl J Med.* 1987;317(21):1315–1321

27. Chiarelli AM, Marrett LD, Darlington G. Early menopause and infertility in females after treatment for childhood cancer diagnosed in 1964–1988 in Ontario, Canada. *Am J Epidemiol.* 1999;150(3):245–254

28. Nicosia SV, Matus-Ridley M, Meadows AT. Gonadal effects of cancer therapy in girls. *Cancer.* 1985;55(10):2364–2372

29. De Bruin ML, Huisbrink J, Hauptmann M, Kuenen MA, Ouwens GM, van't Veer MB, et al. Treatment-related risk factors for premature menopause following Hodgkin lymphoma. *Blood.* 2008;111(1):101–108

30. Schwartz CL, Constine LS, Villaluna D, London WB, Hutchison RE, Sposto R, et al. A risk-adapted, response-based approach using ABVE-PC for children and adolescents with intermediate- and high-risk Hodgkin lymphoma: the results of P9425. *Blood.* 2009;114(10):2051–2059

31. Castellino SM, Geiger AM, Mertens AC, Leisenring WM, Tooze JA, Goodman P, et al. Morbidity and mortality in long-term survivors of Hodgkin lymphoma: a report from the Childhood Cancer Survivor Study. *Blood.* 2010;117(6):1806–1816

32. Weiner MA, Leventhal B, Brecher ML, Marcus RB, Cantor A, Gieser PW, et al. Randomized study of intensive MOPP-ABVD with or without low-dose total-nodal radiation therapy in the treatment of stages IIB, IIIA2, IIIB, and IV Hodgkin's disease in pediatric patients: a Pediatric Oncology Group study. *J Clin Oncol.* 1997;15(8):2769–2779

33. Guerrero Urbano MT, Nutting CM. Clinical use of intensity-modulated radiotherapy: part II. *Br J Radiol.* 2004;77(915):177–182

34. Le Floch O, Donaldson SS, Kaplan HS. Pregnancy following oophoropexy and total nodal irradiation in women with Hodgkin's disease. *Cancer.* 1976;38(6):2263–2268

35. Husseinzadeh N, Nahhas WA, Velkley DE, Whitney CW, Mortel R. The preservation of ovarian function in young women undergoing pelvic radiation therapy. *Gynecol Oncol.* 1984;18(3):373–379

36. Morice P, Castaigne D, Haie-Meder C, Pautier P, El Hassan J, Duvillard P, et al. Laparoscopic ovarian transposition for pelvic malignancies: indications and functional outcomes. *Fertil Steril.* 1998;70(5):956–960
37. Terenziani M, Piva L, Meazza C, Gandola L, Cefalo G, Merola M. Oophoropexy: a relevant role in preservation of ovarian function after pelvic irradiation. *Fertil Steril.* 2009;91(3):935 e15–16
38. Kuohung W, Ram K, Cheng DM, Marcus KJ, Diller LR, Laufer MR. Laparoscopic oophoropexy prior to radiation for pediatric brain tumor and subsequent ovarian function. *Hum Reprod.* 2008;23(1):117–121
39. Williams RS, Littell RD, Mendenhall NP. Laparoscopic oophoropexy and ovarian function in the treatment of Hodgkin disease. *Cancer.* 1999;86(10):2138–2142
40. Critchley HO, Wallace WH. Impact of cancer treatment on uterine function. *J Natl Cancer Inst Monogr.* 2005(34):64–68
41. Siris ES, Leventhal BG, Vaitukaitis JL. Effects of childhood leukemia and chemotherapy on puberty and reproductive function in girls. *N Engl J Med.* 1976;294(21):1143–1146
42. McNatty KP, Smith P, Moore LG, Reader K, Lun S, Hanrahan JP, et al. Oocyte-expressed genes affecting ovulation rate. *Mol Cell Endocrinol.* 2005;234(1–2):57–66
43. Oktay K, Sonmezer M. Ovarian tissue banking for cancer patients: fertility preservation, not just ovarian cryopreservation. *Hum Reprod.* 2004;19(3):477–480
44. Beck-Fruchter R, Weiss A, Shalev E. GnRH agonist therapy as ovarian protectants in female patients undergoing chemotherapy: a review of the clinical data. *Hum Reprod Update.* 2008;14(6):553–561
45. Blumenfeld Z, Avivi I, Eckman A, Epelbaum R, Rowe JM, Dann EJ. Gonadotropin-releasing hormone agonist decreases chemotherapy-induced gonadotoxicity and premature ovarian failure in young female patients with Hodgkin lymphoma. *Fertil Steril.* 2008;89(1):166–173
46. Badawy A, Elnashar A, El-Ashry M, Shahat M. Gonadotropin-releasing hormone agonists for prevention of chemotherapy-induced ovarian damage: prospective randomized study. *Fertil Steril.* 2009;91(3):694–697
47. Waxman JH, Ahmed R, Smith D, Wrigley PF, Gregory W, Shalet S, et al. Failure to preserve fertility in patients with Hodgkin's disease. *Cancer Chemother Pharmacol.* 1987;19(2):159–162
48. Ben-Aharon I, Gafter-Gvili A, Leibovici L, Stemmer SM. Pharmacological interventions for fertility preservation during chemotherapy: a systematic review and meta-analysis. *Breast Cancer Res Treat.* 2010;122(3):803–811
49. Trounson A, Mohr L. Human pregnancy following cryopreservation, thawing and transfer of an eight-cell embryo. *Nature.* 1983;305(5936):707–709
50. Downing BG, Mohr LR, Trounson AO, Freemann LE, Wood C. Birth after transfer of cryopreserved embryos. *Med J Aust.* 1985;142(7):409–411
51. Chen C. Pregnancy after human oocyte cryopreservation. *Lancet.* 1986;1(8486):884–886
52. Yang D, Brown SE, Nguyen K, Reddy V, Brubaker C, Winslow KL. Live birth after the transfer of human embryos developed from cryopreserved oocytes harvested before cancer treatment. *Fertil Steril.* 2007;87(6):1469 e1–4
53. Porcu E, Venturoli S, Damiano G, Ciotti PM, Notarangelo L, Paradisi R, et al. Healthy twins delivered after oocyte cryopreservation and bilateral ovariectomy for ovarian cancer. *Reprod Biomed Online.* 2008;17(2):265–267
54. Oktay K, Cil AP, Bang H. Efficiency of oocyte cryopreservation: a meta-analysis. *Fertil Steril.* 2006;86(1):70–80
55. Smith GD, Serafini PC, Fioravanti J, Yadid I, Coslovsky M, Hassun P, et al. Prospective randomized comparison of human oocyte cryopreservation with slow-rate freezing or vitrification. *Fertil Steril.* 2010;94(6):2088–2095
56. Cobo A, Rubio C, Gerli S, Ruiz A, Pellicer A, Remohi J. Use of fluorescence in situ hybridization to assess the chromosomal status of embryos obtained from cryopreserved oocytes. *Fertil Steril.* 2001;75(2):354–360
57. Porcu E, Bazzocchi A, Notarangelo L, Paradisi R, Landolfo C, Venturoli S. Human oocyte cryopreservation in infertility and oncology. *Curr Opin Endocrinol Diabetes Obes.* 2008;15(6):529–535

58. Ezcurra D, Rangnow J, Craig M, Schertz J. The HOPE Registry: first US registry for oocyte cryo-preservation. *Reprod Biomed Online*. 2008;17(6):743–744
59. Aubard Y, Piver P, Cogni Y, Fermeaux V, Poulin N, Driancourt MA. Orthotopic and heterotopic autografts of frozen-thawed ovarian cortex in sheep. *Hum Reprod*. 1999;14(8):2149–2154
60. Baird DT, Webb R, Campbell BK, Harkness LM, Gosden RG. Long-term ovarian function in sheep after ovariectomy and transplantation of autografts stored at -196 C. *Endocrinology*. 1999;140(1):462–471
61. Gosden RG, Baird DT, Wade JC, Webb R. Restoration of fertility to oophorectomized sheep by ovarian autografts stored at -196 degrees C. *Hum Reprod*. 1994;9(4):597–603
62. Callejo J, Salvador C, Miralles A, Vilaseca S, Lailla JM, Balasch J. Long-term ovarian function evaluation after autografting by implantation with fresh and frozen-thawed human ovarian tissue. *J Clin Endocrinol Metab*. 2001;86(9):4489–4494
63. Radford JA, Lieberman BA, Brison DR, Smith AR, Critchlow JD, Russell SA, et al. Orthotopic reimplantation of cryopreserved ovarian cortical strips after high-dose chemotherapy for Hodgkin's lymphoma. *Lancet*. 2001;357(9263):1172–1175
64. Oktay K, Karlikaya G. Ovarian function after transplantation of frozen, banked autologous ovarian tissue. *N Engl J Med*. 2000;342(25):1919
65. Donnez J, Dolmans MM, Demylle D, Jadoul P, Pirard C, Squifflet J, et al. Livebirth after orthotopic transplantation of cryopreserved ovarian tissue. *Lancet*. 2004;364(9443):1405–1410
66. Roux C, Amiot C, Agnani G, Aubard Y, Rohrlich PS, Piver P. Live birth after ovarian tissue autograft in a patient with sickle cell disease treated by allogeneic bone marrow transplantation. *Fertil Steril*. 2010;93(7):2413.e15–19
67. Seshadri T, Gook D, Lade S, Spencer A, Grigg A, Tiedemann K, et al. Lack of evidence of disease contamination in ovarian tissue harvested for cryopreservation from patients with Hodgkin lymphoma and analysis of factors predictive of oocyte yield. *Br J Cancer*. 2006;94(7):1007–1010
68. Meirow D, Hardan I, Dor J, Fridman E, Elizur S, Ra'anani H, et al. Searching for evidence of disease and malignant cell contamination in ovarian tissue stored from hematologic cancer patients. *Hum Reprod*. 2008;23(5):1007–1013
69. Abir R, Nitke S, Ben-Haroush A, Fisch B. In vitro maturation of human primordial ovarian follicles: clinical significance, progress in mammals, and methods for growth evaluation. *Histol Histopathol*. 2006;21(8):887–898
70. Hovatta O, Silye R, Abir R, Krausz T, Winston RM. Extracellular matrix improves survival of both stored and fresh human primordial and primary ovarian follicles in long-term culture. *Hum Reprod*. 1997;12(5):1032–1036

Adolesc Med 23 (2012) 123–138

Pregnancy in Adolescents

Amanda Y. Black, MD, MPH[a], Nathalie A. Fleming, MD[b],
Ellen S. Rome, MD, MPH[c]*

[a]Department of Obstetrics, Gynecology, and Newborn Care,
The Ottawa Hospital; Division of Pediatric and Adolescent Gynecology,
The Children's Hospital of Eastern Ontario, 501 Smyth Road, Ottawa, Ontario, Canada, K1H 8L6

[b]Department of Obstetrics, Gynecology, and Newborn Care, The Ottawa Hospital; Chief,
Divison of Pediatric and Adolescent Gynecology, The Children's Hospital of Eastern Ontario,
501 Smyth Road, Ottawa, Ontario, Canada, K1H 8L6

[c]Head, Section of Adolescent Medicine, Cleveland Clinic Children's Hospital,
9500 Euclid Avenue, A120, Cleveland, Ohio 44195

INTRODUCTION

Adolescent pregnancy continues to be a social, emotional, and economic challenge for teens and society. Nearly two-thirds of births to women younger than 18 years and more than half of pregnancies to 18–19-year-old girls are unintended.[1] Emotionally, teen mothers are more likely to be depressed, more likely to drop out of school, and at high risk of a repeat pregnancy if they live with the baby's father. Adolescents who choose to have a termination or an adoption have a separate burden to carry, with potential emotional sequelae if they are not given the support and tools with which to process the decision. Fiscally, teen pregnancy can maintain or create a new cycle of poverty, especially if the teen does not complete high school or pursue a college degree. Adolescent fathers remain an understudied group, with a need for interventions preventing teen pregnancy that target girls and boys, as well as services to engage and support parenting adolescents of both genders.

ADOLESCENT PREGNANCY: THE STATS

Every year, 14 million children are born worldwide to women aged 15–19.[2] Globally more women are using contraception, and fewer adolescents are becoming mothers every year; however, declines in adolescent birthrates have

*Corresponding author.
E-mail address: romee@ccf.org (E. S. Rome).

slowed, and in the least developed countries rates may have even increased slightly.[3] In developing countries, 15–33% of pregnant women are younger than 20 years of age. Complications from pregnancy and childbirth are leading causes of death in these adolescent women. Each year, approximately 70,000 adolescent women worldwide die from pregnancy-related causes.[4]

Although some countries have data available on pregnancy rates in younger adolescents (age 10–14 years), most statistical comparisons between countries compare rates among older adolescents (age 15–19 years). Adolescent pregnancy rates are usually expressed as the number of pregnancies (including pregnancies ending in births or abortions) per 1000 women aged 15–19 years. Unintended pregnancy rates are calculated per 1000 women in a specific population. The adolescent abortion rate is the number of induced abortions per 1000 women aged 15–19 years.

Adolescent pregnancy rates vary across developed countries. Some of the highest rates of adolescent pregnancy, abortion, and birth are found in the United States, whereas lower rates are seen in Canada, Australia, and the United Kingdom. The lowest adolescent birthrates are found in the Netherlands, the Scandinavian countries, Japan, Korea, and China. Despite the availability of free abortion in the Scandinavian countries and the Netherlands, pregnancy and abortion rates are low, likely due to better contraceptive accessibility for adolescents.[5]

In the United States, almost 750,000 teens become pregnant each year.[6] The adolescent *pregnancy rate* did decline steadily from 116.9 in 1990 to 69.5 in 2005, the lowest it had been for 30 years. Unfortunately, the most recent comprehensive US data from 2006 showed a 3% increase in adolescent pregnancies with a rate of 71.5 (or about 7% of this age group).[6] There was a wide difference in teen pregnancy rates by state, with the highest rates being in the southern and southwestern states.[6] There was also a wide variation by ethnicity, with black and Hispanic women having the highest teen pregnancy rates (126.3 and 126.6) and non-Hispanic whites having the lowest rates (44.0).[6] The majority of teen pregnancies in the United States end in births (59%), whereas 27% end in abortion.[6] In 2001, *unintended pregnancy rates* in 15–17-year-olds and 18–19-year-olds were 40 and 108, respectively. However, when using only sexually active adolescents in the denominator, the rate of unintended pregnancy is much higher for both 15–17-year-olds (147) and 18–19-year-olds (162)[7] (Figure 1). Between 1991 and 2006, adolescent *birthrates* decreased from a peak of 61.8 to 41.9. Although there was a 4% increase in birthrates between 2005 and 2006, adolescent birthrates in 2009 were at a historic low of 39.1 births per 1000 women aged 15–19, representing a 37% decrease from 1991.[8] Birthrates were highest in the southern states (where access to preventive care, reproductive care, and abortion services are more limited) and were higher in Hispanic (70.1) and black teens (59.9) than in non-Hispanic white teens (25.6)[9,10] (Figure 2). In 2006, the adolescent *abortion rate* was 19.3, which was 56% lower than its peak in 1988 but 1% higher than in 2005. Between 1986 and 2006, the proportion of teen pregnancies ending in abortions decreased from 46% to 32%.[6]

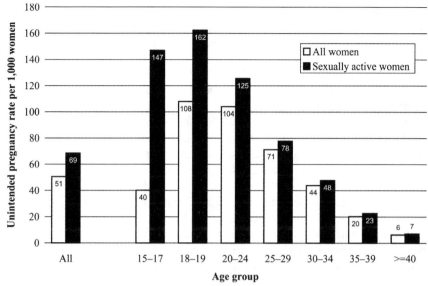

Figure 1. Rates of Unintended Pregnancy for All Women and Sexually Active Women by Age Group, United States, 2001 (Source: Finer LB. Unintended pregnancy among U.S. adolescents: accounting for sexual activity. *J Adolesc Health*. 2010;47(3):312–314. Reprinted with permission from Elsevier.)

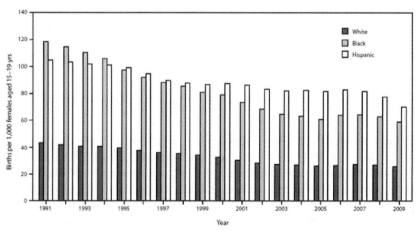

Figure 2. Birthrate for Teens Aged 15–19 Years by Race/Ethnicity,* National Vital Statistics System, United States, 1991-2009 (Sources: Hamilton BE, Martin JA, Ventura SJ. Births: preliminary data for 2009. *Natl Vital Stat Rep*. 2010;59(3); Martin JA, Hamilton BE, Sutton PD, et al. Births: final data for 2008. *Natl Vital Stat Rep*. 2010;59(1); Vital signs: teen pregnancy—United States, 1991-2009. *MMWR*. 2011;60(13):414–420. Available at: http://www.cdc.gov/mmwr/preview/mmwrhtml/mm6013a5.htm?s_cid=mm6013a5_w. Accessed July 26, 2011.)

The decline in teen pregnancies in the United States up until 2002 was largely due to an increase in consistent contraceptive use (86%) and, to a smaller extent, teens choosing to delay sexual activity (14%).[11] The transient increases seen in the 2006 and 2007 teen birthrate may in part have been a delayed reflection of an executive drive for abstinence-only education at the specific expense of comprehensive sexuality education, shifts in the racial and ethnic composition of the population, and changes in the public perception and attitudes toward adolescent pregnancy.[12-14]

Despite having similar levels of sexual activity to their adolescent peers in Canada and Sweden, adolescents in the United States have a pregnancy rate that is more than twice that of Canada (27.9 in 2006) or Sweden (31.4).[15] There has been an overall decline in the Canadian *adolescent pregnancy rate*, from 42.7 in 1997 to 32.1 in 2003.[16] In 2008, live births to adolescents represented 4.1% of all births in Canada,[17] whereas in the United States, 10% of all births were to adolescents.[9] Between 1996 and 2006, *adolescent birthrates* in Canada decreased in a continuous downward trend from 22.1 to 13.7 and *abortion rates* decreased from 22.1 to 14.2.[15,18] The birthrate is higher among older adolescents (23.3, age 18–19) than in younger adolescents (6.5, age 15–17).[19] In Canada, younger adolescents are more likely to have an induced abortion than to give birth, whereas the majority of pregnancies among older teens end in a live birth. In 1997, abortion was the most common outcome of teen pregnancies in Canada.[16]

THE COST OF UNINTENDED PREGNANCY FOR ADULTS AND TEENS

Two recent studies, utilizing different methodological approaches, concluded that the annual cost of unintended pregnancies in the United States is approximately $11 billion.[20,21] These studies likely underestimate the costs, as they are limited to public insurance costs for pregnancy and first year infant care only. In the United Kingdom, the cost to the National Health Service (NHS) alone of adolescent pregnancy was more than £63 million in 2002.[22]

WHICH ADOLESCENT IS AT RISK OF PREGNANCY?

Factors contributing to adolescent pregnancies may differ between developed and developing countries where customs and traditions such as early marriage may be a significant factor. Interestingly, available data from developed countries indicate that variations in the age at first intercourse do not explain differences in adolescent pregnancy rates between countries, particularly between the United Sates and other countries.[5] Adolescent condom use does not differ much between countries; however, use of modern contraceptive methods with low failure rates (pills, injectables, implants, and intrauterine devices [IUDs]) is lower in the United States than in other countries and this is felt to be a more likely cause of higher pregnancy rates.[5,23]

In developed countries, adolescent childbearing is more likely among young women with lower levels of income and education than their peers,[24] with up to a 10-fold increase in low income families.[25] Adolescents who have been victims of abuse or violence have a higher likelihood of becoming pregnant,[25] and high rates of violence before and during pregnancy have been found in American, European, and Australian adolescents.[5,26] Unfortunately, adolescent mothers who have been victims of abuse are at higher risk of seeking late antenatal care, poorer obstetrical outcomes, increased neonatal morbidity, and of committing child abuse during their own child's life.[5,26] In one prospective Australian cohort study, the variable most strongly associated with younger age of motherhood was adverse early life experiences in an adolescent's home.[25] Other factors that contribute to adolescent pregnancies include alcohol and drug use; peer pressure to engage in sexual activity; low self-esteem; lack of education and information about sexual health, including lack of access to contraception; incorrect or inconsistent use of reliable contraceptive methods; and low educational ambitions or goals.[2,5,22] Teen mothers are more likely to have single parent families or have parents who show less interest in their education.[22] Having a mother with low educational attainment and who herself had a teenage pregnancy increases the risk of teenage pregnancy.[22] Younger siblings of adolescent mothers have a higher likelihood of becoming adolescent mothers.[27] Poor academic success has been associated with a lack of career ambition and motivation, which may lead to a desire for pregnancy.[2,25] Conversely, close family relationships, religious beliefs, knowledge of sexuality, strong academic performance, and involvement in extracurricular activities appear to be protective against early sexual activity.

Not all adolescent pregnancies are unplanned. Idealization, in which the positive aspects of pregnancy and parenthood are overestimated and the negative aspects are underestimated, may be a factor in adolescent pregnancies.[28] Unfortunately, adolescents tend to underestimate the amount of support they will receive postpartum.[29] Some studies have found that adolescents plan to conceive due to idealized attitudes toward pregnancy and parenthood rather than by accident or due to negative attitudes toward contraception.[28,30] In one study, 53% of adolescents idealized pregnancy as "the single most exciting and positive event to have occurred in my life."[25] The Millennium Cohort Study suggested that only 15% of teenage mothers plan their pregnancy.[31] This is consistent with the findings of a US study where 17.5% of pregnant adolescents wanted to be pregnant (although a further 20% "didn't mind" becoming pregnant).[32] However, an Australian study found that 77% of adolescents in the adolescent obstetric clinic had planned or semiplanned their pregnancy,[26] and one Canadian study found that 33% of adolescents in an adolescent pregnancy clinic had reported a desire to become pregnant.[33] Another Canadian study found that 15% of adolescents presenting to an abortion clinic had initially intended to conceive.[34] Efforts to promote contraceptive awareness and availability of contraception would not have prevented these pregnancies.

Male partners of pregnant adolescents typically have lower education levels and socioeconomic status, higher unemployment rates, more history of substance abuse, more simultaneous sexual partners, a greater age difference with the pregnant teen, and engage in more aggressive behaviors. An Australian study found that a history of drug use, parental separation/divorce, and exposure to family violence in early childhood were all significant independent factors associated with fatherhood in teenage pregnancy.[35]

THE ROLE OF PARENTS AND SEX EDUCATION

The 2006–2008 US National Survey of Family Growth reported that 65% of female teens and 53% of male teens had received formal sex education that included *both* saying no to sex and information on methods of birth control.[23] Overall, 44% of adolescent girls and 27% of adolescent boys had spoken with their parents about abstinence, contraceptive options, healthy choices, and the ability to say no. Among teens who had already had sexual intercourse, 20% of adolescent girls and 31% of adolescent boys had *never* spoken with their parents about either how to say no to sex or about methods of birth control. Many studies have demonstrated that the quality of the parent-child relationship, maternal discussions about birth control, and perception of maternal disapproval of premarital sex are associated with a delay in first intercourse and increased contraceptive use.[36-38] Adolescents who talk to their parents about sexual issues have been found to be more likely to use condoms and have fewer sexual partners.[37]

Sex education programs have been shown to effectively delay initiation of sexual activity and increase contraceptive use;[39] however, parent-child communication may also delay sexual initiation and reduce sexual risk behaviors.[23] Efforts should be made to provide evidence-based sex education, to encourage parents to talk to their children about sexual and reproductive health, and to provide parents with the information and skills required to increase their comfort and confidence discussing sexual matters openly with their children.[37]

LEVELS OF SEXUAL ACTIVITY AND CONTRACEPTIVE USE

From 1991 to 2009, the percentage of US high school students who had ever had sexual intercourse decreased from 54% to 46%, and the percentage of students who had sexual intercourse in the past 3 months but did not use any method of contraception at last sexual intercourse decreased from 16% to 12%. From 1999 to 2009, the percentage of students who had sexual intercourse in the past 3 months and used dual methods at last sexual intercourse (condoms plus another hormonal method) increased from 5% to 9%.[23] Among sexually active adolescents, the use of hormonal methods (contraceptive pills or Depot medroxyprogesterone acetate [DMPA]), alone or in combination, remained low, whereas the use of long-acting methods of reversible contraception (LARCs) (ie, intrauterine contraceptives or contraceptive implants) was rare.[23] Only 55% of adolescent females received contraceptive methods from a health care provider, and only 56% of these adolescents used LARC or a hormonal method of contraception at last intercourse.[23]

The Canadian Community Health Survey also found a decrease in the percentage of Canadian 15–19-year-olds who had ever had intercourse, from 47% in 1996–1997 to 43% in 2005. Increases in contraceptive use by sexually active teens were also evident, and 70% of adolescent females reported using a condom the last time they had intercourse.[40] A recent Canadian study found the most common methods of contraception in 15–19-year-olds females were the male condom (71.3%), the oral contraceptive pill (66.6%), and withdrawal (17.3%).[41] Although 73% of sexually active Canadian adolescents "always" used a method of contraception, 27% either never used contraception or used contraception inconsistently. In adolescents who had an unplanned pregnancy, 53% stated that they were always using a contraceptive method at the time of conception, whereas 45% admitted to inconsistent use. Condoms were the contraceptive method used most commonly at the time of unintended pregnancy, followed by oral contraceptive pills.

MINOR'S ACCESS TO REPRODUCTIVE AND ANTENATAL CARE

Access to reproductive care for adolescents has improved in the United States over the past 30 years. During this time, states have expanded minors' authority to consent to health care, with a great majority of states and the District of Columbia now allowing a minor to obtain confidential prenatal care that includes prenatal visits and services for labor and delivery.[42] Confidentiality is not absolute in all states, with some states allowing physicians to inform parents that their minor daughter is seeking and/or receiving services when they feel it is in the best interests of the minor. Table 1 outlines US laws relevant to the access of prenatal care in the United States. In Canada, there is no legal age to consent to medical treatment. Under Canadian common law (which applies to all provinces except Quebec), the mature minor doctrine applies. If the adolescent is considered to be a mature minor, the physician can provide medical care and cannot inform the parents without the patient's consent. In Quebec, parents of a child younger than 14 years may access the child's medical record, whereas a child 14 years or older must authorize any disclosure of medical information.[43] The United Kingdom and Australia have similar common law positions with

Table 1.
Access to Prenatal Care in the United States

---

37 states and the District of Columbia (DC) have a law regarding minors' ability to access prenatal care

36 states and DC allow **some** minors to consent to prenatal care

28 states and DC allow **all** minors to consent to prenatal care

4 states require the minor to be a **specific age** before she can consent to prenatal care

4 states allow a "mature minor" to consent to prenatal care (ie, the adolescent can understand nature/consequences of treatment)

1 state requires **parental consent during all but one prenatal visit** during second and third trimesters, but the minor may consent to prenatal care during the first trimester and for the first visit after first trimester

13 states **allow but do not require** physicians to inform parents that their daughter is seeking/receiving prenatal care if deemed in the best interests of the minor

13 states have no explicit policy on minors' authority to consent to prenatal care

---

Source: Guttmacher Institute, Community health centers and family planning, In Brief, New York: Guttmacher, 2001, http://www.guttmacher.org/pubs/ib_6-01.html. Accessed February 10, 2012.

respect to the mature minor, which recognize that an adolescent has the capacity to consent to medical treatment on their own behalf without their parents' knowledge provided that they demonstrate a clear understanding of the nature of the treatment and the treatment is in the best interests of the adolescent.[44]

Complicating the issue of the lack of confidentiality in the United States is the method of billing for medical services.[45] The current "explanation of benefits" forms (EOBs) are routinely mailed to the policy holder whenever care is provided under that policy, thus unintentionally violating an adolescent's confidentiality. Many providers are unaware of the billing practices and do not realize that EOBs that clearly delineate services rendered are being sent to the adolescent's family. In facilities with adolescent medicine expertise, providers may code services in order to best preserve confidentiality, for example using code 626.0 (amenorrhea) rather than 650.0 (pregnancy) at the first antenatal visit. This practice becomes harder when specific prenatal services are being performed.

IMPLICATIONS OF ADOLESCENT PREGNANCY FOR AN ADOLESCENT MOTHER, HER CHILD, HER SIBLINGS, AND THE ADOLESCENT FATHER

Teen pregnancy and motherhood can have detrimental effects on the teen mother and her child. An adolescent mother is more likely to drop out of school and have low educational attainment, live in poor housing conditions, be unemployed or low paid, require social assistance, and suffer from depression.[2,5,22] The child of a teen mother is more likely to live in poverty, grow up without a father, become a victim of neglect or abuse, do less well at school, become involved in crime, abuse drugs and alcohol, and become a teen parent themselves. These children also have an increased risk of cognitive, behavioral, and emotional complications, although these behavioral problems have been attributed more to the mother's mental state rather than young maternal age.[22] The younger sibling of a teen mother is more likely to accept sexual initiation at a younger age, be more accepting of teenage childbearing, have a teen pregnancy themselves, and place less importance on education and employment.[2,27,46] Young fathers are less likely to have finished high school and to have more economically challenged families.[47] Men who become fathers in their teens are more likely to be unemployed, receive benefits, and require social housing even after adjusting for the lower education and income levels that predisposed them to young fatherhood.[22]

OBSTETRICAL OUTCOMES IN ADOLESCENT PREGNANCIES

Some complications of pregnancy may occur more frequently in adolescents than in older women. Teenage pregnancies are at higher risk of adverse outcomes such as preterm and very preterm delivery, low birth weight, small for gestational age (SGA), and neonatal and infant mortality. However, socioeconomic and behavioral factors that are associated with teen pregnancies, such as smoking, alcohol use, drug use, poor nutrition, and poor antenatal care are also risk factors for these adverse outcomes, and thus some have argued that young maternal age is not an independent risk factor. A retrospective cohort study of almost 2 million adolescent births in the United States found that after adjusting for confounding factors (state, race, marital status, smoking, alcohol use, and prenatal care), teenage pregnancy was independently associated with significantly increased risks of very preterm delivery (RR = 1.26), preterm delivery (RR = 1.20), very low birth weight (RR = 1.11), low birth weight (RR = 1.14), small for gestational age (RR = 1.07), and neonatal mortality (RR = 1.15).[48] The results were similar when they limited the findings to white married mothers with age-appropriate education who received adequate prenatal care and did not smoke or drink alcohol during the pregnancy, thus challenging the common assumption that many of the adverse outcomes associated with adolescent pregnancy are attributable to low socioeconomic status. The effect of teen pregnancy on neonatal mortality disappeared after further adjustment for birth weight and gestational age, suggesting the increased risk of neonatal mortality in teenage pregnancy could largely be explained by the higher rates of preterm and low birth weight infants in teenage mothers.[49]

Compared to adult women of the same parity, there does not appear to be a difference in the incidence of hypertension between adolescents and adults.[5] Anemia occurs frequently in younger women, and in a number of studies its prevalence appears to be higher in pregnant adolescents than in older pregnant women. In one study, 50% of pregnant adolescents had hemoglobin levels less than 10.5 g/L.[50] The cause is often nutritional, which can be treated adequately during antenatal care; however, adolescents are at risk of poor maternal weight gain due to poor nutritional intake.[5] Sexually active adolescents have high rates of sexually transmitted infections (STIs). In one Australian adolescent obstetrical clinic, the incidence of chlamydial infection was 27%,[51] and in a Canadian study the incidence of STIs was 25.1%, with 7% having multiple STIs.[52] A prospective Australian study found that screening and treating STIs in pregnant adolescents reduced preterm delivery rates significantly.[50]

Most studies in developed countries have reported a lower rate of caesarean section in adolescents compared to women older than 19 years[5] with rates between 2% and 14%.[48,53] Most studies also show lower percentages of inductions and oxytocin use, a shorter active phase of labor, and a similar length of the second stage of labor.[5]

The impact of paternal age on pregnancy outcomes has also been studied.[54] After adjusting for race, education, maternal smoking and alcohol consumption during the pregnancy, prenatal care, and infant gender, infants fathered by teenagers (younger than 20 years old) had a significantly increased risk of preterm birth (OR 1.15), low birth weight (OR 1.13), SGA babies (OR 1.17), neonatal mortality (OR 1.22), and neonatal mortality between 1 month and 1 year of birth (OR 1.41). The authors concluded that paternal age younger than 20 years is associated with an increased risk of adverse birth outcomes that is independent of maternal confounders.

OUTCOMES FOR INFANTS OF ADOLESCENT PREGNANCIES

The risks for the offspring of an adolescent mother can be classified as risks in the fetal, neonatal, and childhood periods. Not only is the risk of prematurity, low birth weight, and neonatal mortality increased,[48] but some congenital anomalies are more common in adolescent pregnancies. These include central nervous system anomalies (anencephaly, spina bifida, hydrocephaly, and microcephaly), as well as gastrointestinal anomalies (gastroschisis, omphalocele) and musculoskeletal anomalies (cleft lip and palate, polydactyly, syndactyly, adactyly).[48]

In the neonatal period, infants are at increased risk of sudden infant death syndrome (SIDS), accidental death, respiratory infections, abuse, and neglect. A US study found that healthy infants born to young adolescent mothers (15 years of age or younger) had a 3-fold increased risk of neonatal death compared to older mothers.[55] They postulated this was related to child abuse/neglect and SIDS.[55] Other retrospective studies have found that the risk of neonatal mortality is not increased after adjusting for potential confounders, including birth weight and gestational age, thus suggesting that the increased risk of neonatal mortality in teenage pregnancy is largely explained by low birth weight and preterm delivery.[48,49,56] In a German study looking at repeat pregnancies in 8857 adolescent females, adolescents with a repeat delivery had significantly higher odds of perinatal mortality (OR 2.08) and neonatal mortality (OR 4.31), whereas adolescents with a previous abortion had higher odds of stillbirth (OR 3.31) and preterm births (OR 2.21).[57]

ANTENATAL CARE FOR PREGNANT ADOLESCENTS

Antenatal care for adolescents is often inadequate, with adolescents seeking care later in the pregnancy and making fewer visits than older women. Reasons for delay in seeking care in developed countries include financial barriers (cost of medical care and transportation), dissatisfaction with provider services (clinic waiting times and lack of privacy or confidentiality), embarrassment and a desire to keep their pregnancy hidden, contemplation of abortion, and concern about negative or judgmental health care provider attitudes.[5] Adolescents may also find it difficult to miss school for their regular appointments.

Antenatal care is preferably started in the first or second trimester. This allows for accurate determination of gestational age, counseling about pregnancy options, and screening for risky behaviors or conditions that can be addressed or treated during the pregnancy. Pregnant adolescents may engage in higher risk behaviors that can affect perinatal outcomes. Pregnancy is a powerful incentive for many adolescents to reduce tobacco, alcohol, and drug use.[28] One Australian study found that 66% of adolescents stopped using illegal drugs while pregnant.[58] Another study found smoking cessation rates of 60% for smoking, 73% for alcohol use, and 75% for illegal drug use.[25] When substance abuse is identified early in the pregnancy, health care providers may assist by arranging addiction counseling; this harm reduction strategy can significantly impact pregnancy outcomes. Up to 18% of pregnant adolescents have a previous history of a psychological/psychiatric disorder; however, psychopathology is often missed in adolescents assessed in a general obstetrics clinic.[59] These adolescents need to be identified in order to provide them with supportive care. Testing for STIs, including testing in the third trimester and postpartum, should also be performed for pregnant adolescents due to the high incidence of STIs in this age group.

Unfortunately, violence in adolescent pregnancy is not uncommon. Often the violence begins in the first trimester, usually by the partner, and a history of abuse within the last year is predictive of violence during the pregnancy. Pregnant adolescents who have been victims of domestic violence are more likely to smoke, use alcohol or illegal drugs, and have higher incidences of STIs, psychosocial illness, and neonatal morbidity. Adolescent mothers who had been victims of domestic violence have reduced attachment scores to their infants.[60] A multidisciplinary approach to antenatal care can provide counseling opportunities to victims of abuse.

The approaches used to prevent and respond to health problems in adults need to be adapted if they are to meet the special needs of pregnant adolescents because standard obstetrical environments may not do so.[5] The ideal setting for managing adolescent pregnancies is uncertain; however, multidisciplinary adolescent obstetric clinics may help to reduce maternal and perinatal risks. One cohort study found that dedicated multidisciplinary adolescent pregnancy clinics improved screening for infections and psychosocial problems and are associated with a decrease in preterm birth.[50] A recent Canadian study found that adolescents followed in a multidisciplinary adolescent-friendly obstetrical outreach program had a lower risk of preterm delivery (RR_{adj} 0.47) and low birth weight (RR_{adj} 0.41).[53] The authors concluded that multidisciplinary adolescent-focused programs that facilitate early and regular access to obstetrical care and education in a nonthreatening environment should be considered the gold standard for adolescent obstetrical care.

POSTPARTUM CARE AND SUPPORT FOR ADOLESCENT MOTHERS

Support for adolescent mothers and their infants should not be limited to prenatal and perinatal care.[55] Adolescent mothers often have difficult social circumstances and many have been victims of abuse, factors that may lead to abuse and maltreatment of their own children. Adolescent mothers with higher social supports have been found to have fewer postpartum depressive symptoms.[61] Unfortunately, adolescents tend to overestimate the amount of support they have available once the baby is born.[29] This unrealistic expectation has been associated with a higher risk of postpartum depression at 6 months. Indeed, the rate of postpartum depression appears to be lower if the adolescent receives support from her mother or the baby's father. Failure to address the need for postpartum support leads to increased stress and depression and therefore an increased risk for abuse, neglect, and violence.[29]

The preventive effect of postpartum home visits has been studied.[5] An Australian randomized trial found that multiple postpartum visits by nurse-midwives were associated with a reduction of infant deaths, nonaccidental injuries, and child protection notifications. In addition, they reported an improvement in knowledge and use of contraception.[62] Adolescent parenting programs that attempt to improve maternal attitudes have also been evaluated.[63,64] These reviews found positive effects on mother-infant interaction, language development, parental attitudes, and parental knowledge.[63] These programs were also found to have a positive effect on self-esteem, the mother's relationship with her partner, and depression.[64]

Elfenbein hypothesized that adolescent mothers were often unable to respond optimally to their children's needs because of excessive demands on the mother secondary to a low education level and an economically stressed environment that lacks emotional and social support. In addition, adolescent mothers may be consciously choosing to avoid an educational setting in which they were unsuccessful and may have lower cognitive abilities that they pass on to their children. Finally, adolescent mothers may not understand and integrate all of the required tasks for optimal parenting due to cognitive immaturity.[65] Many adolescent mothers are indeed depressed and lack support after their child is born. They may be less sensitive to their children and less aware of their children's needs, leading to more behavioral disturbances in the children. The incidence of depression is high in adolescent mothers and may influence parental behaviors interfering with maternal sensitivity and discipline. The long-term effects, therefore include behavioral problems, higher than average rates of developmental delay, school failure, and substance abuse.

Rapid repeat pregnancy rates for adolescents are high, with up to 25% of adolescent mothers in the United States experiencing a repeat pregnancy within 2 years. Factors that can reduce rapid repeat pregnancy include initiating LARCs, continuing to attend school after a first teen birth, living independently or with a parent (rather than a partner), whereas having a lower cognitive ability, being Hispanic or black, and planning the first teen birth increase the risk of a rapid repeat pregnancy.[66] Young adolescent mothers may not be interested in preventing pregnancy and may lack motivation for contraceptive use. Interventions that focus on providing contraception may be unsuccessful if they do not address motivational issues. One randomized trial found that adolescent mothers who received a computer-assisted motivational intervention had lower rates of rapid repeat pregnancy compared to the usual care group.[67] No method of contraception should be denied to an adolescent on the basis of age alone,[68] and contraceptive options should include LARCs. The Institute of Medicine declared that expanding access to LARCs for young women was a national priority, and the American Congress of Obstetricians and Gynecologists in 2011 stated that we should encourage LARCs for all appropriate candidates, including adolescents.[69] Unfortunately, adolescents may face difficulty accessing reliable and affordable contraception, as well as using it consistently.

IMPLICATIONS FOR PUBLIC HEALTH POLICY AND PRACTICE

Teen pregnancy remains expensive and has many consequences for the teen, her potential offspring, and society; hence, prevention should be a public health priority. Decreasing trends in teen pregnancy reflect improved contraceptive access combined with better access to sex education that discusses both abstinence and family planning counseling. Abstinence-only sex education, similar to DARE programs for substance abuse, have highest applicability with the younger tweens, or the 10–12-year-old age group. Policy can be used to support abstinence only in the youngest age group, shifting to a focus on abstinence combined with contraceptive counseling by the time adolescents reach junior high school and older. Reproductive services need to remain confidential, affordable, and easily accessible to both girls and boys. Pregnancy prevention programs and programs designed to help pregnant and parenting adolescents need to target girls *and* boys. From a policy perspective, adolescents with repeat pregnancies have worse outcomes than their nulliparous adolescent peers,[57] reinforcing the need for programs targeting teen parents that prevent a repeat pregnancy and also focus on building skills and opportunities for improved parenting and life skills. Specific programs that decrease smoking and increase utilization of prenatal and postnatal care can also be beneficial.

CONCLUSIONS

Adolescent pregnancy remains a public health issue with significant medical, emotional, and social consequences for the adolescent mother, her child, and her family. Pregnancy and motherhood during the teenage years are associated with poorer health and well-being for both the mother and baby. Recent declines in teen pregnancy rates reflect an increase in contraceptive use by sexually active teens. Thus, it is important to continue to maintain and enhance access to broadly based sexual health education and reproductive health care services. Teen pregnancy prevention programs should provide evidence-based sex education, support parental efforts to talk with their children about sexual health, and ensure that sexually active teens have ready access to contraception that is effective and affordable.[23] Care of the pregnant adolescent may need to be adjusted to the specific needs of the adolescent and may best be provided in adolescent-focused obstetrical clinics. Postpartum care should include screening for depression, abuse, parenting difficulties, and contraceptive counseling. Exploring motivation for using contraception and ensuring adequate accessibility to contraception may help to decrease the rates of both adolescent pregnancy and rapid repeat pregnancies.

References

1. Hamilton B. Births: preliminary data for 2007. *Natl Vital Stat Rep.* 2009;57(12) (web release)
2. UNICEF. Young People and Family Planning: Teenage Pregnancy. 2008. http://www.unicef.org/malaysia/Teenage_Pregnancies_-_Overview.pdf. Accessed July 25, 2011
3. UNFPA. *State of the World Population.* New York, NY: United Nations Population Fund; 2010
4. Gomez R, Santolaya J. Being mothers too early. *Am J Obstet Gynecol.* 2005;192(2):340–341
5. World Health Organization. *Issues in Adolescent Health and Development: Adolescent Pregnancy.* Geneva, Switzerland: World Health Organization; 2004
6. Kost K, Henshaw S, Carlin L. *U.S. Teenage Pregnancies, Births, and Abortions: National and State Trends and Trends by Race and Ethnicity.* New York, NY: Guttmacher Institute; 2010
7. Finer LB. Unintended pregnancy among U.S. adolescents: accounting for sexual activity. *J Adolesc Health.* 2010;47(3):312–314
8. Ventura S, Hamilton B. U.S. teenage birth rate resumes decline. *NCHS Data Brief.* 2011;(58):1–8
9. Hamilton B, Martin J, Ventura S. Births: final data for 2008. *Natl Vital Stat Rep.* 2010;59(1)
10. Hamilton B, Martin J, Ventura S. Births: preliminary data for 2009. *Natl Vital Stat Rep.* 2010;59(3)
11. Santelli J, Lindberg L, Finer L, Singh S. Explaining recent declines in adolescent pregnancy in the United States: the contribution of abstinence and improved contraceptive use. *Am J Public Health.* 2007;97(1):150–156
12. Santelli JS, Orr M, Lindberg LD, Diaz DC. Changing behavioral risk for pregnancy among high school students in the United States, 1991–2007. *J Adolesc Health.* 2009;45(1):25–32
13. Moore K. *Teen Births: Examining the Recent Increase.* Washington, DC: National Campaign to Prevent Teen and Unplanned Pregnacy; 2008
14. Lindberg LD, Santelli JS, Singh S. Changes in formal sex education: 1995–2002. *Perspect Sex Reprod Health.* 2006;38(4):182–189
15. McKay A, Barret M. Trends in teen pregnancy rates from 1996–2006: a comparison of Canada, Sweden, USA, and England/Wales. *Can J Human Sexuality.* 2010;19(1):43–52
16. Dryburgh H. Teenage pregnancy. *Health Rep.* 2000;12(1):9–19
17. Statistics Canada. Live births, by age of mother, Canada, provinces and territories, annual 2008. CANSIM. http://www.statcan.gc.ca/pub/84f0210x/2008000/related-connexes-eng.htm. Accessed July 27, 2011
18. Statistics Canada. Induced abortion statistics 2005. Ottawa: Statistics Canada, Health Statistics Division. Catalogue No. 82-223-X; 2008
19. Statistics Canada. Pregnancy outcomes by age group (live births). 2005. http://www40.statcan.gc.ca/l01/cst01/hlth65b-eng.htm. Last Update 2010-06-18; Accessed July 27, 2011
20. Sonfield A, Kost K, Gold RB, Finer LB. The public costs of births resulting from unintended pregnancies: national and state-level estimates. *Perspect Sex Reprod Health.* 2011;43(2):94–102
21. Monea E, Thomas A. Unintended pregnancy and taxpayer spending. *Perspect Sex Reprod Health.* 2011;43(2):88–93
22. Paranjothy S, Broughton H, Adappa R, Fone D. Teenage pregnancy: who suffers? *Arch Dis Child.* 2009;94(3):239–245

23. Centers for Disease Control and Prevention. Vital signs: teen pregnancy United States 1991–2009. *MMWR*. 2011;60(13):414–420

24. Singh S, Darroch JE, Frost JJ. Socioeconomic disadvantage and adolescent women's sexual and reproductive behavior: the case of five developed countries. *Fam Plann Perspect*. 2001;33(6):251–258, 89

25. Quinlivan JA, Tan LH, Steele A, Black K. Impact of demographic factors, early family relationships and depressive symptomatology in teenage pregnancy. *Aust N Z J Psychiatry*. 2004;38(4):197–203

26. Quinlivan JA, Evans SF. A prospective cohort study of the impact of domestic violence on young teenage pregnancy outcomes. *J Pediatr Adolesc Gynecol*. 2001;14(1):17–23

27. East PL, Reyes BT, Horn EJ. Association between adolescent pregnancy and a family history of teenage births. *Perspect Sex Reprod Health*. 2007;39(2):108–115

28. Quinlivan JA. Teenagers who plan parenthood. *Sex Health*. 2004;1(4):201–208

29. Quinlivan JA, Luehr B, Evans SF. Teenage mother's predictions of their support levels before and actual support levels after having a child. *J Pediatr Adolesc Gynecol*. 2004;17(4):273–278

30. Condon JT, Donovan J, Corkindale CJ. Australian adolescents' attitudes and beliefs concerning pregnancy, childbirth and parenthood: the development, psychometric testing and results of a new scale. *J Adolesc*. 2001;24(6):729–742

31. Bradshaw J. *Teenage Births*. York, UK: Joseph Rowntree Foundation; 2006

32. Stevens-Simon C, Kelly L, Singer D, Cox A. Why pregnant adolescents say they did not use contraceptives prior to conception. *J Adolesc Health*. 1996;19(1):48–53; discussion 4–5

33. Kives S, Jamieson M. Desire for pregnancy among adolescents in an antenatal clinic. *J Pediatr Adolesc Gynecol*. 2001;14:150–151

34. Golts MM, Black AY, Kives S, Jamieson MA. Original desire for pregnancy among adolescents presenting for pregnancy termination. *J Ped Adolesc Gynecol*. 2003;25(6):S35

35. Tan LH, Quinlivan JA. Domestic violence, single parenthood, and fathers in the setting of teenage pregnancy. *J Adolesc Health*. 2006;38(3):201–207

36. Jaccard J, Dittus PJ, Gordon VV. Maternal correlates of adolescent sexual and contraceptive behavior. *Fam Plann Perspect*. 1996;28(4):159–165, 85

37. Miller K, Fasula A, Poulsen M, et al. Sexual health disparities among African American youth and the need for early prevention approaches: parenting and youth development programs as strategies for pre-risk prevention. *J Equity Health*. 2009;2(1):19–28

38. McNeely C, Shew ML, Beuhring T, Sieving R, Miller BC, Blum RW. Mothers' influence on the timing of first sex among 14- and 15-year-olds. *J Adolesc Health*. 2002;31(3):256–265

39. Oringanje C, Meremikwu MM, Eko H, Esu E, Meremikwu A, Ehiri JE. Interventions for preventing unintended pregnancies among adolescents. *Cochrane Database Syst Rev*. 2009;(4):CD005215

40. Rotermann M. Trends in teen sexual behaviour and condom use. Health Information and Research Division of Statistics Canada. http://www.statcan.gc.ca/pub/82-003-x/2008003/article/10664/5202360-eng.htm. Accessed July 26, 2011

41. Black A, Yang Q, Wen SW, Lalonde A, Guilbert E, Fisher W. Contraceptive use by Canadian women of reproductive age: results of a national survey. *J Soc Obstet Gynecol Can*. 2009;31(7):627–640

42. Guttmacher Institute. State Policies in Brief: Minors' access to prenatal care. 2011. http://www.guttmacher.org/statecenter/spibs/spib_MAPC.pdf. Last Update July 1, 2011. Accessed July 26, 2011

43. The Canadian Medical Protection Association. Age of consent for sexual activity and duty to report. 2010. https://www.cmpa-acpm.ca/cmpapd04/docs/resource_files/perspective/2010/02/pdf/com_p1002_10-e.pdf. Last Update June 2010. Accessed July 26, 2011

44. Bird S. Consent to medical treatment: the mature minor. *Aust Fam Physician*. 2011;40(3):159–160

45. Gold R. Unintended consequences: how insurance processes inadvertently abrogate patient confidentiality. *Guttmacher Policy Review*. 2009;12(4):12–16

46. East PL. Do adolescent pregnancy and childbearing affect younger siblings? *Fam Plann Perspect*. 1996;28(4):148–153

47. Kiernen K. Becoming a young parent: a longitudinal study of associated factors. *Br J Sociol*. 2007;48:406–408

48. Chen XK, Wen SW, Fleming N, Demissie K, Rhoads GG, Walker M. Teenage pregnancy and adverse birth outcomes: a large population based retrospective cohort study. *Int J Epidemiol.* 2007;36(2):368–373

49. Chen XK, Wen SW, Fleming N, Yang Q, Walker MC. Increased risks of neonatal and postneonatal mortality associated with teenage pregnancy had different explanations. *J Clin Epidemiol.* 2008;61(7):688–694

50. Quinlivan JA, Evans SF. Teenage antenatal clinics may reduce the rate of preterm birth: a prospective study. *BJOG.* 2004;111(6):571–578

51. Quinlivan JA, Petersen RW, Gurrin LC. High prevalence of chlamydia and Pap-smear abnormalities in pregnant adolescents warrants routine screening. *Aust N Z J Obstet Gynaecol.* 1998;38(3):254–257

52. Aggarwal A, Spitzer RF, Caccia N, Stephens D, Johnstone J, Allen L. Repeat screening for sexually transmitted infection in adolescent obstetric patients. *J Obstet Gynaecol Can.* 2010;32(10):956–961

53. Fleming N, Tu X, Black A. Evaluation of a unique Canadian community outreach program providing obstetrical care for pregnant adolescents: a matched cohort study. *J Pediatr Adolesc Gynecol.* 2011;24(2):e65

54. Chen XK, Wen SW, Krewski D, Fleming N, Yang Q, Walker MC. Paternal age and adverse birth outcomes: teenager or 40+, who is at risk? *Hum Reprod.* 2008;23(6):1290–1296

55. Phipps MG, Blume JD, DeMonner SM. Young maternal age associated with increased risk of postneonatal death. *Obstet Gynecol.* 2002;100(3):481–486

56. Conde-Agudelo A, Belizan JM, Lammers C. Maternal-perinatal morbidity and mortality associated with adolescent pregnancy in Latin America: cross-sectional study. *Am J Obstet Gynecol.* 2005;192(2):342–349

57. Reime B, Schuckling B, Wenzlaff P. Reproductive outcomes in adolescents who had a previous birth or an induced abortion compared to adolescents' first pregnancies. *BMC Pregnancy Childbirth.* 2008;8(4)

58. Quinlivan JA, Evans SF. The impact of continuing illegal drug use on teenage pregnancy outcomes—a prospective cohort study. *BJOG.* 2002;109(10):1148–1153

59. Quinlivan JA, Petersen RW, Gurrin LC. Adolescent pregnancy: psychopathology missed. *Aust N Z J Psychiatry.* 1999;33(6):864–868

60. Quinlivan JA, Evans SF. Impact of domestic violence and drug abuse in pregnancy on maternal attachment and infant temperament in teenage mothers in the setting of best clinical practice. *Arch Womens Ment Health.* 2005;8(3):191–199

61. Brown JD, Harris SK, Woods ER, Buman MP, Cox JE. Longitudinal study of depressive symptoms and social support in adolescent mothers. *Matern Child Health J.* 2011

62. Quinlivan JA, Box H, Evans SF. Postnatal home visits in teenage mothers: a randomised controlled trial. *Lancet.* 2003;361(9361):893–900

63. Coren E, Barlow J. Individual and group-based parenting programmes for improving psychosocial outcomes for teenage parents and their children. *Cochrane Database Syst Rev.* 2001;(3):CD002964

64. Barlow J, Coren E, Stewart-Brown S. Meta-analysis of the effectiveness of parenting programmes in improving maternal psychosocial health. *Br J Gen Pract.* 2002;52(476):223–233

65. Elfenbein DS, Felice ME. Adolescent pregnancy. *Pediatr Clin North Am.* 2003;50(4):781–800, viii

66. Schelar E, Franzetta K, Manlove J. Repeat teen childbearing: difference across states and by race and ethnicity. *Child Trends Research Brief.* 2007(23)

67. Barnet B, Liu J, DeVoe M, Duggan AK, Gold MA, Pecukonis E. Motivational intervention to reduce rapid subsequent births to adolescent mothers: a community-based randomized trial. *Ann Fam Med.* 2009;7(5):436–445

68. The World Health Organization. *Improving Access to Quality Care in Family Planning: Medical Eligibility Criteria for Contraceptive Use.* 4th ed. Geneva, Switzerland: World Health Organization; 2009

69. ACOG Practice Bulletin No. 121. Long-acting reversible contraception: implants and intrauterine devices. *Obstet Gynecol.* 2011;118(1):184–196

Adolesc Med 23 (2012) 139–163

Premenstrual Syndrome and Dysmenorrhea in Adolescents

Lisa M. Allen, MD, FRCSC*a, Alexandra C. Nevin Lam, MD, FRCSCb

Section Head, Pediatric Gynecology, Hospital for Sick Children; Head, Gynecology, Mt. Sinai Hospital; Site Chief, Department of Obstetrics and Gynecology, Women's College Hospital; Associate Professor, Departments of Obstetrics and Gynecology and Pediatrics, University of Toronto, Toronto, Ontario, Canada

bNorth York General Hospital, Hospital for Sick Children; Lecturer, Department of Obstetrics and Gynecology, University of Toronto, Toronto, Ontario, Canada

INTRODUCTION

Menstrual dysfunction and symptoms commonly affect adolescents. Adolescents may be concerned about whether these symptoms are normal or whether they represent abnormality, especially given their relative inexperience with the pubertal changes that represent their new reproductive capacity. Adolescent health care providers (HCPs) should be able to distinguish symptoms that accompany normal menstruation from those that represent significant pathology and be able to guide young women as to what treatments are available to decrease both symptoms and any impact on their quality of life. This article focuses on the pathophysiology, diagnosis, and management of premenstrual syndrome and dysmenorrhea, both primary and secondary.

PREMENSTRUAL SYNDROME IN ADOLESCENTS

Most females experience premenstrual symptoms as a component of normal ovulatory menstrual cycles. When these symptoms begin to impact on quality of life and result in functional impairment, they then warrant the diagnosis of premenstrual syndrome (PMS), or premenstrual dysphoric disorder (PMDD) at the most severe end of the spectrum. The mean age of presentation for treatment

*Corresponding author.
E-mail address: LAllen@mtsinai.on.ca (L. M. Allen).

of PMS is the late 20s; however, most women recount nearly 10 years of symptoms before this.[1] Retrospective data specific to prevalence in adolescents are provided by several large-scale studies and appear to be comparable to adults, with 20–30% and 5–8% meeting criteria for PMS and PMDD, respectively.[2-5]

Symptoms

The most common symptom endorsed by adolescents is that of negative affect, including mood swings (59%), stress (87.6%), and nervousness (87.6%).[5] Physical symptoms are also quite prominent, with abdominal bloating and pain reported by two-thirds of adolescents in the same study. The impact of these symptoms on quality of life is significant, as more than half of teens attending a primary care gynecology clinic rated their symptoms as moderate to severe, and 59% of this group rated their impairment at home and with family to be moderate to severe.[4]

Diagnosis

The diagnostic criteria for PMDD[6] and PMS[7] are outlined in Box 1 and Box 2, respectively. The hallmark of each diagnosis is its temporal relationship to the menstrual cycle. For the diagnosis, there must be symptom onset in the periovulatory period (after day 13) with continuation until the early follicular phase of the next cycle. The symptoms must then completely abate during the week following menses. In addition, marked functional impairment is required, as is the exclusion of the symptoms as an exacerbation of another disorder. Prospective evaluation of symptoms for at least 2 consecutive cycles is a requirement. It has been documented that 50% of women who complain of PMS do not confirm their retrospective reports when their symptoms are evaluated prospectively.[8] One device to aid with documentation and to establish appropriate cycle timing is the Daily Record of Severity of Problems (DRSP).[9] The importance of an appropriate screening tool in adolescents is key to early identification of those who warrant prospective evaluation, education, and possible treatment. The Premenstrual Symptoms Screening Tool (PSST-A) has been revised for use in adolescents (Table 1), and results from a recent pilot study suggest it is valid for use in this population.[3]

Etiology

The precise pathophysiology of PMS is still unknown. Current knowledge suggests that it is due to a complex set of interactions between periovulatory fluctuating sex steroids and central neurotransmitters, such as serotonin and γ-aminobutyric acid (GABA), in susceptible individuals. A genetic predisposition has been suggested by twin studies.[10] The obvious relationship of PMS to the later phase of the menstrual cycle suggests that periovulatory changes in sex hormones may play a pivotal role. However, there is no difference in the periph-

Box 1. DSM-IV-TR Criteria for Premenstrual Dysphoric Disorder

A. In most menstrual cycles during the past year, 5 (or more) of the following symptoms were present for most of the time during the last week of the luteal phase, began to remit within a few days after the onset of the follicular phase, and were absent in the week postmenses, with at least 1 of the symptoms being either (1), (2), (3), or (4):

  (1) markedly depressed mood, feelings of hopelessness, or self-deprecating thoughts
  (2) marked anxiety, tension, feelings of being "keyed up," or "on edge"
  (3) marked affective lability (eg, feeling suddenly sad or tearful or increased sensitivity to rejection)
  (4) persistent and marked anger or irritability or increased interpersonal conflicts
  (5) decreased interest in usual activities (eg, work, school, friends, hobbies)
  (6) subjective sense of difficulty in concentrating
  (7) lethargy, easy fatigability, or marked lack of energy
  (8) marked change in appetite, overeating, or specific food cravings
  (9) hypersomnia or insomnia
  (10) subjective sense of being overwhelmed or out of control
  (11) other physical symptoms, such as breast tenderness or swelling, headaches, joint or muscle pain, a sensation of "bloating," weight gain

NOTE: In menstruating females, the luteal phase corresponds to the period between ovulation and the onset of menses, and the follicular phase begins with menses. In nonmenstruating females (eg, those who have had a hysterectomy), the timing of luteal and follicular phases may require measurement of circulating reproductive hormones.

B. The disturbance markedly interferes with work or school or with usual social activities and relationships with others (eg, avoidance of social activities, decreased productivity and efficiency at work or school).

C. The disturbance is not merely an exacerbation of the symptoms of another disorder, such as Major Depressive Disorder, Panic Disorder, Dysthymic Disorder, or a Personality Disorder (although it may be superimposed on any of these disorders).

D. Criteria A, B, and C must be confirmed by prospective daily ratings during at least 2 consecutive symptomatic cycles. (The diagnosis may be made provisionally prior to this confirmation.)

Reprinted with permission from the *Diagnostic and Statistical Manual of Mental Disorders,* Fourth Edition, Text Revision (Copyright 2000). American Psychiatric Association.

eral levels of sex steroids between PMS-affected individuals and controls across the menstrual cycle,[11] suggesting that the symptomatology results from an exaggerated response to normal fluctuations in these hormones in predisposed individuals.[12] Sex steroids are further implicated by the fact that treatment with a gonadotropin-releasing hormone (GnRH) agonist for ovulation suppression has been shown in studies to relieve PMS symptoms, as has oophorectomy.[13,14] Evidence for the "susceptible individual" theory is that women with PMS, but not asymptomatic women, experience recurrence of their PMS symptoms when given a physiologic dose of either estrogen or progesterone after induction of medical menopause with a GnRH agonist.[15]

Experimental models have demonstrated that sex steroids modulate serotonin transmission,[16,17] and it is well-established that aberrant serotonin neurotrans-

**Box 2. American College of Obstetricians
and Gynecologists Diagnostic Criteria for Premenstrual Syndrome**

1. The presence by self-report of at least 1 of the following somatic *and* affective symptoms during the 5 days before menses in each of the 3 prior menstrual cycles:

Affective	*Somatic*
Depression	Breast tenderness
Angry outbursts	Abdominal bloating
Irritability	Headache
Anxiety	Swelling of extremities
Confusion	
Social withdrawal	

2. The symptoms are relieved within 4 days of the onset of menses, without recurrence until at least cycle day 13
3. The symptoms are present in the absence of any pharmacologic therapy, hormone ingestion, or drug or alcohol use
4. The symptoms occur reproducibly during 2 cycles of prospective recording
5. Identifiable dysfunction in social or economic performance by 1 of the following criteria:
   Marital or relationship discord confirmed by partner
   Difficulties in parenting
   Poor work or school performance, poor attendance, or tardiness
   Increased social isolation
   Legal difficulties
   Suicidal ideation
   Seeking medical attention for a somatic symptom

Adapted from Mortola JF, Girton L, Yen SSC. Depressive episodes in premenstrual syndrome. *Am J Obstet Gynecol.* 1989;161:1682–1687, with permission from Elsevier.

mission is associated with depression, irritability, anger, and increased cravings for carbohydrates.[18] Women with PMS/PMDD have been shown to have abnormally low serotonin levels during the luteal phase of the menstrual cycle.[19] Further indirect evidence of the association between sex steroids and serotonin are the facts that selective serotonin reuptake inhibitors (SSRIs) rapidly and effectively treat PMS/PMDD,[20-24] treatment with a serotonin-receptor antagonist exacerbates symptoms,[25] and reduced libido is a very common side effect of long-term treatment with SSRIs.[22] Another neurotransmitter implicated in this complex interaction is the GABA-A receptor, which is well recognized to play a regulatory role in affect and is modulated by sex steroids, most notably the progesterone metabolite allopregnanolone.[26] Allopregnanolone binds to the GABA receptor with anxiolytic effects,[27] and studies have shown reduced GABA receptor sensitivity in the luteal phase in women with PMS/PMDD.[28]

Treatment

The treatment of PMS is solely symptom driven, with the goal being improvement in quality of life. It involves supportive care, lifestyle and dietary modifications, and/or pharmacologic interventions. The cornerstone of management of

Table 1.
The Premenstrual Symptoms Screening Tool for Adolescents (PSST-A)
(Please indicate "X" for each symptom under the appropriate rating.)
Do you experience some or any of the following premenstrual symptoms which *START BEFORE* your period and *STOP* within a few days of bleeding?

Symptom	Not at all	Mild	Moderate	Severe
1. Anger/irritability				
2. Anxiety/tension				
3. Tearful/increased sensitivity to rejection				
4. Depressed mood/hopelessness				
5. Decreased interest in work activities				
6. Decreased interest in home activities				
7. Decreased interest in social activities				
8. Difficulty concentrating				
9. Fatigue/lack of energy				
10. Overeating/food cravings				
11. Insomnia				
12. Hypersomnia (needing more sleep)				
13. Feeling overwhelmed or out of control				
14. Physical symptoms (including breast tenderness, headaches, joint/muscle pain, bloating, and weight gain)				

Have your symptoms, as listed above, interfered with:

	Not at all	Mild	Moderate	Severe
A. Your social/work efficiency or productivity				
B. Your relationships with friends or classmates/coworkers				
C. Your relationships with your family				
D. Your social life activities				
E. Your home responsibilities				

Scoring
The following criteria must be present for a diagnosis of PMDD:

1. At least one of #1, #2, #3, or #4 is severe
2. In addition at least four of #1–14 are moderate to severe
3. At least one of A, B, C, D, or E is severe

The following criteria must be present for a diagnosis of moderate to severe PMS:

1. At least one of #1, #2, #3, or #4 is moderate to severe
2. In addition at least four of #1–14 are moderate to severe
3. At least one of A, B, C, D, or E is moderate to severe

Reproduced from Steiner M, Peer M, Palova E, et al. The Premenstrual Symptoms Screening Tool revised for adolescents (PSST-A): prevalence of severe PMS and premenstrual dysphoric disorder in adolescents. *Arch Womens Ment Health*. 2011;14:77–81.

PMS in the adolescent population is education about (1) the menstrual cycle and PMS, (2) self-care measures to reduce symptom severity, and (3) acknowledgment of symptoms and the impact that they may have on overall functioning. One study of an educational program involving secondary school females resulted in a significant reduction in PMS scores in adolescents who received the education versus controls.[29] This response was sustained for 3 months posteducation.

Specific self-care activities that have been advocated include stress management techniques, namely exercise and dietary modification. The role of exercise in treating premenstrual symptoms has been investigated in small interventional studies in adult women only. Of the 4 studies identified by a recent review,[30] all reported a reduction in PMS symptoms following exercise interventions, with one specifically showing symptom improvement following aerobic exercise over strength training.[31]

Many dietary modifications for the treatment of PMS/PMDD have been investigated, including calcium and vitamin D, magnesium, vitamin E, primrose oil, vitamin B6, chaste berry, and carbohydrate-rich diets.[2,12,32] Of these, level 1 evidence only exists in support of calcium supplementation (1200 mg per day in divided doses) for significant improvements in negative affective symptoms, water retention symptoms, food craving, and pain symptoms.[33] Subsequent studies have documented a significant difference in calcium metabolism parameters throughout the menstrual cycle in women with PMDD versus asymptomatic controls.[34] Adequate vitamin D, which is required for calcium absorption, is likely an integral part of this effect, as shown in studies documenting a significant negative relationship between milk consumption and PMS symptoms in adolescents,[5] a cross-sectional study confirming that a higher intake of vitamin D is significantly associated with a lower prevalence of PMS,[35] and a randomized controlled trial (RCT) that demonstrated a significant reduction in PMS symptoms versus placebo.[36]

As one of the presumed underlying mechanisms predisposing an individual to PMS is periovulatory fluctuation in sex steroids, ovulation suppression with a combined oral contraceptive pill (COCP) seems a natural treatment choice. However, past studies have shown inconsistent results for COCPs regardless of the type of progestin or the variable progestin dose used throughout the pack (monophasic vs. triphasic).[37,38] In one study, 71.4% of women stated that the COCP had no effect at all on their PMS symptoms.[39] Recently, the introduction of the novel progestin drospirenone and the established efficacy of a shortened hormone-free interval (HFI) with lower estrogen dosing has resulted in a resurgence of COCP use for the treatment of PMS with significant results. Drospirenone is unique in that it is derived from a compound similar to spironolactone, not testosterone, as are traditional progestins used in COCPs. As a consequence of this, drospirenone has the dual benefit of possessing antimineralocorticoid and antiandrogenic properties. The shortening of the HFI results in constant suppression of gonadotropins such that follicular growth and estradiol production remain arrested,[40] whereas conventional 21-day active/7-day placebo (21/7) dosing regimens are associated with incomplete suppression and often PMS symptom exacerbation with hormone withdrawal.[41] Further maintenance of a more stable hormonal milieu is likely related to the longer half-life of drospirenone.[42]

A lower ethinyl estradiol (EE) dose is also likely important in the prevention of symptoms.[43] Two large multicenter, double-blind RCTs have shown that the drospirenone/20mcg EE-24/4 pill combination is significantly effective in treating the mood, somatic, and behavioral symptoms of PMDD versus controls.[44,45] Furthermore, Pearlstein et al (2005) found a 2-fold improvement in overall quality of life. Evidence in support of extended and continuous cycles is provided by a prospective study, which showed that a 168-day extended cycle of drospirenone/30 mcg EE led to a significant decrease in premenstrual symptoms compared to a 21/7 regimen of the same pill, with the largest effect being seen in the sixth month of continuous use.[46] Recent controversy surrounding the use of drospirenone-containing COCPs and increased venous thromboembolic (VTE) risk has been addressed in clinical practice guidelines, wherein it is concluded that rates are comparable between these and other COCPs on the market.[47] Unfortunately, none of the studies have involved adolescents. The additional benefits of COCPs, including contraception, make this a very attractive option to treat PMS/PMDD in adolescents, when education, lifestyle, and dietary modifications are insufficient.

The use of SSRIs are generally considered to be first-line treatment for severe PMS and PMDD in adult women. Placebo-controlled trials have confirmed a 60–90% response rate with significant improvement versus placebo,[20,24] and a Cochrane systematic review confirmed efficacy in treating physical, functional, and behavioral symptoms.[22] Only fluoxetine, sertraline, and paroxetine have been approved for use in the treatment of PMDD by the US Food and Drug Administration (FDA) (dosing schedule in Table 2). Despite this, a recent meta-analysis including 2964 women concluded that no SSRI was demonstrably better than any other but that the effect size is smaller than previously reported, with an odds ratio of 0.4.[23] The most common adverse effects of SSRIs include nausea,

Table 2.
Dosing of the FDA-Approved SSRIs for Severe PMS/PMDD

SSRI	Dose (once daily or for luteal phase dosing)
Fluoxetine	10–20 mg[20]
Sertraline	Start 25–50 mg up to max 150 mg/day
	Most need 100 mg/day[21]
Paroxetine-CR	12.5–25 mg[24]
Paroxetine	20–30 mg[12]

FDA: Food and Drug Administration;
SSRIs: selective serotonin reuptake inhibitors;
PMS: premenstrual syndrome;
PMDD: premenstrual dysphoric disorder

insomnia, headache, and decreased libido.[22] Studies specific to adolescents are lacking.

Unlike SSRI use in the treatment of mood disorders, clinical response to SSRIs in PMDD occurs within days of exposure. As such, intermittent luteal phase dosing beginning around day 14 of a 28-day cycle (or at symptom onset) and continuing until a few days after the onset of menses (symptom cessation) has been proven to be effective.[48,49] This dosing strategy can be considered for PMS/PMDD-affected women without comorbid mood disorders who experience side effects with conventional daily dosing, and it carries the added benefit of not producing discontinuation symptoms.[32] A recent meta-analysis, however, concluded that although both continuous and intermittent luteal dosing with SSRIs are effective, continuous dosing regimens appear superior.[23]

In the published adolescent literature to date, there is one case report of 3 PMDD-affected adolescents treated successfully with fluoxetine for 2 years.[50] Of the SSRIs approved for the treatment of severe PMS/PMDD, fluoxetine is the only one with FDA approval for use in children and adolescents, and this is for the indication of major-depressive disorder and obsessive-compulsive disorder. In 2004, the FDA issued a "black box warning" for SSRIs based on the results of studies that documented a significant 4% increased rate of suicidal thinking or behavior in youths prescribed SSRIs for treatment of depression versus 2% for placebo. Subsequently, a comprehensive review of trials confirmed that SSRIs are efficacious for the treatment of pediatric mood disorders and that the benefits outweigh the risks regardless of the mood disorder being treated.[51] However, SSRIs are generally not considered first-line treatment as a pharmacologic intervention in adolescents with PMS/PMDD. If required, fluoxetine would be preferable and would require appropriate prospective diagnosis and diligent monitoring, likely under the care of a multidisciplinary team.[2] Fluoxetine is also known to have the least association with a discontinuation syndrome in adolescents, due to its longer half-life than other SSRIs, thereby highlighting it as the SSRI of choice in refractory, severe cases of PMS/PMDD.[52] Other treatment options shown to be effective in adults, such as use of a GnRH-agonist, would not be employed in adolescents due to their associated health implications, including detrimental bone, cardiovascular, and vaginal health effects, unless in absolutely refractory cases. One study suggests that add-back hormonal support concurrent to GnRH-agonist treatment is protective of bone health at the hip, but not at the spine, in adolescents with endometriosis.[53] Theoretically, add-back may cause symptom relapse in the setting of severe PMS/PMDD, thereby limiting its use.

DYSMENORRHEA

Dysmenorrhea is common among women, particularly in middle and late adolescence. Reviewing the literature, a prevalence of 48–93% is reported across multiple countries in this age group.[54-60] The upper prevalence is published both in a Canadian population of 289 high school students and in an Australian cohort of 1055 senior high school girls completing a questionnaire on menstrual disorders.[54,55] United States' data document similar frequencies, from 65% in an urban, primarily black health care population to 85% of 606 Hispanic adolescents in a school-based cohort.[56,61] A recent meta-analysis on factors predisposing women to chronic pelvic pain found no significant difference in dysmenorrhea rates related to ethnicity.[62]

Severe dysmenorrhea affects a smaller proportion of adolescents, 5–42%.[54-56,59] For many, their quality of life is affected. Twenty six percent report missing school due to pain, and this may be even higher (46%) when dysmenorrhea is moderate or severe.[55,63] Fourteen percent usually missed 2 or more days per month due to their pain.[63] Not only is school attendance impacted, but severity of pain also has been shown to significantly affect participation in sports and socialization with peers.[56] Despite the large numbers affected, many do not seek medical attention. Two separate studies, 20 years apart, indicate that only 14% of adolescents with dysmenorrhea consult with a physician.[56,58] Unfortunately, adolescents may not perceive benefit from health care encounters related to this concern; 77% of Hispanic youth who visited a school nurse reported no relief from the encounter.[56] The aforementioned data emphasize to health care providers that menstrual pain is common, and it significantly affects adolescents' quality of life, and yet most adolescents still do not seek out medical care. Inserting questions into routine adolescent health care encounters with regards to menstrual symptoms is essential. Only 2% of adolescents at an urban tertiary adolescent health care center reported having received information on menstruation from their HCP.[61]

Pathophysiology

Dysmenorrhea may be primary or secondary. Primary dysmenorrhea, which comprises 90% of adolescent menstrual pain, is a result of physiologic changes that occur during a menstrual cycle. Secondary dysmenorrhea reflects an underlying pathologic process or disease (eg, endometriosis, Müllerian anomalies, pelvic inflammatory disease, adenomyosis/adenomyotic cysts).

In primary dysmenorrhea, following progesterone withdrawal premenstrually, phospholipids are released from cell membranes, in particular omega-6 fatty acids. The fatty acids are converted to arachidonic acid (AA) by the enzyme phospholipase A2. Prostaglandin (PG) synthesis follows with conversion of AA via cyclooxygenase (COX). The PGs are then transformed to leukotrienes (LTs) via lipoxygenase. Prostaglandin F2 alpha (PGF2 alpha) is a potent vasoconstrictor and stimulates myometrial contractions, leading to uterine ischemia and pain.[64] The PGs and LTs are responsible not only for the cramps in dysmenorrhea but also for the systemic symptoms accompanying menses (nausea, vomiting, bloating, and headaches). Levels of PG activity have been documented to be higher in the menstrual fluid and endometrium of women with dysmenorrhea compared to those who do not have pain. Similarly, LT C4 and D4 levels are correlated with the occurrence of dysmenorrhea, as well as with its severity. Nitrous oxide, a vasodilator may play a role. Transdermal patches of nitrous oxide have been shown to reduce pain in those with dysmenorrhea. The role of vasopressin in the pathogenesis of primary dysmenorrhea remains unclear.[65]

Additional factors that are associated with dysmenorrhea besides young age are a body mass index (BMI) less than 20, smoking, early menarche (younger than 12 years of age), menstrual cycles that are long, heavy, or irregular, and the presence of premenstrual symptoms.[59,62]

Diagnosis

Once one understands the pathophysiology of primary dysmenorrhea, the natural history becomes clear. Primary dysmenorrhea occurs with ovulatory cycles, and hence occurs more frequently in middle and late adolescence when the proportion of ovulatory cycles increases.[58] The normal history is that after a mean of 12 months of relatively symptom-free menses, adolescents may begin to experience pain that occurs transiently with or in close proximity to the onset of menstrual flow. Ninety percent of adolescents report symptoms for less than 48 hours.[55,66] As previously mentioned, PGs mediate systemic symptoms in adolescents with moderate or severe dysmenorrhea. Nausea (55%) and vomiting (24%) are common symptoms.[67] Other reported symptoms are fatigue (67%), headaches (59%), back pain (56%), and dizziness (28%).[56]

The diagnosis of primary dysmenorrhea is made largely on history. If a classic history of primary dysmenorrhea is obtained, a trial of therapy is warranted. History should assess the presenting menstrual symptoms (ie, severity and duration of pain) and the impact of those symptoms on activities such as school performance and attendance and life activities. Severity of pain can be estimated in part from the use of analgesia. Harada et al[68] graded mild, moderate, and severe dysmenorrhea as mild: analgesics required for 1 day; moderate: analgesia required for 2 days; and severe: analgesia required for 3 or more days. Tools such as menstrual calendars or a menstrual distress questionnaire may aid with accurate documentation of symptoms in the adolescent age group.[55] Given that the history is inherent in determining which adolescents would benefit from further investigations, a comprehensive review of the sexual history, the past medical history, and the family history is essential.

Clues obtained on history may lead to a suspicion of secondary dysmenorrhea (Table 3). In an Australian study, the authors aimed to establish not only contemporary data on the teenage experience of menstruation but also features that may identify those requiring management for underlying pathologic disorders. In this study, students were administered a menstrual disorder of teenagers (MDOT) questionnaire. Questions were developed to identify atypical menstrual symptoms (see Table 3). Although 93% of respondents indicated pain with menses, only 15% answered affirmatively with 2 or more atypical symptoms and only 6% with 3 or more. Further research may be able to translate these features into a noninvasive screening tool to assist HCPs in identifying young women at risk for secondary dysmenorrhea.[55]

In nonsexually active adolescents, a pelvic examination is not essential in making a diagnosis of primary dysmenorrhea. In a sexually active adolescent, a pelvic examination should be performed, maintaining awareness that pelvic inflammatory disease may present with the new onset of dysmenorrhea. Endometriosis in adolescents is most often early stage disease, stage 1 or 2 by American Society for Reproductive Medicine (ASRM) classification; therefore, while a bimanual examination may elicit pelvic tenderness, it is rare to palpate evidence of deep infiltrating disease such as uterosacral or cul-de-sac nodularity, uterine fixed retroversion, or endometriomas.[69,70] Müllerian outflow tract anomalies, in particular the asymmetric anomalies such as a uterine didelphys with an obstructing

Table 3.
Clues on History to Consider Secondary Dysmenorrhea in Adolescents

History	Clue	Association
Response to first-line medical therapy	Persistent pain despite NSAID or CHC therapy	Consider secondary dysmenorrhea, up to 69% diagnosis of endometriosis on laparoscopy
Timing of first onset of dysmenorrhea	Dysmenorrhea occurred in close temporal relationship to onset of menarche	PD typically occurs with establishment of ovulatory cycles. Pain that occurs with onset of first menstrual cycles may reflect Müllerian anomalies with outflow tract obstruction
Atypical symptoms	Dyschezia, pain with flatus, dysuria, pain with bladder distension, dyspareunia	These symptoms were reported far less frequently by adolescents and may indicate underlying secondary dysmenorrhea
Family history	Positive family history of a relative with endometriosis	Adolescents have higher rate of first degree relatives affected with endometriosis than adults (30% vs. 8%)
Sexual activity	Sexually active adolescent, may have symptoms of PID (pelvic pain, vaginal discharge), with or without history of STI	PID may present with new-onset dysmenorrhea
Medical history	Known renal tract anomaly	Müllerian anomalies and renal anomalies often coexist; Müllerian anomalies with outflow tract obstruction can present with pelvic pain and secondary dysmenorrhea

NSAID: nonsteroidal anti-inflammatory drug;
CHC: combined hormonal contraception;
PD: primary dysmenorrhea;
PID: pelvic inflammatory disease;
STI: sexually transmitted infection

hemivaginal septum or a noncommunicating uterine horn with a functional endometrium, are a less common but important consideration in the adolescent with secondary dysmenorrhea. Assessing the patency of the outflow tract is important, both by physical examination and by imaging. Initial pelvic imaging should begin with sonography (pelvic, transvaginal, 3D), and subsequently, Müllerian anomalies are often confirmed with magnetic resonance imaging (MRI). Diagnostic laparoscopy may be required when an etiology is not determined, initial treatment modalities have failed, or in combination with surgical management of pathology, such as in endometriosis.

Treatment

Primary Dysmenorrhea Given the high prevalence of dysmenorrhea in adolescents compared to the proportion seeking medical care, it is not surprising that many treat themselves with either nonpharmacologic therapies or over-the-counter (OTC) medications. In fact, 98% of adolescents in one study reported having attempted to relieve their pain with at least one nonpharmacologic method and 91% with OTC medications.[54] HCPs should be aware of what initial modalities adolescents may use to cope during menses, why they select them, and the potential benefits they perceive from these methods.

Adolescents indicate various reasons for their use of alternative strategies. Most commonly cited are that these methods ease discomfort, are convenient or easier than going to a HCP, are preferable to medications, or are used because medication does not provide relief or is not available. Strategies are either physically oriented (rest, heat, exercise, massage, more or less alcohol consumption, change in diet) or psychologically oriented (distraction, imagining, praying/hoping for relief, discussing with others). Most are perceived to be only 30–40% effective, with a large variability in effectiveness scores with each method, suggesting an idiosyncratic response. The least likely to provide relief are those that are psychologically oriented.[54] With OTC medications, young women may unfortunately chose medications that are not effective (ie, acetaminophen, narcotics) or do not maximize use, either by taking less than the recommended dose or less often than the maximum recommended daily frequency.[63,71] In one study, up to 71% of adolescents used less than 50% of the maximum daily dose of analgesia in the first 2 days of their menses.[63] Given that accessible, nonpharmacologic strategies have low to moderate perceived effectiveness, HCPs should be prepared to counsel adolescents on additional strategies for symptom management. In addition, if an OTC therapy is reported to have failed to relieve pain, a thorough history of dose and frequency of use is advised before determining that a change of therapeutic modality is required.

Nonpharmacologic Management Interventions such as exercise/yoga, acupuncture, dietary alterations, and cessation of smoking have been proposed as therapy for dysmenorrhea.[72] Fifteen percent of adolescents use exercise to relieve symptoms.[56] Exercise may exert its beneficial effect by shunting blood flow away from the viscera to the muscles, thereby reducing pelvic congestion; by acting as a mechanism for vasodilation; by suppressing PG release; via release of beta endorphins to act as a nonspecific analgesic; or indirectly by reducing stress.[73,74] The existing literature on exercise and primary dysmenorrhea is conflicting; some smaller observational studies suggest that regular exercise reduces primary dysmenorrhea, whereas others report a lack of association.[73,75,76] A recent meta-analysis of risk factors for dysmenorrhea demonstrated a small protective effect, with an odds ratio of 0.89 (confidence intervals, 0.80 to 0.99).[62] Only a single RCT has been performed to address this question. It included 36 college-aged women with clinically diagnosed primary dysmenorrhea. The young women were randomized to a 12-week walk/jogging program or to no exercise, for 3 cycles. There was a decrease in the Moos Menstrual Distress Questionnaire scores during the menstrual phase for the training group compared to the control group, with a significant linear trend over the 3 cycles.[74] Based on the availability of only this single RCT, the Cochrane Database concluded that there is a lack of evidence to recommend exercise for the treatment of primary dysmenorrhea.[77] Authors unable to demonstrate sufficient evidence that exercise improves primary dysmenorrhea do recognize, however, that there are other broad health benefits of exercise that should be discussed with women.[73,75]

Young smokers have an increase in self-reported menstrual symptoms (pain, premenstrual negative affect, fluid retention) in a dose response relationship, increasing with younger age at onset of smoking, especially for those who start younger than age 13, and the number of cigarettes smoked per day.[62,78,79] The exact mechanism whereby smoking increases severity of dysmenorrhea is unclear. HCPs, however, can use this information in counseling adolescents on smoking risks. The immediate potential benefit of reducing menstrual pain may be a motivator for change that HCPs can promote to adolescents to encourage them to cease smoking.

Dietary modifications to increase consumption of fish/fish oils containing long chain omega-3 polysaturated fatty acids (salmon, tuna, mackerel, herring) may serve as a strategy to reduce pain. The prostaglandins formed from these fatty acids are less potent than those containing omega-6 fatty acids.[65,72] Additional dietary modifications with evidence of benefit over placebo in reducing dysmenorrhea include supplements of vitamins E and B1 and magnesium.[72]

Acupuncture and acupressure as complementary and alternative medicine techniques may assist in the relief of dysmenorrhea. In acupuncture, needles placed at specific skin locations are manipulated, exciting nerve fibers, resulting in the production of endorphins, serotonin, and acetylcholine, which act to enhance analgesia in the central nervous system through dampening or inhibiting of pain impulses.[72,80] Cho reviewed the literature, assessing 27 trials that compared acupuncture/acupressure to a control group (no treatment or placebo treatment using sham acupuncture), nonsteroidal anti-inflammatory drugs (NSAIDs), or herbal medicines for the treatment of primary dysmenorrhea. The studies favored acupuncture/acupressure over indomethacin, ibuprofen, or herbal medicines. Three studies compared acupuncture to sham acupuncture, where needles are placed either via a superficial insertion technique or at nonacupoints. Only one study demonstrated a statistically greater reduction of pain in the acupuncture treatment group. The authors concluded that there is promise for acupuncture but that the conflicting evidence of acupuncture versus sham acupuncture needs further investigation. Sham acupuncture may not be totally inert physiologically, as placement of a needle even minimally through the skin or at nontrigger points may have benefit in itself, or the effect of acupuncture may be attributed to a placebo effect.[80,81]

Pharmacologic Management Pharmacologic therapies aim to reduce the production of PGs and inflammatory cytokines, as well as to reduce menstrual flow, both antegrade and retrograde. When the adolescent seeks assistance from HCPs, the approach to relief of dysmenorrhea is stepwise. First-line therapies to be considered include NSAIDs, combined hormonal contraceptives, and long-acting reversible contraceptives (LARCs), depending on the additional need for contraception.

NSAIDs inhibit the enzymes of the cyclooxygenase pathway (COX-1 and COX-2), preventing conversion of AA into PGs. This class of medications is often considered first-line therapy, unless a woman has a contraindication to their use. NSAIDs fall into 2 classes, those that are nonspecific and inhibit both COX-1 and COX-2 enzymes (eg, ibuprofen, naproxen, diclofenac, meclofenamate) and those that are COX-2 specific inhibitors (celecoxib, rofecoxib, valdecoxib). COX-1 is expressed throughout the body (including the endometrium), is involved in the maintenance of normal hemostasis, and provides gastrointestinal mucosal protection. COX-2 is induced by proinflammatory cytokines and endotoxins at inflammatory sites. Hence the side effects of NSAIDs are related to inhibition of COX-1, whereas the therapeutic and anti-inflammatory effects are related to inhibition of COX-2.[82] COX-2 specific inhibitors are available; however, because they have been linked with an increased risk of cardiac complications, they are no longer indicated for the treatment of primary dysmenorrhea.[64] A Cochrane systematic review has confirmed that NSAIDs are consistently superior to placebo in providing pain relief, with an odds ratio of 4.50 (confidence intervals, 3.85–5.27). Most of the 73 RCTs that have been performed have involved naproxen; however, 21 different NSAIDs have been studied. Equivalent improvement of symptoms has been demonstrated between different products, hence there is insufficient evidence to suggest that any one is superior to the others. Diclofenac and naproxen have demonstrated translation of treatment into improvement of quality of life, as evidenced by less school or work absenteeism.[77]

Many studies of NSAIDs exclude adolescents. One that specifically assessed the adolescent age group included 45 young women, ages 12–18, evaluating the response of symptoms to varying dosing regimens of naproxen. The study determined that a loading dose of 550 mg was more beneficial in 3 treatment cycles compared to a lesser loading dose.[66] When choosing an NSAID for treatment of primary dysmenorrhea in an adolescent, because no single NSAID is superior, choosing one that requires less frequent dosing may be more convenient for the adolescent, particularly during school attendance. Providing a loading dose preemptively may improve success of therapy. Failure of relief of pain with NSAIDs may reflect their failure to inhibit production of other substances involved in the pathophysiology of primary dysmenorrhea, such as LTs. Although the side effects of NSAIDs may include gastrointestinal disturbances, renal failure, and skin reactions, short-term use with menses minimizes these effects. Select suggested NSAID regimens with their effective doses are presented in Table 4.

Combined hormonal contraceptives (CHCs), such as oral contraceptive pills, the transdermal contraceptive patch, and the contraceptive ring, limit the growth of the endometrium, subsequently reducing the amount of PGs and LTs formed and released. Inhibition of ovulation and subsequent progesterone production may be an additional indirect mechanism of effect.[65] The contraceptive benefits of these methods may lead the HCP to prescribe them as first line therapy. Both primary and some causes of secondary dysmenorrhea, in particular endometriosis, may respond to their administration. In 2005 Davis et al reported the first RCT on the effectiveness of oral contraceptives for primary dysmenorrhea in adolescents, despite the widespread clinical use before that time. Adolescents were included if they suffered from moderate or severe dysmenorrhea. Low dose (ethinyl estradiol 20 μg and levonorgestrel 100 mg) therapy was demonstrated to reduce the Moos Menstrual Distress questionnaire pain score, lessen the worst pain experienced, and decrease amount of analgesia required in users compared to placebo therapy, when prescribed cyclically.[67]

Although one would expect similar benefits when administering combined contraceptives either with the transdermal patch (releasing 20 μg of ethinyl estradiol

Table 4.
NSAID Regimens for Adolescent Dysmenorrhea

NSAID	Dosage
Ibuprofen	200–400 mg by mouth every 4–8 hours
Naproxen sodium	550 mg by mouth loading dose, followed by 275 mg every 6–8 hours or 550 mg every 12 hours
Naproxen	250–500 mg by mouth twice a day
Diclofenac	100 mg by mouth loading dose followed by 50 mg every 6–8 hours, maximum 200 mg/day
Mefenamic acid	500 mg by mouth loading dose, then 250 mg every 6 hours or 500 mg every 8 hours

*Usual duration of treatment is with menses for less than or equal to 5 days.
NSAID: nonsteroidal anti-inflammatory drug

and 150 μg of norelgestromin daily) or the vaginal ring (ethinyl estradiol and etonogestrel), the data on relief of dysmenorrhea appear stronger for the vaginal ring than the transdermal patch. In 389 adult women newly starting on a vaginal ring, 26.5% reported improvement in moderate or severe dysmenorrhea, whereas only 1% indicated an increase in pain.[83] In a 1 year randomized, open-labeled, European trial comparing the vaginal ring and a COCP (30 μg ethinyl estradiol and drospirenone), both demonstrated equivalent efficacy in reducing reported moderate or severe dysmenorrhea, from 17.4 to 5.9% for the ring and from 19 to 6.4% for the COC.[84] When the patch was prescribed to 28 US adolescents primarily as a contraceptive, 39% reported a subjective improvement in dysmenorrhea; however, 11% indicated their pain worsened.[85] In a Thai cohort of 58 adolescents and young adult women using contraception, only 13.8% of participants reported a reduction in dysmenorrhea.[57] Comparing side effects of the patch and an OCP in adult women, 13.3% of patch users reported dysmenorrhea as an adverse event, whereas only 9.6% of those prescribed an OCP did so, a statistically significant difference.[86]

Further benefit may be achieved for relief of menstrual symptoms when OCPs are prescribed in extended regimens, reducing the hormone-free interval. In a small study of 32 women randomized to cyclic use of a 20 ug ethinyl estradiol/0.1 mg levonorgestrel OCP or an extended regimen of 168 days without a hormone-free interval, menstrual pain was present on only a mean of 1.9 days in the extended regimen group compared to 13.3 days in the cyclic group over 6 months.[87] Extended regimens can be prescribed for nonoral routes of administration. The vaginal ring prescribed for extended use, 84 days continuously with a 7 day ring-free interval, demonstrated a statistically significant reduction in frequency of dysmenorrhea from a baseline of 56% to 20% in those who continued the method at 1 year.[88]

Further clarification with regards to the optimum mode of administration of CHCs for treatment of dysmenorrhea requires specific studies in adolescents whereby pain is the primary outcome measure and is assessed by standardized methods, rather than by subjective report. The options of nondaily administration may enhance ease of method use in adolescents, although it is unclear if the transdermal patch in adolescents provides equivalent relief of dysmenorrhea as do COCs.

LARCs consist of methods of contraception that require administration less than once per month or cycle. The LARCs that are beneficial in the treatment of either primary or secondary dysmenorrhea include the levonorgestrel-releasing intrauterine system (LNG IUS), depo-medroxyprogesterone acetate (DMPA), or the single-rod progestin contraceptive implant.[89] Not only may these methods provide symptom relief, but for the sexually active adolescent they provide reliable contraception as well. Each has a different mechanism of action, administration, and side effect profile. DMPA may reduce dysmenorrhea; however, it has the concerns of hypoestrogenic loss of bone density with prolonged use and, for some adolescents, a potential side effect of weight gain.[90]

The LNG IUS acts locally within the uterus to cause deciduation of the endometrial stroma, apoptosis in endometrial glands and stroma, and endometrial atrophy.[91] Its primarily local effect limits systemic side effects. In a cohort of 48 adolescents in the United Kingdom (UK) between menarche and age 18, 92% reported improvement in dysmenorrhea at assessments up to 18 months after LNG IUS insertion.[92] Comparing COC to LNG IUS use, one RCT assessing continuation rates of the contraceptive methods suggested superior alleviation of dysmenorrhea with the LNG IUS, when analyzed as a secondary outcome.[93] Usually, LNG IUS use in adolescents for primary dysmenorrhea or endometriosis has not been considered a first-line therapy but has been employed after failure of response to other methods or due to contraindications to standard therapy.[92,94] Previously, barriers to IUS use in adolescents included concern about the possibility of increasing the risk of developing pelvic inflammatory disease (PID). Clarification of the risk demonstrates that PID may be increased briefly around the time of insertion, by transient contamination of the uterine cavity with microorganisms, but then the risk is low over the remaining period of use.[95] There may be a protective effect of LNG IUS compared to a copper IUD, with lower rates of PID reported at 36 months for the LNG IUS.[96] For contraception use, both the World Health Organization (WHO, 2004) and the US Medical Eligibility Criteria (2010), in young women younger than 20 years of age, consider the LNG IUS to be category 2 (ie, the benefits of use generally outweigh the theoretical or proven risks). In nonsexually active adolescents, insertion can be accomplished under general anesthesia, with conscious sedation or with a paracervical block if required.[94] Insertion on or within a few days of menses or with preinsertion treatment with vaginal misoprostol may decrease failure of placement due to an inability to negotiate the cervical os.

The single-rod progestin (etonogestrel) nonbiodegradable implant is an effective method of contraception for 3 years when inserted subdermally. Its mechanism of action is via inhibition of ovulation through maintenance of sufficiently high plasma levels of progestin. When used for contraception, the implant reduces dysmenorrhea, with 81% of 187 women with dysmenorrhea at time of insertion reporting improvement after treatment and only 5% reporting an increase in pain.[97]

Treatments for Specific Causes of Secondary Dysmenorrhea In the adolescent with persistent pelvic pain despite the use of an NSAID and CHC, endometriosis is documented at laparoscopy in up to 69%,[70] making it the most common etiology of secondary dysmenorrhea. Historically there has been a longer delay from onset of symptoms to diagnosis in adolescents compared to adult women, which may result from a different symptom profile.[98] Many young women present with an acyclic component rather than only cyclic pain, and they may not be sexually active or challenging their fertility, hence dyspareunia and infertility are not present to suggest the diagnosis. The youngest reported child to have had a histologically proven diagnosis of endometriosis was 9 years of age.[99] A positive family history of relatives with endometriosis is more common in adolescents than in adult women (30% vs 7.6%).[69]

A suggested approach to the adolescent with dysmenorrhea is demonstrated in Figure 1. In a young woman who has failed initial medical therapy for pain, pelvic imaging and consideration of laparoscopy for diagnosis and treatment of endometriosis is warranted. As endometriosis lesions in adolescents are more

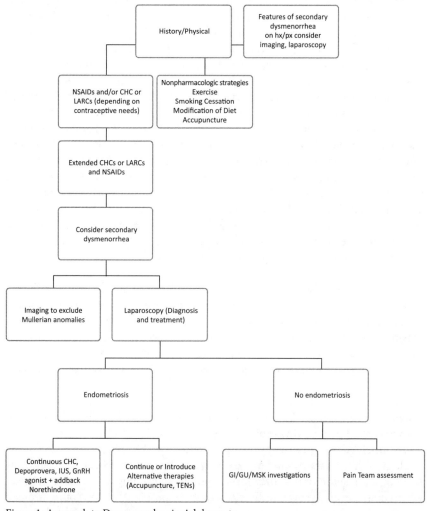

Figure 1. Approach to Dysmenorrhea in Adolescents

often of an atypical form (vesicular or red lesions in approximately 75% of cases), surgery for diagnosis is ideally performed by a surgeon who performs minimally invasive surgery and is familiar with endometriosis in adolescents: The procedure should include an excisional biopsy for histological confirmation.[69]

Early recognition of the symptoms of endometriosis is paramount. A recent study documented that the presence of deep infiltrating endometriosis lesions at laparoscopy in adult women is positively correlated with previous absenteeism from school during menstruation in adolescence, as well as early and prolonged use of OCPs for dysmenorrhea. The authors concluded that early identification of these features could reduce delay in diagnosis.[100]

In many instances, when caring for the adolescent, data regarding the success of therapy are extrapolated from adult populations. Studies of treatment in adolescents are beginning to enhance our knowledge regarding response to therapy in this age group. A recent comparison of adolescents and adults with laparoscopic-proven endometriosis in New Zealand demonstrated a similar positive effect of surgical excision on quality of life questionnaires and visual analogue scales for both populations, one of the first to assess the improvement in pain in adolescents following surgery.[69]

Goals of treatment for the adolescent with endometriosis include establishing a long-term reduction in pain and slowing progression of disease. Once a diagnosis is established, the adolescent should receive medical therapy until a decision is made to pursue conception. It is unclear if the use of medical therapy changes the subsequent development of severe and deeply infiltrating endometriosis.[100,101] The medical therapies previously described for primary dysmenorrhea can be chosen for pain management of the patient with endometriosis with good results (extended use of CHC, Depo-Provera, the LNG IUS).[102,103] GnRH agonists are an additional tool in the management of the pain caused by endometriosis.[104] Theoretical concerns have been expressed regarding their use in younger adolescents, particularly younger than the age of 16, due to concerns about bone health.[101] If prescribed, add-back combined hormone or progesterone-only replacement therapy is advised to minimize symptoms and morbidity while maintaining symptom control.[103]

In order for a Müllerian anomaly to present as secondary dysmenorrhea, there must be partial patency of the outflow tract to allow for visible menarche, whereas cryptomenorrhea leads to the pain. Asymmetric outflow tract obstruction presents as secondary dysmenorrhea, with or without a pelvic mass. The 2 most common variations in Müllerian duct development that result in an asymmetric outflow tract obstruction are a uterine didelphys with a septum obstructing one uterus (OHVIRA syndrome—obstructed hemivagina ipsilateral renal anomaly) or a unicornuate uterus with an associated uterine horn, which both contains an endometrium and is noncommunicating (Figures 2 and 3).

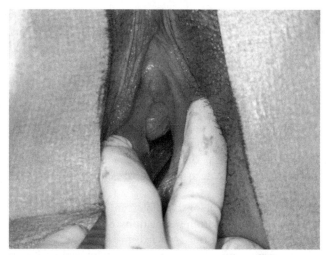

Figure 2. OHVIRA Syndrome The bulge from the left lateral side wall is evident at the time of surgery, and this reflects the hematocolpos behind the obstructing hemivaginal septum in OHVIRA syndrome.

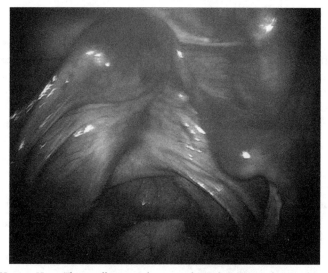

Figure 3. Uterine Horn The small uterine horn on the right contained an endometrium and caused secondary dysmenorrhea.

As uterine didelphys results from a failure of lateral fusion of the Müllerian ducts, 75% of didelphic uteri have an associated longitudinal vaginal septum; a subset of those are obstructing one uterus.[105] OHVIRA syndrome is associated with a renal anomaly in 89% of cases, most commonly renal agenesis ipsilateral to the vaginal obstruction.[106] Uterine horns arise due to an arrest of development of 1 Müllerian duct. A unicornuate uterus is associated with a rudimentary horn in 74% of cases; 26% of horns are both functional and noncommunicating. The treatment of both of these conditions is surgery to relieve the obstruction of the outflow tract by resection of either the obstructing vaginal septum or the uterine horn.[70,107]

SUMMARY

PMS/PMDD is a pervasive problem with a significant impact on the quality of life of affected individuals. This condition most often begins in adolescence with the establishment of normal ovulatory menstrual cycles; however, the underlying pathophysiology has yet to be delineated. Prospective evaluation is key to the confirmation of the diagnosis before the initiation of pharmacotherapy, especially psychotropic therapies, due to the possibly harmful side effect profile for adolescents compared to adults. Similarly, dysmenorrhea is common in adolescents. Although the majority of cases are primary, the HCP must be vigilant to allow for early diagnosis and treatment of secondary causes, thereby preventing long-term sequelae of delayed diagnosis. Stepwise therapy for dysmenorrhea treatment is usually employed; the choice of therapy should account for contraceptive needs of the adolescent in addition to symptom relief. For both PMSS/PMDD and dysmenorrhea, most studies of therapy have been performed in adults and, as such, adolescent-specific trials are required to confirm applicability to this age group.

References

1. Robinson RL, Swindle RW. Premenstrual symptom severity: impact on social functioning and treatment-seeking behaviors. *J Womens Health Gend Based Med.* 2000;9:757–768
2. Rapkin AJ, Mikacich JA. Premenstrual syndrome and premenstrual dysphoric disorder in adolescents. *Curr Opin Obstet Gynecol.* 2008;20:455–463
3. Steiner M, Peer M, Palova E, et al. The Premenstrual Symptoms Screening Tool revised for adolescents (PSST-A): prevalence of severe PMS and premenstrual dysphoric disorder in adolescents. *Arch Womens Ment Health.* 2011;14:77–81
4. Vichnin M, Freeman EW, Lin H, Hillman J, Bui S. Premenstrual syndrome (PMS) in adolescents: severity and impairment. *J Pediatr Adolesc Gynecol.* 2006;19:397–402
5. Derman O, Kanbur NO, Tokur TE, Kutluk T. Premenstrual syndrome and associated symptoms in adolescent girls. *Eur J Obstet Gynecol Reprod Biol.* 2004;116:201–206
6. American Psychiatric Association. *Diagnostic and Statistical Manual of Mental Disorders.* Washington, DC: American Psychiatric Association; 1994
7. Premenstrual Syndrome. *ACOG Practice Bulletin.* 2000;15:1–19
8. Halbreich U. The diagnosis of premenstrual syndromes and premenstrual dysphoric disorder—clinical procedures and research perspectives. *Gynecol Endocrinol.* 2004;19:320–334
9. Borenstein JE, Dean BB, Yonkers KA, Endicott J. Using the daily record of severity of problems as a screening instrument for premenstrual syndrome. *Obstet Gynecol.* 2007;109:1068–1075
10. Treloar SA, Heath AC, Martin NG. Genetic and environmental influences on premenstrual symptoms in an Australian twin sample. *Psychol Med.* 2002;32:25–38
11. Rubinow DR, Hoban MC, Grover GN, et al. Changes in plasma hormones across the menstrual cycle in patients with menstrually related mood disorder and in control subjects. *Am J Obstet Gynecol.* 1988;158:5–11
12. Yonkers KA, O'Brien PM, Eriksson E. Premenstrual syndrome. *Lancet.* 2008;371:1200–1210

13. Hammarback S, Backstrom T. Induced anovulation as treatment of premenstrual tension syndrome. A double-blind cross-over study with GnRH-agonist versus placebo. *Acta Obstet Gynecol Scand.* 1988;67:159–166

14. Casper RF, Hearn MT. The effect of hysterectomy and bilateral oophorectomy in women with severe premenstrual syndrome. *Am J Obstet Gynecol.* 1990;162:105–109

15. Schmidt PJ, Nieman LK, Danaceau MA, Adams LF, Rubinow DR. Differential behavioral effects of gonadal steroids in women with and in those without premenstrual syndrome. *N Engl J Med.* 1998;338:209–216

16. Rubinow DR, Schmidt PJ, Roca CA. Estrogen-serotonin interactions: implications for affective regulation. *Biol Psychiatry.* 1998;44:839–850

17. Bethea CL, Lu NZ, Gundlah C, Streicher JM. Diverse actions of ovarian steroids in the serotonin neural system. *Front Neuroendocrinol.* 2002;23:41–100

18. Meltzer H. Serotonergic dysfunction in depression. *Br J Psychiatry Suppl.* 1989(8):25–31

19. Rapkin AJ, Edelmuth E, Chang LC, et al. Whole-blood serotonin in premenstrual syndrome. *Obstet Gynecol.* 1987;70:533–537

20. Steiner M, Steinberg S, Stewart D, et al. Fluoxetine in the treatment of premenstrual dysphoria. Canadian Fluoxetine/Premenstrual Dysphoria Collaborative Study Group. *N Engl J Med.* 1995;332:1529–1534

21. Yonkers KA, Halbreich U, Freeman E, et al. Symptomatic improvement of premenstrual dysphoric disorder with sertraline treatment. A randomized controlled trial. Sertraline Premenstrual Dysphoric Collaborative Study Group. *JAMA.* 1997;278:983–988

22. Brown J, O'Brien PM, Marjoribanks J, Wyatt K. Selective serotonin reuptake inhibitors for premenstrual syndrome. *Cochrane Database Syst Rev.* 2009:CD001396

23. Shah NR, Jones JB, Aperi J, et al. Selective serotonin reuptake inhibitors for premenstrual syndrome and premenstrual dysphoric disorder: a meta-analysis. *Obstet Gynecol.* 2008;111:1175–1182

24. Cohen LS, Soares CN, Yonkers KA, et al. Paroxetine controlled release for premenstrual dysphoric disorder: a double-blind, placebo-controlled trial. *Psychosom Med.* 2004;66:707–713

25. Roca CA, Schmidt PJ, Smith MJ, et al. Effects of metergoline on symptoms in women with premenstrual dysphoric disorder. *Am J Psychiatry.* 2002;159:1876–1881

26. Sundstrom Poromaa I, Smith S, Gulinello M. GABA receptors, progesterone and premenstrual dysphoric disorder. *Arch Womens Ment Health.* 2003;6:23–41

27. Girdler SS, Straneva PA, Light KC, Pedersen CA, Morrow AL. Allopregnanolone levels and reactivity to mental stress in premenstrual dysphoric disorder. *Biol Psychiatry.* 2001;49:788–797

28. Sundstrom I, Andersson A, Nyberg S, et al. Patients with premenstrual syndrome have a different sensitivity to a neuroactive steroid during the menstrual cycle compared to control subjects. *Neuroendocrinology.* 1998;67:126–138

29. Chau JP, Chang AM. Effects of an educational programme on adolescents with premenstrual syndrome. *Health Educ Res.* 1999;14:817–830

30. Daley A. Exercise and premenstrual symptomatology: a comprehensive review. *J Womens Health (Larchmt).* 2009;18:895–899

31. Steege JF, Blumenthal JA. The effects of aerobic exercise on premenstrual symptoms in middle-aged women: a preliminary study. *J Psychosom Res.* 1993;37:127–133

32. Braverman PK. Premenstrual syndrome and premenstrual dysphoric disorder. *J Pediatr Adolesc Gynecol.* 2007;20:3–12

33. Thys-Jacobs S, Starkey P, Bernstein D, Tian J. Calcium carbonate and the premenstrual syndrome: effects on premenstrual and menstrual symptoms. Premenstrual Syndrome Study Group. *Am J Obstet Gynecol.* 1998;179:444–452

34. Thys-Jacobs S, McMahon D, Bilezikian JP. Cyclical changes in calcium metabolism across the menstrual cycle in women with premenstrual dysphoric disorder. *J Clin Endocrinol Metab.* 2007;92:2952–2959

35. Bertone-Johnson ER, Chocano-Bedoya PO, Zagarins SE, Micka AE, Ronnenberg AG. Dietary vitamin D intake, 25-hydroxyvitamin D3 levels and premenstrual syndrome in a college-aged population. *J Steroid Biochem Mol Biol.* 2010;121:434–437

36. Khajehei M, Abdali K, Parsanezhad ME, Tabatabaee HR. Effect of treatment with dydrogesterone or calcium plus vitamin D on the severity of premenstrual syndrome. *Int J Gynaecol Obstet.* 2009;105:158–161

37. Andersch B. The effect of various oral contraceptive combinations on premenstrual symptoms. *Int J Gynaecol Obstet.* 1982;20:463–469

38. Graham CA, Sherwin BB. A prospective treatment study of premenstrual symptoms using a triphasic oral contraceptive. *J Psychosom Res.* 1992;36:257–266

39. Joffe H, Cohen LS, Harlow BL. Impact of oral contraceptive pill use on premenstrual mood: predictors of improvement and deterioration. *Am J Obstet Gynecol.* 2003;189:1523–1530

40. Willis SA, Kuehl TJ, Spiekerman AM, Sulak PJ. Greater inhibition of the pituitary—ovarian axis in oral contraceptive regimens with a shortened hormone-free interval. *Contraception.* 2006;74:100–103

41. Sulak PJ, Scow RD, Preece C, Riggs MW, Kuehl TJ. Hormone withdrawal symptoms in oral contraceptive users. *Obstet Gynecol.* 2000;95:261–266

42. Rapkin AJ, Winer SA. The pharmacologic management of premenstrual dysphoric disorder. *Expert Opin Pharmacother.* 2008;9:429–445

43. Greco T, Graham CA, Bancroft J, Tanner A, Doll HA. The effects of oral contraceptives on androgen levels and their relevance to premenstrual mood and sexual interest: a comparison of two triphasic formulations containing norgestimate and either 35 or 25 micrograms of ethinyl estradiol. *Contraception.* 2007;76:8–17

44. Yonkers KA, Brown C, Pearlstein TB, et al. Efficacy of a new low-dose oral contraceptive with drospirenone in premenstrual dysphoric disorder. *Obstet Gynecol.* 2005;106:492–501

45. Pearlstein TB, Bachmann GA, Zacur HA, Yonkers KA. Treatment of premenstrual dysphoric disorder with a new drospirenone-containing oral contraceptive formulation. *Contraception.* 2005;72:414–421

46. Coffee AL, Kuehl TJ, Willis S, Sulak PJ. Oral contraceptives and premenstrual symptoms: comparison of a 21/7 and extended regimen. *Am J Obstet Gynecol.* 2006;195:1311–1319

47. Reid R, Leyland N, Wolfman W, et al. SOGC clinical practice guidelines: oral contraceptives and the risk of venous thromboembolism: an update: no. 252, December 2010. *Int J Gynaecol Obstet.* 2010;112:252–256

48. Eriksson E, Ekman A, Sinclair S, et al. Escitalopram administered in the luteal phase exerts a marked and dose-dependent effect in premenstrual dysphoric disorder. *J Clin Psychopharmacol.* 2008;28:195–202

49. Steiner M, Ravindran AV, LeMelledo JM, et al. Luteal phase administration of paroxetine for the treatment of premenstrual dysphoric disorder: a randomized, double-blind, placebo-controlled trial in Canadian women. *J Clin Psychiatry.* 2008;69:991–998

50. Silber TJ, Valadez-Meltzer A. Premenstrual dysphoric disorder in adolescents: case reports of treatment with fluoxetine and review of the literature. *J Adolesc Health.* 2005;37:518–525

51. Bridge JA, Iyengar S, Salary CB, et al. Clinical response and risk for reported suicidal ideation and suicide attempts in pediatric antidepressant treatment: a meta-analysis of randomized controlled trials. *JAMA.* 2007;297:1683–1696

52. Hosenbocus S, Chahal R. SSRIs and SNRIs. A review of the discontinuation syndrome in children and adolescents. *J Can Acad Child Adolesc Psychiatry.* 2011;20:60–67

53. Divasta AD, Laufer MR, Gordon CM. Bone density in adolescents treated with a GnRH agonist and add-back therapy for endometriosis. *J Pediatr Adolesc Gynecol.* 2007;20:293–297

54. Campbell MA, McGrath PJ. Non-pharmacologic strategies used by adolescents for the management of menstrual discomfort. *Clin J Pain.* 1999;15:313–320

55. Parker MA, Sneddon AE, Arbon P. The menstrual disorder of teenagers (MDOT) study: determining typical menstrual patterns and menstrual disturbance in a large population-based study of Australian teenagers. *BJOG.* 2010;117:185–192

56. Banikarim C, Chacko MR, Kelder SH. Prevalence and impact of dysmenorrhea on Hispanic female adolescents. *Arch Pediatr Adolesc Med.* 2000;154:1226–1229

57. Piyasirisilp R, Taneepanichskul S. A clinical study of transdermal contraceptive patch in Thai adolescence women. *J Med Assoc Thai.* 2008;91:137–141

58. Klein JR, Litt IF. Epidemiology of adolescent dysmenorrhea. *Pediatrics.* 1981;68:661–664
59. Ortiz MI, Rangel-Flores E, Carrillo-Alarcon LC, Veras-Godoy HA. Prevalence and impact of primary dysmenorrhea among Mexican high school students. *Int J Gynaecol Obstet.* 2009;107:240–243
60. Farquhar CM, Roberts H, Okonkwo QL, Stewart AW. A pilot survey of the impact of menstrual cycles on adolescent health. *Aust N Z J Obstet Gynaecol.* 2009;49:531–536
61. Houston AM, Abraham A, Huang Z, D'Angelo LJ. Knowledge, attitudes, and consequences of menstrual health in urban adolescent females. *J Pediatr Adolesc Gynecol.* 2006;19:271–275
62. Latthe P, Mignini L, Gray R, Hills R, Khan K. Factors predisposing women to chronic pelvic pain: systematic review. *BMJ.* 2006;332:749–755
63. O'Connell K, Davis AR, Westhoff C. Self-treatment patterns among adolescent girls with dysmenorrhea. *J Pediatr Adolesc Gynecol.* 2006;19:285–289
64. Zahradnik HP, Hanjalic-Beck A, Groth K. Nonsteroidal anti-inflammatory drugs and hormonal contraceptives for pain relief from dysmenorrhea: a review. *Contraception.* 2010;81:185–196
65. Harel Z. Dysmenorrhea in adolescents and young adults: from pathophysiology to pharmacological treatments and management strategies. *Expert Opin Pharmacother.* 2008;9:2661–2672
66. DuRant RH, Jay MS, Shoffitt T, Linder CW, Taylor W. Factors influencing adolescents' responses to regimens of naproxen for dysmenorrhea. *Am J Dis Child.* 1985;139:489–493
67. Davis AR, Westhoff C, O'Connell K, Gallagher N. Oral contraceptives for dysmenorrhea in adolescent girls: a randomized trial. *Obstet Gynecol.* 2005;106:97–104
68. Harada T, Momoeda M, Terakawa N, Taketani Y, Hoshiai H. Evaluation of a low-dose oral contraceptive pill for primary dysmenorrhea: a placebo-controlled, double-blind, randomized trial. *Fertil Steril.* 2011;95:1928–1931
69. Roman JD. Adolescent endometriosis in the Waikato region of New Zealand—a comparative cohort study with a mean follow-up time of 2.6 years. *Aust N Z J Obstet Gynaecol.* 2010;50:179–183
70. Laufer MR, Goitein L, Bush M, Cramer DW, Emans SJ. Prevalence of endometriosis in adolescent girls with chronic pelvic pain not responding to conventional therapy. *J Pediatr Adolesc Gynecol.* 1997;10:199–202
71. Campbell MA, McGrath PJ. Use of medication by adolescents for the management of menstrual discomfort. *Arch Pediatr Adolesc Med* 1997;151:905–913
72. Sanfilippo J, Erb T. Evaluation and management of dysmenorrhea in adolescents. *Clin Obstet Gynecol.* 2008;51:257–267
73. Daley AJ. Exercise and primary dysmenorrhoea: a comprehensive and critical review of the literature. *Sports Med.* 2008;38:659–670
74. Israel RG, Sutton M, O'Brien KF. Effects of aerobic training on primary dysmenorrhea symptomatology in college females. *J Am Coll Health.* 1985;33:241–244
75. Blakey H, Chisholm C, Dear F, et al. Is exercise associated with primary dysmenorrhoea in young women? *BJOG* 2010;117:222–224
76. Wilson C, Emans SJ, Mansfield J, Podolsky C, Grace E. The relationships of calculated percent body fat, sports participation, age, and place of residence on menstrual patterns in healthy adolescent girls at an independent New England high school. *J Adolesc Health Care.* 1984;5:248–253
77. Brown J, Brown S. Exercise for dysmenorrhoea. *Cochrane Database Syst Rev* 2010:CD004142
78. Dorn LD, Negriff S, Huang B, et al. Menstrual symptoms in adolescent girls: association with smoking, depressive symptoms, and anxiety. *J Adolesc Health.* 2009;44:237–243
79. Mishra GD, Dobson AJ, Schofield MJ. Cigarette smoking, menstrual symptoms and miscarriage among young women. *Aust N Z J Public Health.* 2000;24:413–420
80. Cho SH, Hwang EW. Acupuncture for primary dysmenorrhoea: a systematic review. *BJOG.* 2010;117:509–521
81. Liu CZ, Xie JP, Wang LP, et al. Immediate analgesia effect of single point acupuncture in primary dysmenorrhea: a randomized controlled trial. *Pain Med.* 2011;12:300–307
82 Warner TD, Giuliano F, Vojnovic I, et al. Nonsteroid drug selectivities for cyclo-oxygenase-1 rather than cyclo-oxygenase-2 are associated with human gastrointestinal toxicity: a full in vitro analysis. *Proc Natl Acad Sci U S A.* 1999;96:7563–7568
83. Merki-Feld GS, Hund M. Clinical experience with the combined contraceptive vaginal ring in Switzerland, including a subgroup analysis of previous hormonal contraceptive use. *Eur J Contracept Reprod Health Care.* 2010;15:413–422

84. Milsom I, Lete I, Bjertnaes A, et al. Effects on cycle control and bodyweight of the combined contraceptive ring, NuvaRing, versus an oral contraceptive containing 30 microg ethinyl estradiol and 3 mg drospirenone. *Hum Reprod.* 2006;21:2304–2311

85. Harel Z, Riggs S, Vaz R, et al. Adolescents' experience with the combined estrogen and progestin transdermal contraceptive method Ortho Evra. *J Pediatr Adolesc Gynecol.* 2005;18:85–90

86. Sibai BM, Odlind V, Meador ML, et al. A comparative and pooled analysis of the safety and tolerability of the contraceptive patch (Ortho Evra/Evra). *Fertil Steril.* 2002;77:S19–26

87. Kwiecien M, Edelman A, Nichols MD, Jensen JT. Bleeding patterns and patient acceptability of standard or continuous dosing regimens of a low-dose oral contraceptive: a randomized trial. *Contraception.* 2003;67:9–13

88. Barreiros FA, Guazzelli CA, Barbosa R, de Assis F, de Araujo FF. Extended regimens of the contraceptive vaginal ring: evaluation of clinical aspects. *Contraception.* 2010;81:223–225

89. ACOG Practice Bulletin No. 110. Noncontraceptive uses of hormonal contraceptives. *Obstet Gynecol.* 2010;115:206–218

90. Harel Z, Biro FM, Kollar LM. Depo-Provera in adolescents: effects of early second injection or prior oral contraception. *J Adolesc Health.* 1995;16:379–384

91. Fraser IS. Non-contraceptive health benefits of intrauterine hormonal systems. *Contraception.* 2010;82:396–403

92. Aslam N, Blunt S, Latthe P. Effectiveness and tolerability of levonorgestrel intrauterine system in adolescents. *J Obstet Gynaecol* 2010;30:489–491

93. Suhonen S, Haukkamaa M, Jakobsson T, Rauramo I. Clinical performance of a levonorgestrel-releasing intrauterine system and oral contraceptives in young nulliparous women: a comparative study. *Contraception.* 2004;69:407–412

94. Paterson H, Ashton J, Harrison-Woolrych M. A nationwide cohort study of the use of the levonorgestrel intrauterine device in New Zealand adolescents. *Contraception.* 2009;79:433–438

95. Farley TM, Rosenberg MJ, Rowe PJ, Chen JH, Meirik O. Intrauterine devices and pelvic inflammatory disease: an international perspective. *Lancet.* 1992;339:785–788

96. Toivonen J, Luukkainen T, Allonen H. Protective effect of intrauterine release of levonorgestrel on pelvic infection: three years' comparative experience of levonorgestrel- and copper-releasing intrauterine devices. *Obstet Gynecol.* 1991;77:261–264

97. Funk S, Miller MM, Mishell DR Jr, et al. Safety and efficacy of Implanon, a single-rod implantable contraceptive containing etonogestrel. *Contraception.* 2005;71:319–326

98. Ballweg ML. Tips on treating teens with endometriosis. *J Pediatr Adolesc Gynecol.* 2003;16:S27–28

99. Ebert AD, Fuhr N, David M, Schneppel L, Papadopoulos T. Histological confirmation of endometriosis in a 9-year-old girl suffering from unexplained cyclic pelvic pain since her eighth year of life. *Gynecol Obstet Invest.* 2009;67:158–161

100. Chapron C, Lafay-Pillet MC, Monceau E, et al. Questioning patients about their adolescent history can identify markers associated with deep infiltrating endometriosis. *Fertil Steril.* 2011;95:877–881

101. ACOG Committee Opinion No. 310, April 2005. Endometriosis in adolescents. *Obstet Gynecol.* 2005;105:921–927

102. Stavroulis AI, Saridogan E, Creighton SM, Cutner AS. Laparoscopic treatment of endometriosis in teenagers. *Eur J Obstet Gynecol Reprod Biol.* 2006;125:248–250

103. Leyland N, Casper R, Laberge P, Singh SS. Endometriosis: diagnosis and management. *J Obstet Gynaecol Can.* 2010;32:S1–32

104. Gilliam ML. Gonadotrophin-releasing hormone analogues for pain associated with endometriosis. *Obstet Gynecol.* 2011;117:727–728

105. Troiano RN, McCarthy SM. Müllerian duct anomalies: imaging and clinical issues. *Radiology.* 2004;233:19–34

106. Smith NA, Laufer MR. Obstructed hemivagina and ipsilateral renal anomaly (OHVIRA) syndrome: management and follow-up. *Fertil Steril.* 2007;87:918–922.

107. Spitzer RF, Kives S, Allen LM. Case series of laparoscopically resected noncommunicating functional uterine horns. *J Pediatr Adolesc Gynecol.* 2009;22:e23–28

Adolesc Med 23 (2012) 164–177

Adolescent Polycystic Ovary Syndrome

Ellen Lancon Connor, MD*

Associate Professor of Pediatric Endocrinology, University of Wisconsin, Madison, Wisconsin

INTRODUCTION

Once a diagnosis made primarily in fertility clinics, polycystic ovary syndrome (PCOS) was considered to be a condition of the adult female. Now, however, PCOS is recognized as a diagnosis that begins prenatally and manifests itself through early childhood, puberty, and adolescence.[1] Both ovarian and adrenal hyperandrogenism have roles in the signs and symptoms of the syndrome. Ovarian hyperandrogenism can be elucidated by administration of a gonadotropin releasing hormone agonist, with subsequent exaggerated 17-hydroxyprogesterone production with incomplete suppression of testosterone secretion when glucocorticoid-mediated adrenal suppression is performed. Adrenal hyperandrogenism has been documented by 17-hydroxypregnenlone and dehydroepiandrosterone sulfate (DHEAS) surges with adrenocorticopin hormone (ACTH) stimulation.[2,3] How to define PCOS and when the diagnosis of PCOS can be made in adolescence remain topics of controversy; however, associated risk factors can now be recognized in infancy and childhood, and 11–26% of adolescent girls may be affected.[4] Although obesity is commonly associated with adolescent PCOS, some adolescent PCOS patients are lean; both lean and obese PCOS patients, however, may begin to manifest signs of insulin resistance in childhood.[5] As the field of molecular genetics has advanced, our understanding of the heritability of adrenal and ovarian androgen synthesis and insulin metabolism has elucidated the relationship of adolescent PCOS to familial inheritance of type 2 diabetes mellitus and metabolic syndrome. Many questions remain regarding what prenatal or early postnatal interventions might change the pathway leading to adolescent PCOS, and for adolescents with PCOS, many other questions remain regarding appropriate treatment and follow-up.

---

*Corresponding author.
E-mail address: elconnor@pediatrics.wisc.edu (E. L. Connor).

Girls and women with PCOS share a commonality of varying degrees and presentations of menstrual irregularity, clinical and/or biochemical hyperandrogenism, ovarian morphology, increased body mass index (BMI), metabolic syndrome, and insulin resistance. Among adolescents referred to one multidisciplinary clinic, 64% had oligomenorrhea or secondary amenorrhea, 63% had a glucose/insulin ratio less than 4.5, 84% were overweight (BMI > 85th percentile), and 70% were obese.[6] Seventy percent of that same group had acne, 60% were hirsute, and 52% had elevated free testosterone. In another study of adolescents with PCOS, 37% were noted to have metabolic syndrome, with hyperandrogenism being an independent risk factor.[7] Yet another study by Hickey in 2009 identified that girls who had BMIs above average were 10-fold more likely to have adolescent PCOS (using National Institutes of Health [NIH] criteria).[8] Adult surveys have found menstrual abnormalities in 80–100% of patients, polycystic ovarian morphology in 70–95% of some series, obesity in 30–60%, and insulin resistance or hyperinsulinism in 50–70%.[9] Menstrual abnormalities increase the risk of endometrial hyperplasia and uterine cancer. Dyslipidemia is seen in up to 70% of adult PCOS patients[10] and often begins with hypertriglyceridemia and low high density lipoprotein (HDL) in both adolescent and adult patients.

IN THE BEGINNING

Both genetics and environment are involved in the development of adolescent PCOS. Among the factors pointing toward genetics are patterns of disease variability that track through families affected by PCOS, the high penetrance of PCOS among sisters of women with PCOS, and the observation of PCOS in daughters of fathers with type 2 diabetes mellitus. In one study of 93 women with PCOS, 40% of sisters were also affected, as were 35% of mothers.[11] Brothers of women with PCOS have been observed to have elevated levels of DHEAS, and a study of men whose sisters had PCOS documented insulin resistance in those men.[12] Many genes are under scrutiny as candidates in the genetic milieu that predisposes a female to PCOS. These can be broadly classified into (1) genes affecting the synthesis and action of steroids; (2) genes affecting gonadotropic action; (3) metabolism genes that regulate weight and energy use; (4) genes that are a part of the pathway of insulin action; and (5) other genes with unknown function.[13-16]

Environmental influences occur both prenatally and postnatally. Among the prenatal associations are the relationship of adolescent PCOS with high birth weight and mothers with gestational diabetes or metabolic syndrome.[17] The development of PCOS after prenatal hyperandrogenism has been described in other primates. Rhesus monkeys exposed in utero to hyperandrogenism develop a PCOS phenotype of hyperinsulinism, hyperandrogenism, oligo-ovulation, and dyslipidemia, particularly if allowed to become overweight.[18] Another relationship that has been demonstrated is that of intrauterine growth retardation (IUGR) with subsequent premature adrenarche and lean adolescent PCOS.[19] In the latter example, the IUGR state would appear to be a result of in utero insulin resistance because fetal growth is determined by insulin. Interestingly, puberty would seem to be a critical time for intervention if a metabolic syndrome is to be avoided in the IUGR female destined for PCOS. Ibanez has reported the successful use of metformin at puberty to decrease adiposity in key body regions known to have interplay in the development of metabolic syndrome and insulin resistance.[20]

DEFINING ADOLESCENT POLYCYSTIC OVARY SYNDROME

The criteria used to diagnose PCOS have been reviewed and refined through several permutations of consensus groups (Table 1). The 1990 NIH criteria focused on the presence of oligo/anovulation and clinical or biochemical evidence of hyperandrogenism to establish a diagnosis.[21] The 2003 Rotterdam criteria, developed jointly by the European Society for Human Reproduction and Embryology with the American Society for Reproductive Medicine, defined PCOS as being present if 2 of 3 criteria were present: clinical or biochemical hyperandrogenism, oligo/anovulation, and/or radiographic evidence of polycystic ovaries. The Rotterdam criteria introduced some heterogeneity into the population of PCOS patients, as it was now possible to have the diagnosis without having any hyperandrogenism.[22] Considerable disagreement exists in the medical community regarding whether this heterogeneity is helpful in following the evolution of PCOS in some patients or simply muddies the waters in trying to evaluate the efficacy of therapies in patients identified as having PCOS. Certainly, the Rotterdam criteria may actually identify several genetically distinct groups, including some with fewer tendencies toward metabolic syndrome and insulin resistance. Androgen Excess-PCOS (AE-PCOS) Society criteria attempted in 2009 to define PCOS with more attention to hyperandrogenism by defining PCOS as hyperandrogenism plus either oligo/anovulation or radiographic evidence of polycystic ovaries.[23,24] A polycystic ovary was defined in both the Rotterdam criteria and the AE-PCOS criteria as one which contains at least 12 or more follicles (2–9 mm) in a peripheral pattern, or an ovary with a volume greater than 10 mL[22] (Figure 1).

The use of any of the previously described criteria is difficult in the evaluation of a young adolescent patient. Puberty is known to be a state of physiologic insulin

Table 1. Comparison of Diagnostic Criteria for Polycystic Ovary Syndrome

Criteria	Hyperandrogenism	Anovulation	Polycystic ovaries	Lack of other diagnoses
NIH Criteria	Required	Required	Not required	+
Rotterdam Criteria (2 of first 3 required)	+/−	+/−	+/−	+
AE-PCOS Society Criteria (1st and either 2nd or 3rd findings required)	Required	+/−	+/−	+

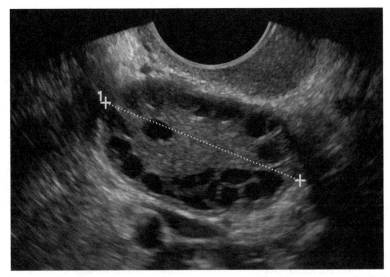

Figure 1. Ultrasonography of Polycystic Ovary with "String of Pearls" Appearance of Follicles

resistance, and insulin is known to have roles in ovarian and adrenal metabolism, as well as hepatic sex hormone binding globulin (SHBG) production. Specifically, insulin decreases hepatic SHBG production, leading to increased free
testosterone in the serum. Oligo-ovulation with subsequent menstrual irregularity is a common finding in the first 18 months following menarche. Furthermore, recent studies have found considerable overlap between polycystic ovaries
and normal ovaries in both adolescents and adults. Chinese adolescents who
had PCOS were found to have a mean ovarian volume of 6.7 mL, rather than the
10 mL traditionally used in the definition of polycystic ovarian volume in adult
women.[25] Further complicating the evaluation of PCOS in puberty is the fact
that ovarian volume continues to increase for 2–3 years following menarche, and
although measurements are more accurate with transvaginal rather than transabdominal ovarian ultrasound, most sonographic data obtained on adolescents
are transabdominal. Hyperandrogenism diagnosed clinically by acne may actually reflect increased free androgen production in puberty rather than a pathologic state. With these unique aspects of adolescence in mind, Carmina et al has
recommended that adolescent PCOS be defined much more stringently, requiring all components of the Rotterdam criteria for absolute diagnosis, waiting at
least 2 years postmenarche to evaluate for the diagnosis, and considering girls
with hyperandrogenism and oligomenorrhea as having "probable but uncon-
firmed PCOS."[26] The advantage of these criteria is prevention of inclusion of girls
who do not have PCOS from temporarily having a stigmatizing or pessimistic
diagnosis that is ultimately disproved after a transient period of irregular menses
or androgen excess. The disadvantage of the use of Carmina's criteria could be a
delay in definitive treatment of girls who have hirsutism or oligomenorrhea due
to PCOS but do not yet have polycystic ovaries and delayed evaluation of these

girls for the insulin resistance of PCOS, known to be a significant risk factor for metabolic system and cardiovascular disease.

The diagnosis of PCOS at any age must be made only after absolute exclusion of the diagnoses of Cushing syndrome, hypothyroidism, prolactinoma, an androgen-secreting tumor, congenital adrenal hyperplasia, and exogenous androgen exposure. In adolescent girls, the diagnosis of Cushing syndrome is best excluded by obtaining 11 PM salivary cortisol measurements, as the normal diurnal variation of cortisol results in extremely low late night salivary cortisol levels in patients without Cushing syndrome. Urinary free cortisol measurements are second best, but are difficult to obtain in adolescent girls who find the collections cumbersome, unpleasant, and intrusive. Thyroid abnormalities should be ruled out with a third generation thyroid-stimulating hormone (TSH) assay, and serum prolactin rules out hyperprolactinemia. Some patients with PCOS will have prolactin levels in the 20s or 30s but not in the greater than 100 ng/mL range typical of a pituitary tumor. Total testosterone levels greater than 200 ng/dL may indicate an androgen-secreting tumor, but the variability of both total and free testosterone assays in women and children requires consideration in interpretation.[27] Testosterone secreting tumors do not always lead to clitoromegaly, so the assay should always be obtained regardless of physical findings. Congenital adrenal hyperplasia screening should be carried out by assessing 17 OH progesterone, DHEAS, and androstenedione between 8 AM and 9 AM, taking advantage of the ACTH secretion peak. Elevated follicle stimulating hormone (FSH) levels should alert the clinician to the differential diagnosis of premature ovarian failure. Lastly, pregnancy should always be considered as a cause of amenorrhea, even in an adolescent with acne or hirsutism.

Some laboratory measurements are suggestive but not absolutely diagnostic of PCOS. An LH/FSH ratio greater than 2 suggests PCOS, as the luteinizing hormone (LH) increases in response to both hyperinsulinemia and hyperandrogenism, as well as to elevated estrogen. However, a woman may meet diagnostic criteria for PCOS without having such a ratio. Similarly, low sex hormone binding globulin production by the liver may be seen as a result of hyperinsulinism. Low sex hormone binding globulin can produce an elevated free testosterone level. Some patients with PCOS, however, exhibit signs consistent with hyperandrogenism without having biochemical hyperandrogenism, probably as a result of receptor responsiveness. Thus, the laboratory evaluation is essential for excluding other diagnoses but not necessarily diagnostic of PCOS.

If an adolescent is diagnosed with PCOS by Rotterdam criteria, AE-PCOS criteria, or the more stringent criteria proposed by Carmina et al, subsequent laboratory studies should include assessment of metabolic syndrome risk factors, including hyperinsulinism/insulin resistance, glucose tolerance, and hyperlipidemia. Fasting glucose values are of less value in assessing the stage of glucose tolerance than are values of an oral glucose tolerance test, carried out with ingestion of 75 g of a glucose drink after a 12 hour fast; impaired glucose tolerance as evidenced by a 2 hour glucose greater than 140 mg/dL is present before impaired fasting glucose. Obtaining an insulin value with the fasting glucose allows calculation of the glucose/insulin ratio, another surrogate marker of insulin resistance. Although some studies have used a glucose/insulin ratio less than 7 in nondiabetic subjects as indicative of insulin resistance, such a cutoff will include some normal adolescents with physiologic resistance of puberty; therefore, a cutoff of less than 4.5 in a nondiabetic subject is preferable.[28,29] The fasting lipid profile of an insulin resistant patient with PCOS may reveal an elevated triglyceride level and low high density lipoprotein (HDL), with relatively mild increases in total or low density lipoprotein (LDL) cholesterol, reflecting the initial changes due to insulin resistance.

THERAPEUTIC CONSIDERATIONS

The approach to the adolescent with PCOS must address each of the following concerns[30]:

1. Menstrual dysfunction, risk of endometrial cancer, and future fertility
2. Hyperandrogenism, including acne, hirsutism, and alopecia
3. Metabolic syndrome risks
4. Psychological concerns impeding or influencing the patient's perception of therapy, quality of life, and likelihood of success with recommended treatments
5. Risk of other comorbidities

Menstrual Dysfunction and Future Fertility

Adolescent PCOS may present with secondary amenorrhea, menorrhagia, metrorrhagia, or menometrorrhagia. Excessive bleeding may result in missed schooldays and extracurricular activities, anemia, or even a need for transfusion. Primary amenorrhea has been described as a historical feature in some women eventually diagnosed with PCOS. Dysmenorrhea and oligomenorrhea (fewer than 6 menstrual cycles per year) are common findings in adolescent PCOS. In the patient with excessive bleeding, a careful family history of bleeding diatheses should be sought, and evaluation for clotting deficiencies considered. Patients with amenorrhea, oligomenorrhea, and menorrhagia may benefit from menstrual regulation with a combined estrogen and progesterone tablet in the form of an oral contraceptive pill (OCP), unless the patient has a personal or family history of clotting disorders. Individual OCP selection should begin with a low to moderate estrogen component (usually 20–35 mcg estradiol) and less androgenic progesterone. Dysmenorrhea may also respond well to these therapeutic choices, and the more favorable progesterone component OCPs can be useful in the management of hirsutism and acne. Some patients may opt for the vaginal contraceptive ring, particularly those who have difficulty remembering to take daily oral medications. Patients with oligomenorrhea who have a clotting disorder history in themselves or in their families can regulate menses with progesterone-only therapies, including monthly, bimonthly, or trimonthly use of 5–10 days of medroxyprogesterone 10 mg, norethindrone 5 mg, or prometrium 200 mg. Some girls may opt for protection from endometrial cancer risk with the levonorgestrel intrauterine system (IUS); this option may be particularly favorable to those who are sexually active. Girls choosing to use an IUS should be advised of the frequent development of secondary amenorrhea with this method. Advantages of the use of OCP therapy in those patients without contraindications include improvements in both the menstrual and hyperandrogenism symptoms. A combined OCP decreases pituitary LH production, which subsequently decreases ovarian theca cell stimulation and ovarian hyperandrogenism.

Some controversy has arisen regarding newer contraceptives containing the fourth generation progestin drospirenone. These OCPs have seen a sharp rise in prescriptions filled due to the popularity both of the low dose estrogenic component and of the androgen receptor blockade action, similar to about 25 mg of spironolactone. Some increase in serum potassium is possible, but more concern has been expressed about a possible increase in the incidence of thromboembolic events in users of pills containing drospirenone as opposed to levonorgestrel.[31] A recent British Medical Journal editorial made the observation that, although the studies have been small, have not been prospective controlled studies, and have not controlled for obesity and the inclusion of new contraceptive users, no study has demonstrated a lower incidence of thromboembolism with drospirenone than levonorgestrel.[32] The use of an OCP that does not contain drospirenone would seem advisable in girls with PCOS presenting for institution of OCP therapy.

Care should be taken when prescribing OCPs to the adolescent with PCOS to discuss the risk of thromboembolic events with OCP use, and OCPs should not be prescribed if there is a known history of clots in the patient and should be used with caution if the history is in family members. Girls should also be counseled that the risk of thromboembolic events increases with obesity, a sedentary lifestyle, and cigarette use.

Patients and parents often have numerous questions about future fertility. Girls must be counseled that a diagnosis of PCOS is not a guarantee of protection from pregnancy if they have unprotected sex. At the same time, if a young woman does have difficulty conceiving when pregnancy is desired, numerous methods of improving the likelihood of conception do exist. Patients with a diagnosis of PCOS should also be counseled that having a healthy BMI improves the likelihood of achieving a successful pregnancy.

Hyperandrogenism

Hyperandrogenism can manifest differently in each girl with PCOS, even in the same family. A history of early, severe, scarring acne may be described in some patients. Thus, dermatologists considering isotretinoin use in adolescent girls should screen clinically and biochemically for PCOS. Other girls may have little or no acne but may have hirsutism beginning in the peripubertal or postpubertal periods. Hirsutism must be distinguished from hypertrichosis, which is fine, vellus hair in nonandrogen-dependent regions. By contrast, hirsutism is androgen dependent and is characterized by terminal hairs, often described as being "central" in location: The face, chin, center of the breasts, periareolar area, lower abdomen, central thighs, and lower back areas are often involved. The Ferriman-Gallwey score (FGS) is often utilized in studies assessing hirsutism, although interpretation should consider ethnicity and the fact that many of the regions considered are areas of potential hypertrichosis.[33] Eight or higher on the FGS is considered hirsute in Caucasians, yet some ethnic groups with less body hair may be hirsute with a lower score, and some ethnicities known for hypertrichosis should have their FGS interpreted cautiously.

Antiandrogen therapy for acne and hirsutism may begin with OCPs that have low androgenic potential. A gradual decrease in new hair growth and acne can be seen in some patients with OCPs alone over the first year of therapy. Hair that is already present must be removed by conventional methods. For patients not responding to OCPs alone, and those in whom OCPs are not an option, spironolactone can be used as an effective antiandrogen that blocks the androgen receptors. An initial dose of 50 mg twice daily may gradually be increased to 100 mg twice daily as needed. Use of the drug requires attention to hydration status, avoidance of dehydration, and avoidance of high potassium containing foods. Serum potassium should be checked at least annually. Spironolactone's effect may not be fully seen for 6 months. Girls must be counseled regarding the teratogenicity of spironolactone. (As an antiandrogen, spironolactone causes ambiguity of the genitalia of male infants.) Therefore, contraception must be used at all times by a patient taking spironolactone, and spironolactone must be discontinued before conception if pregnancy is planned or immediately if an unplanned pregnancy occurs.

During the initial period of use of spironolactone, other acne treatments and methods of hair removal should be continued. One topical treatment for hirsutism is eflornithine, which blocks the enzyme ornithine decarboxylase in hair follicles; it must be applied twice daily and is generally not covered by medical insurance policies.[34]

Successful treatment for hirsutism stops or significantly slows terminal hair production. Treatment does not change hypertrichosis, which has a familial inheritance and is more noticeable in girls with dark hair. Furthermore, treatment does not remove hair already present. Terminal hairs can be removed by waxing, shaving, sugaring, depilatory use, laser treatments, electrolysis, or threading. If laser therapy is chosen, a girl should have a test treatment in a small area of hair not readily visible to be certain skin color changes do not occur.

Metabolic Syndrome

PCOS is associated with an increased incidence of metabolic syndrome, and metabolic syndrome significantly increases a woman's risk for future cardiovascular disease through increased insulin resistance, glucose intolerance/diabetes mellitus, hypertension, and dyslipidemia. Independent from BMI, adiponectin levels are lower in adolescent girls with PCOS than in age-matched controls.[35] Adiponectin is well-recognized as an "anti-inflammatory marker" in adolescents and adults, and low adiponectin levels are predictive of metabolic syndrome risk.

The diagnosis of PCOS mandates an evaluation of BMI, resting blood pressure, a fasting lipid panel, HgbA1c, glucose tolerance, and the glucose/insulin ratio. For adolescent girls, blood pressure and BMI should be assessed using sex and age-related normative data. A BMI percentile greater than or equal to the 85th percentile (overweight) or greater than or equal to the 95th percentile (obese) requires immediate lifestyle interventions; these should include recommendations for 150 minutes per week of aerobic activity and dietary modifications. Dietary modifications include elimination of juice, regular soda, and high carbohydrate energy drinks; use of skim milk; avoidance of intake of large amounts of high fructose corn syrup; and the implementation of a meal plan in which roughly 50% of the solid meal consists of fruits and vegetables with the remaining 50% composed of equal amounts of protein and whole grain carbohydrates.

Specific weight loss goals should be discussed specifically with each adolescent with PCOS, as even a modest weight loss of 5–10% can be associated with significant improvements in multiple components of PCOS, including ovulatory function, menstrual patterns, lipid profiles, testosterone levels, and insulin sensitivity.[36,37] Weight loss of 6.5% in one study was associated with improvement of menstrual function in an adolescent cohort, with those who achieved weight loss being 3.4 times more likely to have improved menstrual function than those who did not.[38]

Metformin has been frequently prescribed in an off-label use for PCOS among adult women and adolescents to address the role of insulin resistance in the syndrome and to attempt to decrease the risk of metabolic syndrome and the development of further abnormalities in glucose metabolism. Studies in adolescents with PCOS have documented safety and some variable efficacy in improving menstruation, reducing hyperandrogenism, and improving insulin sensitivity at metformin doses of 1500 to 2000 mg per day.[39]

The most common side effects of metformin are gastrointestinal in the form of loose stools, flatulence, loss of appetite, and/or abdominal pain; these can be minimized by beginning therapy with a single 500 mg daily dose with food, which is increased over 2–4 weeks to doses of 500–1000 mg twice daily. Some patients tolerate the extended release form of the tablet better than the conventional form. All patients should be advised to avoid taking metformin if consuming alcoholic beverages and to omit metformin therapy if receiving radiologic contrast or if there is vomiting. To date, although the risk of lactic acidosis was considered a concern when metformin first entered the market, it has been an extremely rare event. Patients receiving metformin should have annual laboratory studies for serum creatinine and B12 levels. Liver enzymes should be evaluated before initiation of therapy and then every 4–6 months thereafter.

Psychological Concerns

The physical stigma of disfiguring acne or worsening hirsutism can be associated with significant social distress for adolescents and can result in school phobia or avoidance. Obesity and acanthosis nigricans pose similar problems, and some girls are reluctant to exercise in public for fear of taunting. Worries about future fertility can be significant for older adolescent girls and for the parents of girls with PCOS. PCOS and obesity often affect many family members, and families may approach diagnostic evaluation and prescribed therapies with some trepidation, shame, or guilt. Furthermore, depression, anxiety, and other psychiatric diagnoses including attention deficit disorder (ADD) may complicate a girl's adherence to or her family's support of recommended therapies. Recognition of all of these psychological concerns and provision of referrals to appropriate psychological or psychiatric services can improve outcomes for adolescent girls with PCOS.

Goals of therapy should be discussed at the initial visit with each girl. In having such discussions, the practitioner may learn that the goals and desires of the adolescent are very different than that of the practitioner or the parents. For example, the pediatrician may want to address hypertriglyceridemia, the risks associated with long-standing secondary amenorrhea, and the long-term risk of metabolic syndrome with dietary modification, an exercise prescription, and a trial of oral medroxyprogesterone or an OCP, whereas the 16-year-old's goals might involve rapid weight loss before the prom and elimination of mild hirsutism (which she views as disfiguring) but avoidance of any menses.[40] Validation of the patient's and parent's concerns, education regarding PCOS and metabolic syndrome, and use of motivational interviewing to identify and set realistic goals can be a turning point in improving the adolescent girl's health.

Other Associated Comorbidities

A number of comorbidities may accompany PCOS in an obese adolescent and worsen insulin resistance and the risk for metabolic syndrome and subsequent cardiovascular complications.[41] Among these comorbidities are obstructive sleep apnea, steatohepatitis, renal insufficiency, and orthopedic complications.

Obstructive sleep apnea (OSA) is seen in a significant number of girls with PCOS. Neuroendocrine responses to hypoxia and hypercapnia from OSA may worsen insulin resistance, hypertension, and hyperinsulinism,[42] and OSA is a risk factor for type 2 diabetes mellitus. Treatment of OSA has been associated with improvements in insulin sensitivity, norepinephrine release, and diastolic blood pressure in young obese women with PCOS.[42,43,44]

Nonalcoholic fatty liver disease (NAFLD), or steatohepatitis, is common in PCOS and is a marker of insulin resistance and inflammation in girls and women with PCOS.[45,46] NAFLD-induced cirrhosis is expected to become the leading diagnosis in patients awaiting hepatic transplantation. Current gold standard methods of detecting NAFLD are quantitative liver enzyme measurements and hepatic biopsy, both of which can miss the heterogeneous early stages of the disease. Better accuracy is possible with quick hepatic MRI techniques that measure total hepatic triglyceride content.[47,48] Diagnosing NAFLD sooner may prevent the progression of NAFLD to a need for hepatic transplantation.

Renal insufficiency can occur with obesity[49] and is a significant problem for the adolescent with PCOS, particularly because of the use of medications for the components of PCOS. Many of these medications require renal clearance or affect volume delivery to the kidney. Metformin, which may be desirable for type 2 diabetes or insulin resistance, cannot be used in adolescents with renal insufficiency. The presence of hirsutism may require the use of spironolactone, which would not be acceptable in the patient with renal insufficiency. Hypertension accompanying the metabolic syndrome in an adolescent patient with PCOS is often treated with angiotensin converting enzyme (ACE) inhibitor therapy; again, this would not be recommended for the patient with renal insufficiency. Thus, careful monitoring of serum creatinine, as well as urine protein to creatinine ratios, would seem prudent in the obese adolescent with PCOS.

CONCLUSIONS

The management of the adolescent with PCOS must address multiple health care issues, both short-term and long-term. The practitioner must navigate the current social climate of health care coverage to advocate for the services the adolescent with PCOS needs. Judicious use of a multidisciplinary team or "medical PCOS home" to address the menstrual dysfunction, hyperandrogenism, long-term psychological concerns, metabolic syndrome, insulin resistance, and other comorbidities of adolescent PCOS is indicated. Such a team may include a primary care provider, pediatric gynecologist, dietician, psychologist, social worker, pediatric endocrinologist, radiologist, and/or dermatologist in meeting the needs of the girl with PCOS. Addressing insulin sensitivity and dyslipidemia without improving hirsutism and its perceived stigma does not achieve the quality of life the adolescent is seeking. Regulating menses without achieving weight loss in the girl with a BMI above the 99th percentile does not prevent metabolic syndrome sequelae. Addressing adolescent PCOS and its comorbidities requires a multitasking approach by the clinician, the patient, and the parents.

References

1. Rosenfield R. Clinical review: identifying children at risk for polycystic ovary syndrome. *J Clin Endocrinol Metab.* 2007;92:787–796
2. Ehrmann DA, Barnes RB, Rosenfield RL. Polycystic ovary syndrome as a form of functional ovarian hyperandrogenism due to dysregulation of androgen secretion. *Endocr Rev.* 1995;16:322–353
3. Rosenfield RL. Ovarian and adrenal function in polycystic ovary syndrome. *Endocrinol Metab Clin North Am.* 1999;28:265–293
4. Driscoll DA. Polycystic ovary syndrome in adolescence. *Ann NY Acad Sci.* 2003;997:49–55
5. Lewy VD, Danadian K, Witchel SF, et al. Early metabolic abnormalities in adolescent girls with polycystic ovary syndrome. *J Pediatr.* 2001;138:38
6. Bekx MT, Connor EL, Allen DB. Characteristics of adolescents presenting to a multidisciplinary clinic for polycystic ovarian syndrome. *J Pediatr Adolesc Gynecol.* 2010;23:7–10
7. Coviello AD, Legro RS, Dunaif A. Adolescent girls with polycystic ovary syndrome have an increased risk of the metabolic syndrome associated with increasing androgen levels independent of obesity and insulin resistance. *J Clin Endocrinol Metab.* 2006;91:492–497
8. Hickey M, Sloboda DM, Atkinson HC, et al. The relationship between maternal and umbilical cord androgen levels and ovarian function in adolescence: a prospective cohort study. *J Clin Endocrinol Metab.* 2009;94:3714–3720
9. Goodarzi MO, Azziz R. Diagnosis, epidemiology, and genetics of the polycystic ovary syndrome. *Best Pract Res Clin Endocrinol Metab.* 2006;20(2):193–205
10. Diamanti-Kandarakis E, Papavassiliou AT, Kandarakis SA, et al. Pathophysiology and types of dyslipidemia in PCOS. *Trends Endocrinol Metab.* 2007;18:280
11. Azziz R, Kashar-Miller MD. Family history as a risk factor for the polycystic ovary syndrome. *J Pediatr Endocrinol Metab.* 2000;13(Suppl 5):1303–1306
12. Yildiz BO, Yarali H, Oguz H, Bayraktar M. Glucose intolerance, insulin resistance, and hyperandrogenemia in first degree relatives of women with polycystic ovary syndrome. *J Clin Endocrinol Metab.* 2003;88:2031–2036
13. Escobar-Morreale HF, Luque-Ramirez M, San Millan JL. The molecular genetic basis of functional hyperandrogenism and the polycystic ovary syndrome. *Endocr Rev.* 2005;26:251–282
14. Rosencratz MA, Coffler MS, Haggan A, et al. Clinical evidence for predominance of delta-5 steroid production in women with polycystic ovary syndrome. *J Clin Endocrinol Metab.* 2011;96:1106–1113
15. Urbanek M, Sam S, Legro RS, Dunaif A. Identification of a polycystic ovary syndrome susceptibility variant in fibrillin-3 and association with a metabolic phenotype. *J Clin Endocrinol Metab.* 2007;92:4191–4198
16. Ewens KG, Stewart DR, Ankener W, et al. Family-based analysis of candidate genes for polycystic ovary syndrome. *J Clin Endocrinol Metab.* 2010;95:2306–2315
17. Leibel NI, Baumann EE, Kocherginsky M, Rosenfield RL. Relationship of adolescent polycystic ovary syndrome to parental metabolic syndrome. *J Clin Endocrinol Metab.* 2006;91:1275–1283
18. Abbott DH, Tarantal AF, Dumesic DA. Fetal, infant, adolescent, and adult phenotypes of polycystic ovary syndrome in prenatally androgenized female rhesus monkeys. *Am J Primatol.* 2009;71:776–784
19. Ibanez L, Potau N, Francois I, de Zegher F. Precocious pubarche, hyperinsulinism, and ovarian hyperandrogenism in girls: relation to reduced fetal growth. *J Clin Endocrinol Metab.* 1998;83:3558–3662
20. Ibanez L, Valls C, Potau N, Marcos MV, de Zegher F. Sensitization to insulin in adolescent girls to normalize hirsutism, hyperandrogenism, oligomenorrhea, dyslipidemia, and hyperinsulinism after precocious pubarche. *J Clin Endocrinol Metab.* 2000;85(10):3526–3530
21. Zawadski JK, Dunaif A. Diagnostic criteria for polycystic ovary syndrome: toward a rational approach. In: Dunaif A, Givens JR, Haseltine FP, Merriam GR, eds. *Polycystic Ovary Syndrome.* Boston, MA: Blackwell Science Publications; 1992:377–384
22. The Rotterdam ESHRE/ASRM-sponsored PCOS consensus workshop group. Revised 2003 consensus on diagnostic criteria and longterm health risks related to polycystic ovary syndrome (PCOS). *Human Reprod.* 2004;19:41–47

23. Azziz R, Carmina E, Dewailly D, et al. Positions statement: criteria for defining polycystic ovary syndrome as a predominantly hyperandrogenic syndrome: an Androgen Excess Society guideline. *J Clin Endocrinol Metab.* 2006;91:4237–4245

24. Azziz R, Carmina E, Dewailly D, et al. The Androgen Excess and PCOS Society criteria for the polycystic ovary syndrome: the complete task force report. *Fertil Steril.* 2009;91(2):456–488

25. Chen Y, Yang D, Li L, Chen X. The role of ovarian volume as a diagnostic criterion for Chinese adolescents with polycystic ovary syndrome. *J Pediatr Adolesc Gynecol.* 2008;21(6):347–350

26. Carmina E. The diagnosis of polycystic ovary syndrome in adolescents. *Am J Obstet Gynecol.* 2010;203(3):201.e1–5

27. Vieira JG. The importance of methodology in serum testosterone measurement: comparison between a direct immunoassay and a method based on a high performance liquid chromatography and tandem mass spectroscopy. *Arq Brs Endocrinol Metab.* 2008;52(6):1050–1055

28. Legro RS, Finegood D, Danaif A. A fasting glucose to insulin ratio is a useful measure of insulin sensitivity in women with polycystic ovary syndrome. *J Clin Endocrinol Metab.* 1998;83:2694–2698

29. Vuguin P, Saenger P, diMartino-Nardi J. Fasting glucose insulin ratio: a useful measure of insulin resistance in girls with premature adrenarche. *J Clin Endocrinol Metab.* 2001;86:4618–4621

30. Berlan ED, Emans SJ. Managing polycystic ovarian syndrome in adolescent patients. *J Pediatr Adolesc Gynecol.* 2009;22:137–140

31. Parkin L, Sharples K, Hernandez RK, Jick SS. Risk of thromboembolism in users of oral contraceptives containing drospirenone or levonorgestrel: nested, case-control study based on UK General Practice Research Database. *Br Med J.* 2011;342:d2139

32. Dunn N. The risk of deep venous thrombosis with oral contraceptives containing drospirenone. *BMJ.* 2011;342:d2519

33. Ferriman D, Gallwey JD. Clinical assessment of body hair growth in women. *J Clin Endocrinol Metab.* 1961;21:1440

34. Malhotra B, Noveck R, Behr D, Palmisano M. Percutaneous absorption and pharmacokinetics of Eflornithine Hcl 13.9% cream in women with unwanted facial hair. *J Clin Pharmacol.* 2001;41:972–978

35. Yasar L, Ekin M, Gedikbasi A, Erturk AD, Savan K, Ozdemir A, Temur M. Serum adiponectin levels in high school girls with polycystic ovary syndrome and hyperandrogenism. *J Pediatr Adolesc Gynecol.* 2011;24:85–89

36. Hoeger KM. Role of lifestyle modification in the management of polycystic ovary syndrome. *Best Pract Res Clin Endocrinol Metab.* 2006;20:293

37. Wabitsch M, Hauner H, Heinze E, et al. Body fat distribution and steroid hormone concentrations in obese adolescent girls before and after weight reduction. *J Clin Endocrinol Metab.* 1995;80:3469

38. Ornstein RM, Copperman NM, Jacobson MS. Effect of weight loss on menstrual function in adolescents with polycystic ovary syndrome. *J Pediatr Adolesc Gynecol.* 2011;24:161–165

39. Allen HF. Randomized controlled trial evaluating response to metformin versus standard therapy in the treatment of adolescents with polycystic ovary syndrome. *J Pediatr Endocrinol Metab.* 2005;18(8):761–768

40. Trent ME, Rich M, Austin SB, et al. Quality of life in adolescent girls with polycystic ovary syndrome. *Arch Pediatr Adolesc Med.* 2002;156:556

41. Somers VK, White DP, Amin R, et al. Sleep apnea and cardiovascular disease: an American Heart Association/American College of Cardiology Foundation Scientific Statement from the American Heart Association Council for High Blood Pressure Research Professional Education Committee, Council on Clinical Cardiology, Stroke Council, and Council on Cardiovascular Nursing. *J Am Coll Cardiol.* 2008;52:686–717

42. Tasali E, Ip MS. Obstructive sleep apnea and metabolic syndrome: alterations in glucose metabolism and inflammation. *Proc Am Thorac Soc.* 2008;5:207–217

43. Fogel RB, Malhotra A, Pillar G, Pittman SD, Dunaif A, White DP. Increased prevalence of obstructive sleep apnea in obese women with polycystic ovary syndrome. *J Clin Endocrinol Metab.* 2001;86:1175–1180

44. Tasali E, Chapotot F, Leproult R, Whitmore H, Ehrmann DA. Treatment of obstructive sleep apnea improves cardiometabolic function in young obese women with polycystic ovary syndrome. *J Clin Endocrinol Metab.* 2011;96(2):365–374

45. Ma RCW, Liu KH, Lam PM et al. Sonographic measurement of mesenteric fat predicts presence of fatty liver among subjects with polycystic ovary syndrome. *J Clin Endocrinol Metab.* 2011;96(3):799–807

46. Setji TL, Holland ND, Sanders LL, et al. Nonalcoholic steatohepatitis and nonalcoholic fatty liver disease in young women with polycystic ovary syndrome. *J Clin Endocrinol Metab.* 2006;91:1741

47. Reeder SB, Robson PM, Yu H, et al. Quantification of hepatic steatosis with MRI: the effects of accurate fat spectral modeling. *Mag Reson Imaging.* 2009;29(6):1332–1339

48. Rehm JL, Connor EL, Reeder SB. Nonalcoholic fatty liver disease in an adolescent with polycystic ovarian syndrome. *J Pediatr Adolesc Gynecol.* 2011;24(2):e61 [Abstract]

49. Reisen E. Obesity and hypertension: mechanisms, cardio-renal consequences, and therapeutic approaches. *Med Clin North Am.* 2009;93(3):733–751

Adolesc Med 23 (2012) 178–191

Ovarian Cysts in Adolescents: Medical and Surgical Management

Yolanda A. Kirkham, MA, MD, FRCSC[a],
Sari Kives, MD, MSc, FRCSC[a]*

[a]Section of Pediatric Gynaecology, Hospital for Sick Children, University of Toronto, Toronto, Ontario, Canada

INTRODUCTION

Contemporary management of ovarian cysts in the adolescent consists of conservative management whether expectant, medical, or surgical. An understanding of ovarian physiology in the perimenarcheal and postpubertal patient supports ovarian preservation surgery as the rate of malignancy is low and the alternative can be devastating. The most common ovarian cysts in adolescents are functional, which often regress without further treatment.[1] The rates of germ cell neoplasms, such as teratomas, are also high in adolescents, but often benign. Symptomatic ovarian cysts warrant further investigation. Endometriomas arising from endometriosis are extremely uncommon. Tubo-ovarian abscesses are managed medically and rarely by drainage or surgery. Ovarian torsion is a surgical emergency, and prompt conservative operative management is indicated. Consideration for additional imaging, tumor markers, and surgical management of persistent or complex masses with ultrasound findings suspicious for malignancy is appropriate. For surgical management of presumed benign masses, a laparoscopic approach is advocated and preservation of ovarian tissue and function is of utmost importance. A conservative surgical treatment approach with unilateral salpingo-oophorectomy and staging is appropriate for suspected malignancies.

Similar to the adult population, adnexal masses in the adolescent may be physiologic or neoplastic. Physiologic cysts include those with ovarian, paratubal, or tubal origin. Functional ovarian cysts are the most common ovarian lesion in children and adolescents, constituting 33% of surgically treated ovarian abnor-

---

*Corresponding author.
E-mail address: kivess@smh.ca (S. Kives).

malities.[2] Neoplastic masses may be benign, malignant, or of borderline malignant potential. In sexually active adolescents, masses may be of inflammatory or infectious origin (tubo-ovarian abscesses, pyosalpinges, or hydrosalpinges) or secondary to pregnancy (ectopic pregnancies). Pelvic masses may present emergently, with ovarian cyst rupture, hemorrhage, or torsion; or electively, with incidental diagnosis. Appendicitis, other gastrointestinal disorders, endometriomas, and obstructive gynecological anatomy also constitute the complex differential diagnosis of ovarian cysts (Table 1).

PRESENTATION

The most common presenting symptom for adnexal masses is abdominal pain in 60–80% of children and adolescents.[2-6] Pain may be intermittent, constant, or

Table 1.
Differential Diagnosis of Ovarian Cysts in Adolescents

Ovarian		Torsion
	Benign	
		Functional or physiologic cysts
		Mature cystic teratoma (dermoid cyst)
		Polycystic ovarian syndrome (PCOS)
		Endometrioma
		Serous and mucinous cystadenoma
	Malignant	
		Germ cell tumors
		Epithelial tumors
		Sex cord stromal tumors
		Metastatic tumors
		Other (lymphoma, leukemia)
Tubal		Paraovarian/paratubal cysts
		Hydrosalpinx
Infectious		Pelvic inflammatory disease (PID)
		Tubo-ovarian abscess (TOA)
		Pyosalpinx
Obstetrical		Ectopic pregnancy
		Corpus luteal cysts
		Theca lutein cysts
		Luteoma
Obstructive		Imperforate hymen
		Transverse vaginal septum
		Noncommunicating uterine horn
		Hematometrocolpos
Gastrointestinal		Appendicitis
		Appendiceal abscess
		Diverticular abscess
Urinary		Adrenal cyst
		Renal cyst
		Ureteric stone
Other		Peritoneal inclusion cyst

acute. Presentation also includes abdominal distention, menstrual irregularity, precocious puberty, virilization, urinary frequency, or constipation. Acute pain associated with nausea, vomiting, and pallor, with or without fever, warrants immediate attention and surgical intervention with high suspicion for torsion. An incidental finding of an ovarian cyst in asymptomatic patients is also common, particularly with the increased availability and use of sonography.[7]

FUNCTIONAL CYSTS

Among adolescents, the most common ovarian masses are functional cysts and benign neoplasms.[8,9] There is a bimodal distribution of functional cysts, peaking during the fetal/neonatal and perimenarcheal ages.[10,11] Although fetal and neonatal cysts develop due to exposure to maternal hormones, functional cysts increase at perimenarche due to increasing hormonal activity of the ovary. Functional cysts are the result of dysfunctional ovulation and failed involution of maturing follicles. Follicular, corpus luteal, or theca lutein cysts represent 18–60% of surgically managed ovarian and adnexal masses,[4,12] and 45% of all pediatric adnexal abnormalities.[2] As these cysts are usually benign and resolve spontaneously, every effort should be made to manage these cysts expectantly with serial ultrasound. Simple cysts on ultrasound in one series were shown to be benign in 100% of premenopausal women.[13]

Although there are no published data to support recommendations regarding specific follow-up intervals for simple cysts,[14] 2 to 3 months of observation is appropriate as up to 60% generally resolve by this time. Predictive factors for resolution are right-sided cysts and cysts less than 7 cm in size.[15] Oral contraceptive pills with 35 micrograms of ethinyl estradiol may be prescribed for suppression of further large cyst development[16] but not for cyst regression.[17] Persistence of any cyst should warrant re-evaluation of the differential diagnosis.

Bleeding into the cyst may result in a hemorrhagic cyst that presents with pain or is visualized on ultrasound. The bleeding can be self-limited but occasionally may result in hemoperitoneum in cases of cyst rupture. Serial hemoglobin levels, ordered in the emergency room, may be useful in determining the need for surgery. Laparoscopy or laparotomy, depending on surgeon skill and resources, with minimal use of electrocautery is appropriate for treating persistent cysts with a goal of preserving ovarian tissue with ovarian cystectomy if necessary. Doret reviewed rates of surgical removal of functional cysts in adults and found that operative management occurred in less than 30% of patients with non-neoplastic ovarian cysts.[18] Surgical series in children and adolescents within the past 10 years[2,6] have shown similar surgical rates for functional cysts, with some as low as 18%.[4]

Paratubal and paraovarian cysts may mimic simple ovarian cysts in presentation and on imaging. Remnants of the paramesonephric or Wolffian ducts, Hydatids of Morgagni, and paraovarian cysts are commonly asymptomatic, benign, and range from 1 to 8 cm, with the former rarely growing beyond 2 cm.[19] Surgical management may be required for cysts greater than 4 cm in size, torsion, and/or failure to regress.[19,20] The principles of untwisting the adnexa, cyst excision, and preservation of tissue apply.

Complex masses in the reproductive-aged female are most commonly hemor-rhagic cysts and endometriomas. The former resolve, whereas the latter persist. Hemorrhagic cysts regress as early as 2 weeks but typically within 8 weeks.[21] Optimal sonographic follow-up 6 weeks later should be arranged during the first 7–10 days following the onset of menses, before development of additional hem-orrhagic cysts.[14] Ovarian torsion, tubo-ovarian abscesses, and ectopic pregnan-cies may also appear as complex masses. Pregnancy and pelvic inflammatory disease must be considered in the sexually active adolescent.

Laparoscopy is useful for both treatment and diagnosis of benign masses. Mül-lerian anomalies, hemorrhagic cysts, and torsion may be diagnosed visually through laparoscopy. Ovarian or paraovarian cystectomy also permits a patho-logic confirmation. The advantages of laparoscopy for surgical management of benign ovarian cysts include reduced hospital convalescence, operative time, postoperative pain, intraoperative blood loss, adhesion formation, and adverse events.[9,22] The shift toward minimally invasive surgery for management of pre-sumed benign ovarian disease is apparent in a 15-year review of children and adolescents.[9] A laparoscopic approach has clearly become the standard of care.[23] Laparoscopy is also a safe and feasible option for excision of masses larger than 10 cm,[24] particularly with the advent of innovative approaches (vaginal, lower quadrant, or umbilical port) for aspiration of suspected benign masses. Broach[23] and Mansuria[25] summarize techniques and clinical pearls for the laparoscopic approach in the pediatric and adolescent population.

NEOPLASMS

Neoplastic ovarian masses in the pediatric and adolescent population include tumors of germ cell, epithelial, sex cord stromal, and metastatic or other origins. Germ cell tumors are the most common histological subtype in adolescents. They include the mature (benign) and immature (malignant) cystic teratoma, dysgerminoma, gonadoblastoma, endodermal sinus tumor, polyembryoma, embryonal carcinoma, and choriocarcinoma. Epithelial tumors in the adoles-cent population are composed, most commonly, of serous and mucinous cystad-enomas. Sex cord stromal tumors may exhibit hormonal activity and include juvenile and adult-variant granulosa cell tumors, Sertoli-Leydig cell tumors, and thecomas and fibromas. Malignancies such as adenocarcinomas of the colon, leukemia, and lymphoma may also metastasize to the ovary.[26,27] Because nonepi-thelial masses predominate in the adolescent, the following discussion focuses on the benign germ cell tumor, the mature cystic teratoma.

Mature cystic teratomas, or dermoid cysts, arise from ectodermal, mesodermal, and endodermal tissue. Derivatives of these cell types, such as skin, hair, teeth, bone, and sebaceous and thyroid glands, can be found within the teratoma. Dermoids grow slowly at a rate of 1.8 mm per year[28] and are usually asymptomatic, although diagnosis may also result from incidental discovery, pain, or symptoms of torsion.[29] Bilateral dermoids occur in 10–15% of cases.[26,29] The recurrence rate of dermoids is approximately 3–4%.[30]

Laparoscopy provides a safe and effective surgical management strategy for dermoid cysts. When laparoscopy is unavailable or unsuitable for a large cyst, mini-laparotomy offers an alternative approach for complex ovarian cysts.[31] Exteriorization followed by aspiration of the teratoma, for example, avoids difficulties in grasping and manipulating the cyst. This technique may prevent cyst rupture; accidental spillage of debris; and rarely, chemical peritonitis.[32] However, despite higher rates of rupture in laparoscopic cases, spillage of contents by any route of surgery is rarely if ever related to postoperative complications.[33] A laparoscopic approach is also associated with a significantly higher recurrence rate of 7.6% versus 0%,[34] possibly due to incomplete resection or unrecognized smaller cysts at the time of surgery. Although new techniques for dermoid cyst excision, such as laparoscopic enucleation within an endoscopic bag,[35] continue to be explored, expectant management of asymptomatic dermoids less than 5 cm in diameter[36] remains the standard of care. The risks of surgical intervention (surgical risks, follicular damage, asynchronous recurrence) must be weighed against the risks of expectant management. Patients should be made aware of the possibility of torsion, spontaneous rupture, and a 1–2% risk of malignancy.[37,38]

MALIGNANT NEOPLASMS

The incidence of ovarian malignancy in the adolescent population is relatively low as compared to the incidence in children (10–14%).[37,39] Surgical case series have described adolescent malignancy rates of less than 4.2–7%.[20,37,39] The most common ovarian malignancy in adolescence is the germ cell tumor,[40] which represents 55% of ovarian cancers.[41] This is followed by epithelial and sex cord stromal tumors.[20] Surgical staging for germ cells tumor by the Children's Oncology Group (COG)[42] is less aggressive and extirpative than International Federation of Gynecology and Obstetrics (FIGO)[43] staging for epithelial and sex cord stromal tumors. By eliminating the need for removal of the contralateral ovary and uterus for surgical staging of germ cell tumors, the adoption of COG guidelines reflects advocacy for fertility preservation in pediatric and adolescent patients. However, there continues to be controversy on the extent of surgical resection for staging of the less common but potentially more morbid nongerm cell subtypes in this population.

Because some neoplasms secrete protein tumor markers, drawing blood samples for these markers is valuable in diagnosis, disease monitoring, and identification of recurrence (Table 2). Useful markers to order in the adolescent patient and the neoplasms corresponding to their elevation are: alpha-fetoprotein (AFP) (endodermal sinus tumors, embryonal carcinoma, mixed germ cell tumors); human chorionic gonadotropin (HCG) (pregnancy, choriocarcinomas, embryonal carcinomas, mixed germ cell tumors); CA-125 (epithelial tumors); lactate dehydrogenase (LDH) (dysgerminoma, mixed germ cell tumors); carcinoembryonic antigen (CEA) (mucinous epithelial ovarian carcinomas); estradiol (thecomas and adult granulosa cell tumor); and testosterone (Sertoli-Leydig cell tumors).[27,44] AFP, HCG, and LDH are particularly helpful for germ cell tumors. CA-125 is less specific and may be elevated in premenopausal women with pregnancy, pelvic inflammatory disease, endometriosis, Crohn's disease, pancreatitis, and intra-abdominal malignancy.[45] Preoperative serum testosterone and estradiol are appropriate for hormonally active masses contributing to virilization or precocious puberty. Tumor markers in the normal range do not exclude the possibility of an ovarian malignancy (Table 2).[46]

Table 2.
Serum Tumor Markers

Serum Marker	Associated Tumor
CA-125	Epithelial tumors (especially serous)
	Immature teratoma (rare)
Alpha-fetoprotein (AFP)	Endodermal sinus tumors
	Embryonal carcinomas
	Mixed germ cell tumors
	Immature teratoma (rare)
	Polyembryoma (rare)
Human chorionic gonadotropin (HCG)	Choriocarcinoma
	Embryonal carcinomas
	Mixed germ cell tumors
	Polyembryoma
	Dysgerminoma (rare)
Carcinoembryonic antigen (CEA)	Serous tumors
	Mucinous tumors
Lactate dehydrogenase (LDH)	Dysgerminoma
	Mixed germ cell tumors
Estradiol	Thecomas
	Adult granulosa cell tumors
Testosterone	Sertoli cell tumors
	Leydig (hilus) cell tumors
F9 embryoglycan	Embryonal carcinoma
	Yolk sac tumor
	Choriocarcinoma
	Immature teratoma
Inhibin	Granulosa-theca cell tumor
Müllerian inhibiting substance	Granulosa-theca cell tumor

Source: Laufner MR. Adnexal masses. In: Emans SJH, Laufner MR, eds. *Emans, Laufner, Goldstein's Pediatric and Adolescent Gynecology*, 6th ed. Philadelphia, PA: Lippincott Williams & Wilkins; 2012:392. Reprinted with permission from Wolters Kluwer Health.

Ultrasound is the preferred imaging modality for evaluation of adnexal masses.[47] Sonography differentiates between cystic, complex, or solid lesions. Features suspicious for malignancy include mural nodules, internal septations, wall thickness, and vascularity.[14] Ultrasound also allows for identification of ancillary features such as ascites; hydronephrosis; lymphadenopathy; pleural effusions; and liver, peritoneal, or omental metastases.[14] Masses greater than 8 cm or with a solid component are predictive of a malignancy in children and adolescents. A presenting complaint of precocious puberty is also highly suspicious for an underlying neoplasm.[48]

Surgical planning for a suspected malignancy includes preoperative investigation; discussion of the risks, benefits, indications, and alternatives of the planned procedure; and discussion of possible necessity for a second operation or adjuvant therapy. In pediatric and adolescent patients, conservative surgical management with respect to both the approach and procedure is always a priority. An initial laparoscopic approach is acceptable for inspection, with conversion to laparotomy if necessary. Intraoperative frozen section may direct management. Conservative surgery with unilateral adnexal removal (ovary with or without tube) is recommended, even in proven histological cases of a malignancy. In cases of malignancy, however, surgical staging should also be performed. Midline laparotomy is the appropriate surgical approach for any highly suspected malignancy.

As adolescent malignancy is rare and germ cell tumors are the most common in this age group, further discussion pertains to germ cell neoplasms. According to the COG surgical procedural guidelines for staging ovarian germ cell tumors,[46] staging should include (1) collection of peritoneal washings or ascites, (2) examination of the peritoneal surfaces with biopsy or excision of suspicious nodules, (3) examination and palpation of retroperitoneal lymph nodes with sampling of firm or enlarged nodes, (4) inspection and palpation of the omentum with biopsy of abnormal areas, (5) inspection and palpation of the contralateral ovary with biopsy of abnormal areas, and (6) complete resection of the tumor-containing ovary with sparing of the fallopian tube if not involved. Despite the assistance of preoperative tumor markers, imaging, and staging guidelines, surgical decision-making is inconsistent and occurs intraoperatively before pathological diagnosis.[46] Involvement of gynecology, general surgery, and oncology is therefore recommended to optimize the initial treatment and organize appropriate postoperative follow-up. Adjuvant treatment with chemotherapy for the pediatric and adolescent population is multiagent and platinum-based.

ENDOMETRIOMA

Although the rate of endometriosis in adolescents with pelvic pain is very high in patients with no sonographic evidence of pathology,[49] endometriomas are rare in adolescents. Endometriosis diagnosed in the adolescent is usually of early stage and rarely progresses to endometriomas (endometriosis within the ovary). Prior to a recent case report of bilateral endometriomas in an adolescent,[50] there had been no case reports of endometriomata in women younger than 18 years of age. In one case series,[20] endometrioid cysts comprised 12.8% of resected ovarian masses, but this study included patients up to the age of 21. A 6–12 week ultrasound follow-up is appropriate to differentiate an endometrioma from a functional cyst.[47] The tumor marker CA-125 may also be elevated from the presence of endometriosis and these "chocolate cysts."[51] In adults, there is support for resection of the cyst wall in endometriomata of more than 3 cm to decrease dysmenorrhea, dyspareunia, recurrence, and requirement for further surgery.[52] However, there is also increasing evidence that cystectomy may decrease ovarian reserve.[53] Thus, primary expectant management should be considered and laparoscopic management by cystectomy should aim to preserve the ovarian cortex. Hormonal suppression of endometriosis, particularly after excision, is a widely accepted treatment strategy to prevent symptoms and possibly disease progression.

TUBO-OVARIAN ABSCESS

In adolescents who are sexually active, the possibility of an ovarian mass of infectious origin should be considered. Adolescents with pelvic inflammatory disease often fulfill criteria for hospitalization due to age and the high likelihood of noncompliance with the outpatient regimen. The presence of a tubo-ovarian abscess warrants admission. Presenting symptoms may include pelvic pain, pelvic mass, adnexal tenderness, leukocytosis, and fever. Causative agents include *Chlamydia trachomatis*, *Neisseria gonorrhea*, or anaerobic and facultative bacteria,[54] which demonstrate the polymicrobial nature of this ascending infection. Ultrasound, computed tomography, and laparoscopy may aid in diagnosis.[55] Two inpatient parenteral treatments are recommended by the Centers for Disease Control and Prevention in the United States:[56] cefotetan 2 g IV every 12 hours or cefoxitin 2 g IV every 6 hours, plus doxycycline 100 mg orally or IV every 12 hours; or clindamycin 900 mg IV every 8 hours plus gentamicin 2 mg/kg loading dose IV followed by a maintenance dose of 1.5 mg/kg every 8 hours or 3–5 mg/kg every 24 hours. In cases where severe disease is suspected, adding metronidazole 500 mg every 8 hours IV may be indicated in either regimen. Intravenous antibiotics are recommended until 24 hours after clinical improvement is noted. Patients should then be transitioned to an oral regimen of clindamycin 450 mg orally 4 times a day or doxycycline 100 mg twice a day (+/- metronidazole 500 mg orally twice per day) to complete a total of 14 days of therapy. Occasionally, ultrasound-guided percutaneous drainage or surgical intervention is necessary.[57] Long-term sequelae are hydrosalpinges, chronic pelvic pain, ectopic pregnancy, and infertility.

TORSION

Torsion is rare with an incidence of 4.9 per 100,000 females aged 1 to 20 years.[58] Although less frequent in adolescents than in children, early recognition is important for both ovarian function and future fertility. Ovarian torsion is usually associated with adnexal pathology, or occasionally, a pathologic or long utero-ovarian ligament. The rate of malignancy in cases of ovarian torsion is very low (0.5–1.8%).[58,59] Benign ovarian neoplasms have a 13-fold increased risk of adnexal torsion as compared to malignant neoplasms,[60] likely secondary to the absence of adhesions.

In ovarian torsion, flow of the ovarian vein within the infundibulopelvic ligament becomes obstructed first, leading to congestion of the ovary through continued impaired arterial flow. Compromise of the venous flow is followed by compromised central, and then finally peripheral arterial flow.[61] Thus, the presence of arterial flow does not rule out ovarian torsion. Due to stromal edema and engorgement of the vasculature within the ovary, with or without torsion of the tube, a solid, complex, or cystic pelvic mass may be visualized on ultrasound.[14] One must retain a high index of suspicion for torsion in adolescents with a pelvic mass and pain.

Diagnosis of torsion is commonly delayed or misdiagnosed. Unilateral pain, nausea, vomiting, and/or low-grade fever are the most common presenting symptoms. Both appendicitis and ovarian torsion may present with right-sided pain and peritoneal signs. Ovarian torsion involves the right adnexa more frequently.[62] It is prudent to inform patients with expectantly managed ovarian cysts of the previously described symptoms and to remind them to seek immediate medical attention should they arise. Surgical management should proceed without delay at the time of suspected diagnosis.

There is growing support for untwisting procedures as both short-term and long-term data on follicular development and successful fertility following untwisting emerge.[63] Contemporary management includes untwisting and ovarian cystectomy if an ovarian cyst is present. The cystectomy can also be delayed and performed at a second surgery to avoid injury to the ovary and follicular loss.[62] Traditionally, unilateral salpingo-oophorectomy was performed. Epidemiologic data from 2001 to 2006 show high oophorectomy rates of 58–61% in the United States.[58] Oophorectomy was associated with lower socioeconomic status and more common in younger children than adolescents. As future viability of the blue-black ovary is unpredictable, adnexa-preserving surgical management is becoming standard of care. Furthermore, intraoperative inspection of the ovary is unreliable and necrotic-appearing ovaries have demonstrated follicular activity on sonography weeks after conservative management.[64] Previous fears of reperfusion injury or embolization have been unfounded as there is no difference in ovaries that undergo untwisting, with or without adnexectomy.[65] Following untwisting, a bivalve procedure of the ovary may further relieve vascular congestion of the ovary by decreasing the arterial blood pressure and facilitating reperfusion.[66] Visible bleeding on the ovary after bivalving is a reassuring sign. Persistent postoperative pain, fever, and leukocytosis may suggest ovarian necrosis, although postoperative pain also occurs in patients with subsequent normal ovaries.[67]

Ovarian-preserving surgery with prophylactic oophoropexy of the untwisted and contralateral ovaries may be considered for prevention of torsion with no appreciable complications.[67] Adnexal fixation remains a controversial technique as long-term consequences have not been studied, and differing opinions exist among surgeons. Oophoropexy of the contralateral ovary can be considered in cases when torsion occurs in a normal ovary without need for ovarian or para-tubal cystectomy or when oophorectomy is performed. Surgical techniques include suturing of the ovary to the pelvic sidewall, round ligament, or uterosac-ral ligament[68] or plication of the utero-ovarian ligaments by suturing,[69] laparo-scopic endoloop,[70] or surgical clips.[71] With the increased use of reproductive techniques, ideal placement of the ovary should aim to accommodate future access for transvaginal egg retrieval and in vitro fertilization, should the need arise for patients with compromised fertility.[71] In the literature, follow-up sonog-raphy of ovaries following conservative untwisting shows decreased ovarian vol-ume proportional to the number of revolutions of torsion.[72] No recommenda-tions have been made as to optimal timing for postoperative ultrasound follow-up, although 6 weeks is convenient and practical for review at the time of the postoperative visit. Sonography permits identification of a persistent patho-logic cyst in conservatively managed ovarian torsion.[63] Persistent ovarian cysts may require reoperation, although malignancy is extremely rare and presenta-tion is usually stage 1.[46]

MULTIMODAL MANAGEMENT

A multimodal approach to investigation of the ovarian mass is essential (Figure 1). In addition to a thorough history including sexual activity, the physical examination should include a general, abdominal, pelvic, and/or rectal exami-nation. Constitutional symptoms, signs of virilization or precocity, menstrual irregularity, and/or dysmenorrhea can direct further evaluation. A complete blood count for assessment of acute bleeding and leukocytosis, a pregnancy test, and transabdominal or transvaginal ultrasound imaging are useful initial inves-tigations. Ultrasound remains the primary modality for diagnosis, as well as an important modality for expectant management with serial ultrasounds.[14] Mag-netic resonance imaging (MRI) assists in delineation of the origin of a mass, as well as differentiating complex Müllerian anomalies from ovarian cysts[73] and benign from malignant lesions.[14] MRI is particularly useful, and is the gold stan-dard for selecting the appropriate operative procedure for Müllerian anoma-lies.[73] Computed tomography may be used for assessment of malignancy, lymph adenopathy, metastases, and nongynecologic cases (such as appendicitis), but the higher risks of radiation exposure due to organ sensitivity and longer life expectancy in the adolescent should be considered.[14] Tumor markers are also an important adjunct in investigating the malignant ovarian mass.

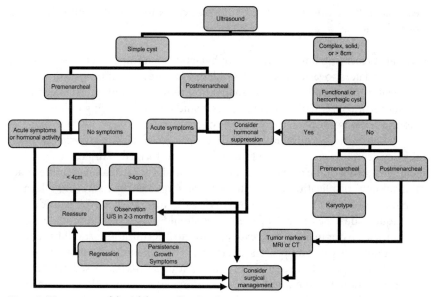

Figure 1. Management of the Adolescent Ovarian Cyst

Appropriate referral to a pediatric gynecologist or a gynecologic surgeon experienced in the management of young patients is recommended for either expectant or surgical management. If unavailable, consultation with a general gynecologist or pediatric surgeon is also appropriate. Trends in surgical management support ovarian-sparing surgery, such as ovarian cystectomy rather than oophorectomy whenever possible. Advocacy for and surgical conservation of the ovary is more likely among pediatric gynecologists compared to pediatric surgeons.[74] With the increasing number of available pediatric gynecologists, referrals have increased, compared to previous years when younger children were managed solely by general surgeons.[37] However, access to gynecologists remains more likely in postmenarcheal females older than the age of 16.[74] Fertility preservation through expectant management or conservative surgical management by laparoscopy for suspected benign ovarian cysts should be a priority.

References

1. Porcu E, Venturoli S, Dal Prato L, et al. Frequency and treatment of ovarian cysts in adolescence. *Arch Gynecol Obstet.* 1994;255:69–72
2. Spinelli C, Di Giacomo M, Cei M, Mucci N. Functional ovarian lesions in children and adolescents: when to remove them. *Gynecol Endocrinol.* 2009;25(5):294–298
3. Al Jama FE, Al Ghamdi AA, Gasim T, Al Dakhiel SA, Rahman J, Rahman MS. Ovarian tumors in children and adolescents—a clinical study of 52 patients in a university hospital. *J Ped Adol Gynecol.* 2011;24(1):25–28

4. Kirkham YA, Lacy JA, Kives S, Allen L. Characteristics and management of adnexal masses in a Canadian paediatric and adolescent population. *J Obstet Gynecol Can.* 2011;33(9):935-943
5. Ryoo U, Lee DY, Bae DS, Yoon BK, Choi D. Clinical characteristics of adnexal masses in Korean children and adolescents: retrospective analysis of 409 cases. *J Minim Invasive Gynecol.* 2010;17(2):209-213
6. Kocak M, Beydilli G, Dilbaz S, Tasci Y, Haberal A. Adnexal masses in adolescent girls with pelvic pain: report on 63 cases. *Gynecol Surg.* 2008;5(3):203-207
7. Balan P. Ultrasonography, computed tomography and magnetic resonance imaging in the assessment of pelvic pathology. *Eur J Radiol.* 2006;58:147-155
8. Skiadas VT, Koutoulidis V, et al. Ovarian masses in young adolescents: imaging findings with surgical confirmation. *Eur J Gynaecol Oncol.* 2004;25(2):201-206
9. Michelotti B, Segura BJ, Sau I, Perez-Bertolez S, Prince JM, Kane TD. Surgical management of ovarian disease in infants, children, and adolescents: a 15-year review. *J Laparoendosc Adv Surg Tech.* 2010;20(3):261-264
10. Ziereisen F, Guissard G, Damry N, Avni EF. Sonographic imaging of the paediatric female pelvis. *Eur Radiol.* 2005;15:1296-1309
11. Strickland JL. Ovarian cysts in neonates, children and adolescents. *Curr Opin Obstet Gynecol.* 2002;14:459-465
12. De Silva KS, Kanumakala S, Grover SR, Chow CW, Warne GL. Ovarian lesions in children and adolescents—an 11-year review. *J Pediatr Endocrinol Metab.* 2004;17:951-957
13. Gerber B, Müller H, Külz T, Krause A, Reimer T. Simple ovarian cysts in premenopausal patients. *Int J Gynaecol Obstet.* 1997; 57(1):49-55
14. American College of Radiology. ACR appropriateness criteria: clinically suspected adnexal masses. http://www.acr.org/SecondaryMainMenuCategories/quality_safety/app_criteria/pdf/ExpertPanelonWomensImaging/SuspectedAdnexalMassesDoc11.aspx. Accessed July 2011
15. McCormick TC, Underwood L, Ciari M, Strickland J. Ovarian cysts in adolescence. An evaluation of spontaneous resolution or need for intervention. A retrospective analysis. *J Pediatr Adolesc Gynecol.* 2010;23(2):e82-e83
16. Powell JK. Benign adnexal masses in the adolescent. *Adolesc Med.* 2004;15:535-547
17. Grimes DA, Jones LB, Lopez LM, Schulz KF. Oral contraceptives for functional ovarian cysts. *Cochrane Database Syst Rev.* 2011;9:CD006134
18. Doret M, Raudrant D. Functional ovarian cysts and the need to remove them. *Eur J Obstet Gynecol Reprod Biol.* 2001;100:1-4
19. Perlman S, Hertweck P, Fallat ME. Paratubal and tubal abnormalities. *Semin Pediatric Surg.* 2005;14:124-134
20. Deligeoroglou E, Eleftheriades M, Shiadoes V, et al. Ovarian masses during adolescence: clinical, ultrasonographic and pathologic findings, serum tumor markers and endocrinological profile. *Gynecol Endocrinol.* 2004;19:1-8
21. Okai T, Kobayashi K, Ryo E, Kagawa H, Kozuma S, Taketani Y. Transvaginal sonographic appearance of hemorrhagic functional ovarian cysts and their spontaneous regression. *Int J Gynaecol Obstet.* 1994;44(1):47-52
22. Medeiros LRF, Rosa DD, Bozzetti MC, et al. Laparoscopy versus laparotomy for benign ovarian tumour. *Cochrane Database Syst Rev.* 2009;(2):CD004751
23. Broach AN, Mansuria SM, Sanfilippo JS. Pediatric and adolescent gynecologic laparoscopy. *Clin Obstet Gynecol.* 2009;52(3):380-389
24. Eltabbakh GH, Charboneau AM, Eltabbakh NG. Laparoscopic surgery for large benign ovarian cysts. *Gynecol Oncol.* 2008;108(1):72-76
25. Mansuria MS, Sanfilippo JS. Laparoscopy in the pediatric and adolescent population. *Obstet Gynecol Clin N Am.* 2004;31:469-483
26. Schultz KAP, Ness KK, Nagarajan R, Steiner ME. Adnexal masses in infancy and childhood. *Clin Obstet Gynecol.* 2006;49(3):464-479
27. Lara-Torre E. Ovarian neoplasias in children. *J Pediatr Adolesc Gynecol.* 2002;15:47-52
28. Caspi B, Appelman Z, Rabinerson D, Zalel Y, Tulandi T, Shoham Z. The growth pattern of ovarian dermoid cysts: a prospective study in premenopausal and postmenopausal women. *Fertil Steril.* 1997;68:501-505

29. Milingos S, Protopapas A, Drakakis P, et al. Laparoscopic treatment of ovarian dermoid cysts: eleven years' experience. *J Am Assoc Gynecol Laparosc.* 2004;11(4):478–485
30. Anteby EY, Ron M, Revel A, Shimonovitz S, Ariel I, Hurwitz A. Germ cell tumors of the ovary arising after dermoid cyst resection: a long-term follow-up study. *Obstet Gynecol.* 1994;83(4):605–608
31. Ferro F, Iacobelli BD, Zaccara A, Spagnoli A, Trucchi A, Bagolan P. Exteriorization-aspiration minilaparotomy for treatment of neonatal ovarian cysts. *J Pediatr Adolesc Gynecol.* 2002;15:205–207
32. Clément D, Barranger E, Benchimol Y, Uzan S. Chemical peritonitis: a rare complication of an iatrogenic ovarian dermoid cyst rupture. *Surg Endosc.* 2003;17(4):658
33. Savasi I, Lacy JA, Gerstle JT, Stephens D, Kives S, Allen L. Management of ovarian dermoid cysts in the pediatric and adolescent population. *J Pediatr Adolesc Gynecol.* 2009;22:360–364
34. Laberge PY, Levesque S. Short-term morbidity and long-term recurrence rate of ovarian dermoid cysts treated by laparoscopy versus laparotomy. *J Obstet Gynecol Can.* 2006;28:789–793
35. Campo S, Campo V. A modified technique to reduce spillage and operative time: laparoscopic ovarian dermoid cyst enucleation 'in a bag'. *Gynecol Obstet Invest.* 2011;71:53–58
36. O'Neill KE, Cooper AR. The approach to ovarian dermoids in adolescents and young women. *J Pediatr Adolesc Gynecol.* 2011;24(3):176–180
37. Templeman C, Fallat ME, Blinchevsky A, Hertweck SP. Noninflammatory ovarian masses in girls and young women. *Obstet Gynecol.* 2000;96:229–233
38. Cass DL, et al. Surgery for ovarian masses in infants, children, and adolescents: 102 consecutive patients treated in a 15-year period. *J Pediatr Surg.* 2001;36(5):693–699
39. Van Winter JT, Simmons PS, Podratz KC. Surgically treated adnexal masses in infancy, childhood, and adolescence. *Am J Obstet Gynecol.* 1994;170(6):1780–1789
40. Fabro MA, Costa L, Spata E, et al. Ovarian tumors in children. *Pediatr Med Chir.* 1996; 18:151–154
41. Wu XC, Chen VW, Steele B, et al. Cancer incidence in adolescents and young adults in the United States, 1992-1997. *J Adolesc Health.* 2003;32:405
42. Billmire D, Vinocur C, Rescorla F, et al; Children's Oncology Group (COG). Outcome and staging evaluation in malignant germ cell tumors of the ovary in children and adolescents: an intergroup study. *J Pediatr Surg.* 2004;39(3):424–429
43. Creasman WT. New gynecologic cancer staging. *Obstet Gynecol.* 1990;75:287–288
44. Laufer MR. Adnexal masses. In: Emans SJH, Laufer MR, eds. *Emans, Laufer, Goldstein's Pediatric and Adolescent Gynecology,* 6th ed. Philadelphia, PA: Lippincott Williams & Wilkins; 2012:381–404
45. Jacobs I, Oram D, Fairbanks J, Turner J, Frost C, Grudzinskas JG. A risk of malignancy index incorporating CA-125, ultrasound and menopausal status for the accurate preoperative diagnosis of ovarian cancer. *Br J Obstet Gynaecol.* 1990;97:922–929
46. Oltmann SC, Garcia NM, Barber R, Hicks B, Fischer AC. Pediatric ovarian malignancies: how efficacious are current staging practices? *J Pediatr Surg.* 2010;45(6):1096–1102
47. Levine D, Brown DL, Andreotti RF, et al. Management of asymptomatic ovarian and other adnexal cysts imaged at US: Society of Radiologists in Ultrasound Consensus Conference Statement. *Radiology.* 2010;256:943–954
48. Oltmann SC, Garcia N, Barber R, Huang R, Hicks B, Fischer A. Can we preoperatively risk stratify ovarian masses for malignancy? *J Pediatr Surg.* 2010;45(1):130–134
49. Kho K, Nezhat C, Zurawin J. Adolescent endometriosis: the journey to diagnosis. *Fertil Steril.* 2009;92(3):S59
50. Wright KN, Laufer MR. Endometriomas in adolescents. *Fertil Steril.* 2010;94(4):1527–1529
51. Templeman CL, Fallat ME. Benign ovarian masses. *Semin Pediatr Surg.* 2005;14:93–99
52. Hart RJ, Hickey M, Maouris P, Buckett W. Excisional surgery versus ablative surgery for ovarian endometriomata. *Cochrane Database Syst Rev.* 2008;2:CD004992
53. Iwase A, Hirokawa W, Goto M, et al. Serum anti-Mullerian hormone level is a useful marker for evaluating the impact of laparoscopic cystectomy on ovarian reserve. *Fertil Steril.* 2010;94(7):2846–2849

54. Jossens MO, Schachter J, Sweet RL. Risk factors associated with pelvic inflammatory disease of differing microbial etiologies. *Obstet Gynecol.* 1994;83(6):989–997
55. Lee DC, Swaminathan AK. Sensitivity of ultrasound for the diagnosis of tubo-ovarian abscess: a case report and literature review. *J Emerg Med.* 2011;40(2):170–175
56. Workowski KA, Berman S; Centers for Disease Control and Prevention (CDC). Sexually transmitted diseases treatment guidelines, 2010. *MMWR Recomm Rep.* 2010; 59(RR-12):1–110. Erratum in: *MMWR Recomm Rep.* 2011;60(1):18. Dosage error in article text.
57. Yang CC, Chen P, Tseng JY, et al. Advantages of open laparoscopic surgery over exploratory laparotomy in patients with tubo-ovarian abscess. *J Am Assoc Gynecol Laparosc.* 2002;9:327–332
58. Guthrie BD, Adler MD, Powell EC. Incidence and trends of pediatric ovarian torsion hospitalizations in the United States, 2000–2006. *Pediatrics.* 2010;125(3):532–538
59. Oltmann SC, Fischer A, Barber R, Huang R, Hicks B, Garcia N. Pediatric ovarian malignancy presenting as ovarian torsion: incidence and relevance. *J Pediatr Surg.* 2010;45(1):135–139
60. Sommerville M, Grimes DA, Koonings PP, et al. Ovarian neoplasms and the risk of adnexal torsion. *Am J Obstet Gynecol.* 1991;164:577–578
61. Breech LL, Hillard PJ. Adnexal torsion in pediatric and adolescent girls. *Curr Opin Obstet Gynecol.* 2005;17:483–489
62. Cass DL. Ovarian torsion. *Semin Pediatr Surg.* 2005;14:86–92
63. Oelsner G, Cohen SB, Soriano D, et al. Minimal surgery for the twisted ischaemic adnexa can preserve ovarian function. *Hum Reprod.* 2003;18(12):2599–2602
64. Aziz J, Davis V, Allen L, Langer JC. Ovarian torsion in children: is oophorectomy necessary? *J Pediatr Surg.* 2004;39(5):750–753
65. McGovern PG, Noah R, Koenigsberg R, Little AB. Adnexal torsion and pulmonary embolism: case report and review of the literature. *Obstet Gynecol Surv.* 1999;54(9):601–608
66. Styer AK, Laufer MR. Ovarian bivalving after detorsion. *Fertil Steril.* 2002;7:1053–1055
67. Celik A, Ergün O, Aldemir H, et al. Long-term results of conservative management of adnexal torsion in children. *J Ped Surg.* 2005;40(4):704–708
68. Crouch NS, Gyampoh B, Cutner AS, Creighton SM. Ovarian torsion: to pex or not to pex? Case report and review of the literature. *J Pediatr Adolesc Gynecol.* 2003;16:381–384
69. Fuchs N, Smorgick N, Tovbin Y, et al. Oophoropexy to prevent adnexal torsion: how, when, and for whom? *J Minim Invasive Gynecol.* 2010;17(2):205–208
70. Weitzman VN, DiLuigi AJ, Maier DB, Nulsen JC. Prevention of recurrent adnexal torsion. *Fertil Steril.* 2008;90(5):2018
71. Rollene N, Nunn M, Wilson T, Coddington C. Recurrent ovarian torsion in a premenarchal adolescent girl: contemporary surgical management. *Obstet Gynecol.* 2009;114(2):422–424
72. Weber-LaShore A, Reid J, Bates J, Huppert JS. Resolution of ovarian cysts and torsion. *J Pediatr Adolesc Gynecol.* 2010;23(2):e91–e92
73. Minto CL, Hollings N, Hall-Craggs M, Creighton S. Magnetic resonance imaging in the assessment of complex Müllerian anomalies. *BJOG.* 2001;108:791–797
74. Bristow RE, Nugent AC, Zahurak ML, Khouzhami V, Fox HE. Impact of surgeon specialty on ovarian-conserving surgery in young females with an adnexal mass. *J Adolesc Health.* 2006;39(3):411–416

Adolesc Med 23 (2012) 192–206

Human Papillomavirus Disease in Adolescents: Management and Prevention

Lea E. Widdice, MD*

*Division of Adolescent Medicine, Cincinnati Children's Hospital Medical Center,
University of Cincinnati College of Medicine, 3333 Burnet Ave., Cincinnati, Ohio 45229*

INTRODUCTION

Human papillomavirus (HPV) is the most common sexually transmitted infection (STI). Although most infections do not cause clinical disease, the virus can cause both benign and malignant epithelial tumors. Evaluation and treatment of HPV depends on the clinical manifestation of the viral infection. Although the most concerning clinical manifestations of HPV disease are rare in adolescents, primary prevention measures, such as vaccination, need to begin before the onset of sexual activity. Cervical cancer screening, a well-established and effective secondary prevention measure, was previously universally recommended to start in adolescence. However, the age at which to initiate cervical cancer screening has been shifting away from adolescents to young adult women. This article describes the clinical manifestations, evaluation, treatment, and epidemiology of HPV and associated diseases in adolescents, as well as prevention options for HPV infection and HPV-associated diseases in adolescents.

HPV CLASSIFICATION AND INFECTION

Human papillomaviruses are a family of viruses that infect the skin and mucous membranes of humans and are categorized based on the location of infection and potential to cause cancer. Papillomaviruses are species specific such that bovine or canine papillomaviruses do not infect humans and vice versa. The virus contains a capsid made of 2 proteins, L1 and L2, and genetic material of DNA. There are more than 140 identified HPV genotypes that infect humans. Genotypes are distinguished from each other based on the DNA sequence for

---

*Corresponding author.
E-mail address: lea.widdice@cchmc.org (L. E. Widdice).

the oncoproteins E6 and E7, and L1 protein genes.[1] A unique HPV type is defined as a virus with greater than 10% difference in the DNA sequence of the L1 protein. HPVs are grouped based on their most common site of infection, either mucosal or cutaneous epithelium. Cutaneous HPVs infect cutaneous epithelium. A subset of these types causes plantar and palmar warts in children, adolescents, and adults. Mucosal HPVs, the topic of this article, infect mucosal epithelium including the cervix, anus, and oral cavity. Mucosal HPVs are further classified into groups, based on epidemiological and molecular association with cervical cancer, designating their oncogenic potential. High-risk, or oncogenic, HPV types are known to cause cancer. Probable high-risk types have evidence to suggest they are oncogenic, but the evidence is not conclusive. Low-risk, nononcogenic, HPV types are not associated with cancer. Although low-risk HPV types are not associated with cancer, they may be related to other HPV-associated diseases. See Table 1 for classification of HPV types.

HPV infection occurs in human epithelium. Viral reproduction requires epithelial differentiation. The virus initially infects cells of the epithelial basal layer. Microtrauma or microabrasions expose basal cells to HPV infection and may provide easier access to infection. After becoming intracellular, the virus loses the protein capsid and the viral DNA enters the host cell nucleus. Viral replication requires 2 viral proteins, E1 and E2, and host cell DNA replication machinery. Other viral proteins stimulate division of the infected basal cells. After host cell differentiation, cells continue to replicate, viral genes are amplified, and infectious virions are assembled and released from host cells during exfoliation. This process relies on expression of viral genes E6 and E7. Actions of E6 and E7 proteins include inhibition of apoptosis and reactivation of cellular DNA synthesis. In infections with high-risk HPV types, actions of E6 and E7 can lead to the development of cancer.

CLINICAL MANIFESTATIONS OF HPV INFECTION

Asymptomatic Infection

HPV infection can be asymptomatic and occur without visible signs or symptoms of disease. The majority of HPV infections are transient in adolescents. The average duration of infection is 7 to 10 months.[2] About 90% of infections clear

Table 1.
Classification of HPV Types

Common Site of Infection	Classification	HPV Types
Mucosal	High-risk	16, 18, 31, 33, 35, 39, 45, 51, 52, 56, 58, 59, 68, 73, 82
	Probable high-risk	26, 53, 66
	Low-risk	6, 11, 40, 42, 43, 44, 81
Cutaneous		1, 2, 3, 4, 10, 26, 27, 28, 29, 48, 49,50, 57, 60, 63, 65

within 3 years.[3] Whether infections are completely cleared by the immune system or whether the virus remains latent in host cells is debated.[4] However, it is persistent infections with high-risk HPV types detectable by current HPV DNA testing methods that are associated with cancers. Currently, there is no indication to test for asymptomatic HPV in patients unless the testing is part of cervical cancer screening in patients older than the age of 30. Screening for subclinical or asymptomatic infections, such as for routine STI screening, is not indicated and is discouraged.

Genital Warts and Other Papillomas

HPV can cause genital warts and other papillomas. These are reviewed in the article on sexually transmitted infections.

HPV infection can cause papillomas of mucosal epithelium in nongenital sites such as on the conjunctiva, gingiva, and nasal mucosa. Recurrent respiratory papillomatosis (RRP) is a rare manifestation of infection with low-risk HPV types 6 and 11. RRP is characterized by recurrent papillomas in the respiratory tract. Presentation is bimodal with the most common presentation occurring in children younger than 18 years of age, with a median age of diagnosis of 4 years. A second peak in presentation occurs in adults between the ages of 20–30 years. Infections leading to juvenile onset RRP are thought to result from vertical transmission of HPV from mother to baby. Adult onset RRP may be related to increased sexual risk behaviors, including number of partners and oral sex,[5] or reactivation of infection acquired as a neonate. Although tumors of RRP are not malignant, their potential to obstruct the airway and recurrence after treatment make them potentially fatal. The prevalence of juvenile and adult-onset RRP is generally estimated to range between 1 to 4 per 100,000.[6]

Dysplasia

Dysplasia of mucosal epithelium is one of the most common manifestations of HPV infection and may occur in response to infection with high-risk or low-risk HPV types. Natural history studies have confirmed that cervical dysplasia can regress to normal or progress to cervical cancer. Investigation to describe the natural history of anal dysplasia is ongoing. Dysplasia usually causes no symptoms. Expression of viral proteins results in specific pathologic changes described as squamous intraepithelial lesions (SIL). Low-grade SIL (LSIL) encompasses mild basal cell proliferation and perinuclear halos. These changes are considered benign. High-grade squamous intraepithelial lesions (HSIL) have more cytologic abnormalities, including aneuploidy, altered chromatin texture, and increased nuclear volume.

Dysplasia is often diagnosed as part of routine screening for cervical cancer. It may be detected on a clinical examination if a gross lesion is seen during the pelvic examination. Treatment depends on the grade of the lesion and should occur as part of a cervical screening program or in consultation with a specialist. Dysplasia can occur at sites other than the cervix. However, the natural histories of dysplasia at other anatomic sites have not been well described. At this time, only recommendations for cervical cancer screening and treatment of cervical dysplasia are based on well-established, evidence-based guidelines and algorithms. In cervical cancer screening, cytological categories are used for triage with biopsy to determine histological diagnoses of dysplasia or cancer. Histological diagnoses of cervical intraepithelial neoplasia (CIN) 1, 2, 3 and carcinoma in situ are used in treatment algorithms. One of the 3 major cervical cancer screening guidelines has changed its recommendation for routine screening of healthy adolescents and recommends waiting to initiate screening until the age of 21 years.[7] This change is based on improved understanding of the natural history of HPV infection, LSIL, and HSIL in adolescents; the low impact of cervical cancer screening in adolescents; and the risk of treatment of low grade lesions. (See the section on prevention.)

Cancers

HPV-associated cancers occur in the anogenital and oropharyngeal areas. These include virtually all cervical cancers, the majority of anal cancers, and a large proportion of vaginal, vulvar, and penile cancers.

Multiple factors influence the development of cervical cancer. Persistent infection with high-risk HPV is a necessary but not sufficient cause of cervical cancer. Persistence refers to detection of the same HPV type 2 or more times over a given time period. There is not a standard definition of persistence,[8] although the risk of developing cancer increases with increasing duration of HPV infection. Viral protein E2 regulates viral proteins E6 and E7. If loss of E2 occurs, E6 and E7 are overexpressed and inhibit cell cycle arrest and prevent apoptosis by binding to host cell tumor suppressor genes. E6 and E7 are expressed by both high- and low-risk HPV types; however, high-risk E6 and E7 bind with higher affinity than low-risk E6 and E7. In low-grade lesions, E6 and E7 expression is limited compared to expression in high-risk lesions.[9]

EPIDEMIOLOGY

HPV Detection

HPV infection is the most common viral STI in the United States. Seventy-five percent to 80% of adult men and women have been exposed to genital HPV at some point in their lives;[10] and about 6 million new infections occur each year.[11] Prevalence rates are usually based on detection of viral DNA from exfoliated epithelial samples. Rates of cervical HPV vary by age and geographic region. HPV is more commonly detected in younger women compared to older women.

In nationally representative data from the United States, the highest prevalence of cervical HPV occurs in women 20–24 years old, with 45% of women in this age group having detectable HPV.[12] Epidemiological studies examining HPV prevalence in adolescent populations with high rates of sexual activity report a 70–80% HPV prevalence among sexually active adolescents. About one-fourth of adolescents and women in their late 20s, 30s, and 40s have HPV. The prevalence among older women is lower; about one-fifth of women in their 50s and older have HPV. Among women with cervical HPV detected, high-risk types are detected in a higher proportion of infections than low-risk types. HPV 16 is generally the most commonly detected type, regardless of cytology findings.[13]

The prevalence of subclinical HPV in genital sites other than the cervix is lower than rates detected in the cervix. Prevalence of HPV in the anal and penile anal area of men ranges from 26–35%.[14-16] The prevalence of HPV in the oral mucosa of healthy adolescents and young adults is around 3%.[17,18]

Risk factors associated with incident HPV infection include behavioral and biological factors. Early age of sexual initiation, higher number of sexual partners, higher number of partner's partners, having a new partner, and inconsistent condom use are all associated with incident HPV infection. Immunosuppression, cervical ectopy, a history of genital herpes simplex virus or *Chlamydia trachomatis*, and smoking are also associated with incident HPV infection. Condom use does reduce the risk of HPV infection.[19]

Adolescents may be more vulnerable to HPV infection due to the epithelial structure of the cervix and a naive mucosal immune response. The adolescent cervix is notable for ectopy, a fragile, columnar, rapidly differentiating, metaplastic epithelium. The epithelium of the cervix in most adult women is a thicker, more protective, squamous epithelium. The columnar epithelium that lines the endocervix and ectocervix of the adolescent epithelium gradually transforms into squamous epithelium. The transformation zone is where this squamous metaplasia occurs. Cervical cancers arise in the transformation zone. It is also possible that adolescents may be more vulnerable to HPV because of a naïve mucosal immune response. However, this is not well understood. It is possible that women develop cell-mediated immunity to HPV over time.

Sexual activity is the most important risk factor for the acquisition of HPV in women and men. Acquisition of cervical HPV occurs soon after the onset of sexual activity. In sexually active adolescent females with only 1 male sexual partner, the median time from first intercourse to HPV infections is about 3 months.[20] Among women reporting only 1 lifetime partner, 50% became HPV positive within 3 years of sexual debut. [21] In addition, the sexual history of a woman's partner is a factor in cervical HPV acquisition; women whose male partners had at least 1 previous partner were more likely to have HPV compared to women whose partners had no previous partners.[22] In both men and women, a greater number of lifetime and recent sexual partners is associated with increased risk of acquisition of HPV. Circumcision and condom use may be protective factors against HPV acquisition.[19,23]

HPV transmission can occur with any direct skin-to-skin contact. Penetrative vaginal or anal sex is the most common route of transmission. Kissing, oral sex, and hand-genital contact can result in transmission. In infants and children, perinatal, horizontal, and vertical transmission can occur. External genital warts can be found in infants and toddlers and are often associated with a history of genital warts in the mother. When oral or cervical HPV is detected in the mother or father, an increased rate of HPV is detected in the genitalia of infants,[24] suggesting that skin-to-skin contact with caregivers may be another route of transmission.

Abnormal Cytology

Prevalence of abnormal cytology is lower than but parallels the prevalence of HPV detection. This is because SIL is a manifestation of HPV infections. As with HPV infection, SIL is more common in younger women compared to older women. In a study of almost 80,000 cytology slides from women age 10–39, the rate of abnormal cytology was highest in 10–19-year-olds (3.8% of 10–19-year-olds had LSIL, HSIL or SIL of uncertain grade) compared to 20–29-year-olds (3.3% had SIL) and 30–39-year-olds (1.4% had SIL). Although the overall rate of abnormal cytology is highest in adolescent women, the proportion of HSIL among the abnormal cytology is lowest in adolescent women (18% of abnormal cytology smears in younger women were HSIL compared to 36% of abnormal cytology in older women).[25] Thus when abnormal cytology is detected in younger women, it is less likely to lead to a diagnosis of a precancerous or cancerous lesion. In addition, most older women referred for LSIL have CIN 2/3 detected, unlike adolescent women in whom most women referred for LSIL will have CIN 1 or CIN 2 detected.

LSIL is considered benign when detected in adolescent women. In a study of 13–22-year-old women, 61% of LSIL regressed to normal cytology after 1 year and 91% of LSIL regressed to normal after 3 years.[26] In this study, the time between detection of LSIL and regression to normal was 8 months. LSIL is not considered benign when detected in older women, in part due to misclassifications of HSIL as LSIL on cytology. LSIL does often regress in older women, but at a lower rate (64–88%) than in adolescent women.[27,28] CIN 1 is often considered benign, with 70–90% of CIN 1 lesions regressing to normal. The natural history of CIN 2 has been difficult to describe. CIN 2 is heterogeneous in its biological properties, with some CIN 2 being caused by nononcogenic HPV types and some being caused by oncogenic HPV types. CIN 2 is a difficult diagnosis with low reproducibility between pathologists, and many studies have combined CIN 2 and CIN 3 as an outcome. It is believed that CIN 2 more often regresses to CIN 1 or normal and less often progresses to CIN 3 or cancer in adolescent women compared to adult women. A longitudinal study in women 13–24 years of age reported 63% regression of CIN2 to normal by 2 years and 12% progression to CIN 3 by 2 years.[29] In a study that included older women, the reported rate of CIN 2 regression was 53% and the reported rate of CIN 2 progression was 21% after 72 months of follow-up. In this study, 14% of CIN 3 regressed and 69% of CIN 3 progressed to cancer.[27,30]

Factors associated with the development and regression of abnormal cytology are thought to be related to HPV acquisition. Studies consistently show a strong association between HPV persistence and the development of CIN 1/LSIL and CIN 2/CIN 3/HSIL/invasive cancer.[8] The association between persistent HPV and high-grade cervical lesions is stronger than the association between persistent HPV and low-grade cervical lesions. This is consistent with the belief that CIN 1/LSIL represents transient HPV infections that often regress. Persistent HPV, especially high-risk types, is the strongest risk factor associated with development of HSIL.[2] The relative risk of developing HSIL after persistent infection was increased by 14 in one study.[3] Additional risk factors are associated with the development of high-grade cervical lesions. The most consistent risk factor associated with high-grade cervical lesions among women with high-risk HPV infection is smoking.[30,31] Inconsistent evidence exists that suggests that oral contraceptive use and *Chlamydia trachomatis* infection may increase the risk of high-grade cervical lesions.[32,33] Condom use appears to be a protective factor. It has been associated with a reduced risk of high-grade lesions in HPV-positive women and regression of CIN.[34,35]

Cancers

HPV-associated cancers are the rarest form of HPV-associated disease. HPV is a necessary, but not sufficient, cause of virtually all cervical cancers, as well as a large proportion of anal, vaginal, vulvar, penile, and oropharyngeal cancers. HPV-associated cancers usually occur in adults and rarely occur in adolescents or children. In the United States, the age adjusted incidence of cervical cancer from 2000–2004 was 8.7 per 100,000 women. The incidence of cervical cancer among children and adolescents 19 years and younger was 0.1 per 100,000. The incidence of cervical cancer among 20–29-year-olds was 4.5 per 100,000 and among 30–39-year-olds was 13.0 per 100,000. Incidence rates peaked among 40–49-year-olds (16.5 per 100,000) and declined slightly among older women (50–64-year-olds, 15.4 per 100,000, and 64 and older, 14.6 per 100,000).[36] These data came from large, anonymous cancer registries where it is impossible to determine the risk factors associated with adolescents with cervical cancer. As already discussed, persistent infection with a high-risk HPV type causes squamous cell carcinoma of the cervix. HPV 16 and HPV 18 cause approximately 70% of cervical cancers; the remaining cervical cancers are caused by other high-risk types.[37] Additional factors have been found to be associated with cervical cancer; these include cigarette smoking, high parity, coinfection with another STI such as *Chlamydia trachomatis,* and immunosuppression.[4,38] Prolonged use (> 5 years) of oral contraceptives has also been associated with cervical cancer. However, the risk of cervical cancer after cessation of oral contraceptives declines so that no increased risk is detectable 10 years after cessation of oral contraceptives.[39]

Anal cancer occurs in women and men. The age adjusted rate of anal cancer in the United States from 2000–2004 was 1.6 per 100,000 women. This rate is higher than that found among all men, 1.3 per 100,000 men. Rates of anal cancer have increased over the past 3 decades, with the highest increase noted among men. Among men, the highest incidence is among men who have sex with men. HPV is associated with about 85–90% of anal cancers. HPV 16 and 18 are the most common causes of anal cancer. Risk factors for anal cancer among women include a high-grade cervical lesion, cervical and vulvar cancers, and human immunodeficiency virus (HIV). Risk factors for anal cancer among men include HIV and a history of sex with men.[40]

A number of other anogenital cancers are strongly associated with HPV infection. Most, 64–91%, of vaginal cancers are HPV positive.[41] The age adjusted incidence of vaginal cancer in the United States is low, 0.7 per 100,000 women.[42] HPV 16 is the most commonly detected HPV type in HPV-associated vaginal cancers. Other risk factors include sexual behaviors and a history of treatment for other anogenital cancers.[4]

Among vulvar cancers, a subgroup most often diagnosed in young women is associated with HPV infection. The rate of vulvar cancers is 2.2 per 100,000 women.[42] Sixty to ninety percent of warty and basaloid carcinomas are HPV positive, mostly with HPV 16. High-risk sexual behaviors are associated with these cancers.[4]

HPV is also associated with penile cancers. The age adjusted incidence rate of penile cancer in the United States is 0.81 per 100,000 men. HPV is present in 80–100% of warty and basaloid carcinomas but only about one-third of verrucous and keratinizing types. HPV 16 and 18 are detected most often in penile cancers caused by HPV. In addition to HPV infections, risk factors associated with penile cancer include phimosis, lack of neonatal circumcision, and anogenital warts.[43]

A subset of head and neck cancers (approximately 25–35%) are caused by HPV. The age adjusted incidence rate of head and neck cancers between 1998–2003 was estimated to be 5.2 per 100,000 men and 1.3 per 100,000 women.[44] HPV 16 is the most commonly detected type in HPV positive head and neck cancers.[43] These HPV-positive cancers are associated with sexual activity and are not associated with alcohol or tobacco use.

PREVENTION

Condoms, Screening, and Partner Notification

Condom use has been shown to reduce the risk of HPV transmission, acquisition, and HPV-associated disease.[19,45] Among sexually active college-aged women, consistent condom use decreased HPV infections by 70%.[19] The prevalence of HPV infections are so high that neither asymptomatic screening nor partner notification is useful for HPV prevention.[46]

Vaccination

Vaccines to protect against HPV infection and HPV related diseases are available for use in both girls and boys. The antigens of HPV vaccines are virus-like particles (VLPs). VLPs are viral surface proteins encoded by the L1 gene. Each VLP is specific for 1 HPV type. These proteins are morphologically identical to the HPV L1 protein and form a capsid that produces an antibody response. They cannot infect cells and cannot replicate; therefore, they are not infectious nor could they be oncogenic. The vaccines contain no DNA or RNA and do not contain the preservative thimerosal.

Two vaccines are currently available for clinical use. The quadrivalent vaccine (GARDASIL™, manufactured by Merck and Co., Inc.) has VLPs from high-risk HPV types 16 and 18 and low-risk HPV types 6 and 11. It was licensed by the Food and Drug Administration (FDA) in the United States in June 2006 for use in women aged 9–26 years old and in October 2009 for use in men aged 9–26 years. The bivalent HPV vaccine (Cervarix, GlaxoSmithKline) has VLPs from high-risk HPV types 16 and 18. It was licensed by the FDA in October 2009 for use in women.

The Advisory Committee on Immunization Practices (ACIP) recommends universal routine immunization with HPV vaccine. Based on the different impact of HPV-associated disease in women and men, recommendations differ for girls and boys. Routine immunization for girls may occur with either the bivalent or quadrivalent vaccine. The target age population is 11–12 year olds. Nine to 10 year olds may be vaccinated at their clinician's discretion. Routine immunization should occur for unvaccinated girls and women aged 13–26 years old. Routine immunization for boys may occur with the quadrivalent vaccine, which prevents genital warts in addition to HPV-associated cancers. The bivalent HPV vaccine has not received a recommendation for boys in the United States. As with girls, the target age population for boys is 11–12 years old. Nine to 10 year olds may be vaccinated at their clinician's discretion. Routine immunization should occur for unvaccinated boys aged 13–21 years old. Routine immunization with quadrivalent HPV is also recommended for men aged 22–26 years old with risk factors including immunosuppression and men who have sex with men.[47]

The quadrivalent and bivalent vaccines prevent HPV-related diseases, including cervical, vulvar, vaginal, and anal cancers and precancers. In addition, the quadrivalent vaccine protects against genital warts. Vaccination may also offer some protection from cervical precancers from nonvaccine high-risk HPV types.

The two vaccines are not interchangeable and should not be given to the same individual. Both vaccines require 3 doses to build long-term immunity. The second dose should be given 1–2 months after the first and the third dose should be given 6 months after the first dose but no sooner than 12 weeks after the second dose or 24 weeks after the first dose. Research is currently under way to examine the immunogenicity of a 2 dose vaccine schedule and the impact of receiving the second or third dose off schedule. However, if a patient is late getting the second dose, current recommendations are to administer the second dose as soon as possible followed by the third dose no sooner than 12 weeks after the second. If the third dose is late, current recommendations are to give the dose as soon as possible. The three dose series does not need to be restarted if 1 or more doses are late.

The vaccines have been evaluated in separate, randomized clinical trials with more than 50,000 young women and 4,000 young men. More than 97% of participants seroconverted for HPV vaccine types and, overall, high antibody titers were produced. Antibody titers were higher in children and adolescents compared to young women.[48-51] Among women in clinical trials who were not infected with HPV 16 or 18 and who received vaccine according to protocol, efficacy of the vaccines in preventing cervical precancers was greater than 90%.[52,53] Among men in the clinical trial to evaluate the quadrivalent vaccine who were not infected with HPV and received all 3 doses of vaccine, efficacy of the vaccine in preventing genital warts was 89%.[54] The duration of protection is still under investigation. Large clinical trials remain ongoing to monitor the immunogenicity of the vaccine, the presence of precancerous disease, and genital warts in vaccinated women. A strong amnestic response, suggesting the development of immune memory, was observed in one study that provided an antigen challenge 5 years after vaccination.[55]

Safety of the vaccine has been evaluated in clinical trials and postlicensing surveillance data. In clinical trials, most participants experienced mild to moderate pain, swelling, or erythema at the injection site. Less than 0.1% of participants experienced a vaccine-related serious adverse event, and the rate was similar between vaccine and placebo groups. Safety of the vaccine was reviewed by the FDA and the Centers for Disease Control and Prevention (CDC) and reported in 2009.[56] The review used information from the Vaccine Adverse Event Reporting System (VAERS). This is a voluntary system for health care providers, vaccine manufacturers, and the public to report vaccine adverse events. At the time of the review, more than 23 million doses of the quadrivalent vaccine had been administered in a 2.5 year period. Nearly 12,500 adverse events were reported. Ninety-four percent of the VAERS reports were classified as nonserious. The most common of these nonserious events were syncope, pain at the injection site, dizziness, nausea, and headaches. None of the serious adverse events appeared to be causally linked to the vaccine. All reported deaths that had adequate medical records for review were attributable to causes other than vaccination. There did appear to be an increase in reported rates of blood clots compared with what has been found for other vaccines given to females of the same age. No causal association between blood clots and the vaccine was found in the review. There was an increase in syncopal episodes reported compared to what has been found for other vaccines given to females of the same age. Because of the risk of head injury from a syncopal event, it is recommended that patients receiving HPV vaccine sit or lie for 15 minutes after the injection. Overall, the vaccine is considered to have a very safe record.

Targeting 11–12 year olds for vaccination is important. The vaccine is a prophylactic vaccine that protects against HPV infection; the vaccine does not clear an infection in a person that is already infected with HPV. Almost one-third of ninth-grade girls (age 14–15 years) in the United States are already sexually experienced, and nearly 10% of girls have initiated sexual intercourse before age 13.[57] Children are at risk for HPV infection at a young age. In addition, although intercourse is the most efficient means of transmission, girls who have never had sexual intercourse can acquire HPV infections. This is most likely due to sexual experimentation. Thus the recommended age of vaccination needs to be early enough to protect most of the target population.

HPV vaccine can be given to individuals who are sexually active, have had HPV-related disease, or may be immunocompromised due to disease or medications. If an individual is infected with a vaccine HPV type, has had dysplasia caused by a vaccine HPV type, or has had genital warts, the vaccine can prevent infections from other vaccine types. Thus, there is no reason to withhold vaccination from sexually active individuals or individuals with a history of genital warts or dysplasia. Studies of safety and efficacy of HPV vaccines in HIV-infected individuals are currently under way. Current recommendations are to immunize those who may be immunocompromised due to disease or medications.

HPV vaccines are not recommended in pregnancy. Neither vaccine has been shown to be causally associated with adverse outcomes in pregnant women or fetuses. Despite this, clinicians should avoid the vaccine in pregnant girls and young women. A pregnancy test need only be completed before vaccination in girls and women whose clinical history suggests a risk for pregnancy, for example, for women whose last menstrual period is longer than 4 weeks before the intended HPV vaccine dose and who are sexually active without using birth control. If an HPV vaccine is inadvertently administered during pregnancy, no intervention is needed. Patients or clinicians should call to enter the patient in the vaccines in pregnancy registry (Merck, 800-986-8999; GlaxoSmithKline, 888-452-9622).

Cervical Cancer Screening

Cervical cancer screening with cervical cytology (Pap smear) testing has been highly effective in reducing the incidence of cervical cancer over the past 6 decades. However, for the nearly 30 years that adolescents have been screened for cervical cancer, the already extremely low rate of cancer in this age group was not affected. Thus, unlike adult women, cytology and HPV testing are not effective screening tests in adolescents. In addition to not impacting cancer rates in adolescent girls, screening of adolescents has resulted in unnecessary evaluation and treatment of dysplasia. This is consistent with the recognition of the commonness and benign nature of LSIL in adolescents. An unfortunate risk of these unnecessary treatments includes negative pregnancy outcomes, including an increased risk of preterm delivery after ablative or excisional procedures to remove dysplasia.[58] Recent cervical cancer screening guideline updates have recognized these findings, which have led the American College of Obstetricians and Gynecologists (ACOG) to change the recommended age of onset for cervical cancer screening in healthy young women. The newest guidelines recommend that screening begins at 21 years of age, regardless of previous sexual experience.[7] Other organizations continue to recommend that screening begin within 3 years of onset of sexual activity and not later than 21 in women who may not be disclosing their onset of sexual activity.[59,60] Referral and treatment of abnormal cytology and histology remain conservative for adolescents if screening was undertaken before 21. Abnormal cytology and dysplasia in adolescents should be followed by someone familiar with these conservative guidelines to prevent unnecessary procedures.

Cervical cancer screening remains a critical part of cervical cancer prevention, even in young women currently being vaccinated. The impact of vaccination on the rates of cervical cancer in the population will not be witnessed for at least 2 to 3 decades. Given the poor uptake of the vaccine, with more than one-half of adolescents having not initiated the vaccine and one-third having not completed the 3-dose vaccine series once the series was started, the full impact of the vaccine on cervical cancer screening programs will take many decades to be realized. Until then, women should continue to be screened for cervical cancer regardless of immunization status.

CONCLUSION

In summary, HPV is the most common STI. Infection with HPV can be transient or can lead to diseases of the mucosa including genital warts, dysplasia, and cancers. Prevention of infection with HPV types most commonly associated with dysplasia and cancer can be obtained by vaccination with HPV vaccines. Until the impact of widespread immunization is attained and its impact on rates of cervical cancer precursors is known, cervical cancer screening according to clinical guidelines is still recommended.

References

1. Barrasso R, De Brux J, Croissant O, Orth G. High prevalence of papillomavirus-associated penile intraepithelial neoplasia in sexual partners of women with cervical intraepithelial neoplasia. *N Engl J Med.* 1987;317(15):916–923
2. Ho GY, Bierman R, Beardsley L, Chang CJ, Burk RD. Natural history of cervicovaginal papillomavirus infection in young women. *N Engl J Med.* 1998;338(7):423–428
3. Moscicki AB, Shiboski S, Broering J, et al. The natural history of human papillomavirus infection as measured by repeated DNA testing in adolescent and young women. *J Pediatr.* 1998;132(2):277–284
4. Trottier H, Burchell AN. Epidemiology of mucosal human papillomavirus infection and associated diseases. *Public Health Genomics.* 2009;12(5–6):291–307
5. Kashima HK, Shah F, Lyles A, et al. A comparison of risk factors in juvenile-onset and adult-onset recurrent respiratory papillomatosis. *Laryngoscope.* 1992;102(1):9–13
6. Larson DA, Derkay CS. Epidemiology of recurrent respiratory papillomatosis. *APMIS.* 2010;118(6–7):450–454
7. ACOG Committee on Practice Bulletins—Gynecology. ACOG Practice Bulletin No. 109. Cervical Cytology Screening. *Obstet Gynecol.* 2009;114:1409–1420
8. Koshiol J, Lindsay L, Pimenta JM, Poole C, Jenkins D, Smith JS. Persistent human papillomavirus infection and cervical neoplasia: a systematic review and meta-analysis. *Am J Epidemiol.* 2008;168(2):123–137
9. Motoyama S, Ladines-Llave CA, Luis Villanueva S, Maruo T. The role of human papilloma virus in the molecular biology of cervical carcinogenesis. *Kobe J Med Sci.* 2004;50(1–2):9–19
10. Cates W Jr. Estimates of the incidence and prevalence of sexually transmitted diseases in the United States. American Social Health Association Panel. *Sex Transm Dis.* 1999;26(4 Suppl):S2–7
11. Koutsky LA, Galloway DA, Holmes KK. Epidemiology of genital human papillomavirus infection. *Epidemiol Rev.* 1988;10:122–163
12. Dunne EF, Unger ER, Sternberg M, et al. Prevalence of HPV infection among females in the United States. *JAMA.* 2007;297(8):813–819
13. Clifford GM, Gallus S, Herrero R, et al. Worldwide distribution of human papillomavirus types in cytologically normal women in the International Agency for Research on Cancer HPV prevalence surveys: a pooled analysis. *Lancet.* 2005;366(9490):991–998
14. Weaver BA, Feng Q, Holmes KK, et al. Evaluation of genital sites and sampling techniques for detection of human papillomavirus DNA in men. *J Infect Dis.* 2004;189(4):677–685
15. Partridge JM, Koutsky LA. Genital human papillomavirus infection in men. *Lancet Infect Dis.* 2006;6(1):21–31
16. Chin-Hong PV, Vittinghoff E, Cranston RD, et al. Age-Specific prevalence of anal human papillomavirus infection in HIV-negative sexually active men who have sex with men: the EXPLORE study. *J Infect Dis.* 2004;190(12):2070–2076
17. Smith EM, Swarnavel S, Ritchie JM, Wang D, Haugen TH, Turek LP. Prevalence of human papillomavirus in the oral cavity/oropharynx in a large population of children and adolescents. *Pediatr Infect Dis J.* 2007;26(9):836–840
18. D'Souza G, Agrawal Y, Halpern J, Bodison S, Gillison ML. Oral Sexual Behaviors Associated with Prevalent Oral Human Papillomavirus Infection. *J Infect Dis.* 2009;199(9):1263–1269
19. Winer RL, Hughes JP, Feng Q, et al. Condom use and the risk of genital human papillomavirus infection in young women. *N Engl J Med.* 2006;354(25):2645–2654
20. Collins S, Mazloomzadeh S, Winter H, et al. High incidence of cervical human papillomavirus infection in women during their first sexual relationship. *BJOG.* 2002;109(1):96–98
21. Winer RL, Feng Q, Hughes JP, O'Reilly S, Kiviat NB, Koutsky LA. Risk of female human papillomavirus acquisition associated with first male sex partner. *J Infect Dis.* 2008;197(2):279–282
22. Winer RL, Lee SK, Hughes JP, Adam DE, Kiviat NB, Koutsky LA. Genital human papillomavirus infection: incidence and risk factors in a cohort of female university students. *Am J Epidemiol.* 2003;157(3):218–226

23. Castellsague X, Munoz N. Chapter 3: Cofactors in human papillomavirus carcinogenesis—role of parity, oral contraceptives, and tobacco smoking. *J Natl Cancer Inst Monogr.* 2003(31):20–28
24. Rintala MA, Grenman SE, Puranen MH, et al. Transmission of high-risk human papillomavirus (HPV) between parents and infant: a prospective study of HPV in families in Finland. *J Clin Microbiol.* 2005;43(1):376–381
25. Mount SL, Papillo JL. A study of 10,296 pediatric and adolescent Papanicolaou smear diagnoses in northern New England. *Pediatrics.* 1999;103(3):539–545
26. Moscicki AB, Shiboski S, Hills NK, et al. Regression of low-grade squamous intra-epithelial lesions in young women. *Lancet.* 2004;364(9446):1678–1683
27. Syrjanen K, Kataja V, Yliskoski M, Chang F, Syrjanen S, Saarikoski S. Natural history of cervical human papillomavirus lesions does not substantiate the biologic relevance of the Bethesda System. *Obstet Gynecol.* 1992;79(5 (Pt 1)):675–682
28. Schlecht NF, Platt RW, Duarte-Franco E, et al. Human papillomavirus infection and time to progression and regression of cervical intraepithelial neoplasia. *J Natl Cancer Inst.* 2003;95(17):1336–1343
29. Moscicki AB, Ma Y, Wibbelsman C, et al. Rate of and risks for regression of cervical intraepithelial neoplasia 2 in adolescents and young women. *Obstet Gynecol.* 2010;116(6):1373–1380.
30. Wheeler CM. Natural history of human papillomavirus infections, cytologic and histologic abnormalities, and cancer. *Obstet Gynecol Clin North Am.* 2008;35(4):519–536; vii
31. Castle PE, Wacholder S, Lorincz AT, et al. A prospective study of high-grade cervical neoplasia risk among human papillomavirus-infected women. *J Natl Cancer Inst.* 2002;94(18):1406–1414
32. Moscicki AB, Schiffman M, Kjaer S, Villa LL. Chapter 5: Updating the natural history of HPV and anogenital cancer. *Vaccine.* 2006;24 Suppl 3:S42–51
33. Castle PE, Giuliano AR. Chapter 4: Genital tract infections, cervical inflammation, and antioxidant nutrients—assessing their roles as human papillomavirus cofactors. *J Natl Cancer Inst Monogr.* 2003(31):29–34
34. Hildesheim A, Herrero R, Castle PE, et al. HPV co-factors related to the development of cervical cancer: results from a population-based study in Costa Rica. *Br J Cancer.* 2001;84(9):1219–1226
35. Hogewoning CJ, Bleeker MC, van den Brule AJ, et al. Condom use promotes regression of cervical intraepithelial neoplasia and clearance of human papillomavirus: a randomized clinical trial. *Int J Cancer.* 2003;107(5):811–816
36. Saraiya M, Ahmed F, Krishnan S, Richards TB, Unger ER, Lawson HW. Cervical cancer incidence in a prevaccine era in the United States, 1998–2002. *Obstet Gynecol.* 2007;109(2 Pt 1):360–370
37. Munoz N, Bosch FX, de Sanjose S, et al. Epidemiologic classification of human papillomavirus types associated with cervical cancer. *N Engl J Med.* 2003;348(6):518–527
38. Appleby P, Beral V, Berrington de Gonzalez A, et al. Carcinoma of the cervix and tobacco smoking: collaborative reanalysis of individual data on 13,541 women with carcinoma of the cervix and 23,017 women without carcinoma of the cervix from 23 epidemiological studies. *Int J Cancer.* 2006;118(6):1481–1495
39. Smith JS, Green J, Berrington de Gonzalez A, et al. Cervical cancer and use of hormonal contraceptives: a systematic review. *Lancet.* 2003;361(9364):1159–1167
40. Markowitz LE, Dunne EF, Saraiya M, Lawson HW, Chesson H, Unger ER. Quadrivalent Human Papillomavirus Vaccine: Recommendations of the Advisory Committee on Immunization Practices (ACIP). *MMWR Recomm Rep.* Vol 562007:1–24
41. Munoz N, Castellsague X, de Gonzalez AB, Gissmann L. Chapter 1: HPV in the etiology of human cancer. *Vaccine.* 2006;24S3:S1–S10
42. Ries L, Melbert D, Krapcho M, et al. SEER Cancer Statistics Review, 1975–2004, National Cancer Institute. 2007; http://seer.cancer.gov/csr/1975_2004/
43. Giuliano AR, Anic G, Nyitray AG. Epidemiology and pathology of HPV disease in males. *Gynecol Oncol.* 2010;117(2 Suppl):S15–19
44. Ryerson A, Peters E, Coughlin S, et al. Burden of potentially human papillomavirus-associated cancers of the oropharynx and oral cavity in the US, 1998–2003. *Cancer.* 2008;113

45. Kjaer SK, Munk C, Winther JF, Jorgensen HO, Meijer CJ, van den Brule AJ. Acquisition and persistence of human papillomavirus infection in younger men: a prospective follow-up study among Danish soldiers. *Cancer Epidemiol Biomarkers Prev.* 2005;14(6):1528–1533

46. Workowski KA, Berman S. Sexually transmitted diseases treatment guidelines, 2010. *MMWR Recomm Rep.* 2010;59(RR-12):1–110

47. Centers for Disease Control and Prevention. VFC: The ACIP-VFC Vaccine Resolutions. http://www.cdc.gov/vaccines/programs/vfc/acip-vfc-resolutions.htm. Accessed November 11, 2011

48. Block SL, Nolan T, Sattler C, et al. Comparison of the Immunogenicity and Reactogenicity of a Prophylactic Quadrivalent Human Papillomavirus (Types 6, 11, 16, and 18) L1 Virus-Like Particle Vaccine in Male and Female Adolescents and Young Adult Women. *Pediatrics.* 2006;118(5):2135–2145

49. Garland SM, Hernandez-Avila M, Wheeler CM, et al. Quadrivalent vaccine against human papillomavirus to prevent anogenital diseases. *N Engl J Med.* 2007;356(19):1928–1943

50. Paavonen J, Jenkins D, Bosch FX, et al. Efficacy of a prophylactic adjuvanted bivalent L1 virus-like-particle vaccine against infection with human papillomavirus types 16 and 18 in young women: an interim analysis of a phase III double-blind, randomised controlled trial. *Lancet.* 2007;369(9580):2161–2170

51. Reisinger KS, Block SL, Lazcano-Ponce E, et al. Safety and persistent immunogenicity of a quadrivalent human papillomavirus types 6, 11, 16, 18 L1 virus-like particle vaccine in preadolescents and adolescents: a randomized controlled trial. *Pediatr Infect Dis J.* 2007;26(3):201–209

52. Food and Drug Administration. Product approval-prescribing information [package insert]. Cervarix [human papillomavirus bivalent (types 16 and 18) vaccine, recombinant]. 2009; http://www.fda.gov/biologicsbloodvaccines/vaccines/approvedproducts/ucm186957.htm Accessed May 25, 2010

53. Gardasil [Package Insert]. Whitehouse Station, NJ: Merck & Co., Inc.; 2006

54. Food and Drug Administration. Product approval-prescribing information [package insert]. Human Papillomavirus Quadrivalent (Types 6, 11, 16, 18) Vaccine, Recombinant. 2011; http://www.fda.gov/BiologicsBloodVaccines/Vaccines/ApprovedProducts/UCM094042. Accessed October 25, 2011

55. Villa LL, Ault KA, Giuliano A, et al. Immunologic responses following administration of a vacine targeting human papillomavirus Types 6, 11, 16, and 18. *Vaccine.* 2006;24:5571–5583

56. Slade B, Leidel L, Vellozzi C, et al. Postlicensure safety surveillance for quadrivalent human papillomavirus recombinant vaccine. *JAMA.* 2009;302(7):750

57. Centers for Disease Control and Prevention. Youth risk behavior surveillance—United States, 2009. *MMWR Surveill Summ.* 2010;59(No. SS-5):1–142

58. Kyrgiou M, Koliopoulos G, Martin-Hirsch P, Arbyn M, Prendiville W, Paraskevaidis E. Obstetric outcomes after conservative treatment for intraepithelial or early invasive cervical lesions: systematic review and meta-analysis. *Lancet.* 2006;367(9509):489–498

59. American Cancer Society. Early detection of cervical cancer. *CA Cancer J Clin.* 2002 2002;52:375–376

60. U.S. Preventive Services Task Force. Screening for Cervical Cancer, Topic Page. http://www.ahcpr.gov/clinic/uspstf/uspscerv.htm. Accessed October 26, 2011

Note: Page numbers of articles are in **boldface** type. Page references followed by "*f*" and "*t*" denote figures and tables, respectively.